BACTERIAL DIARRHEAL DISEASES

NEW PERSPECTIVES IN CLINICAL MICROBIOLOGY

Other volumes in this series:

Bacterial Diarrheal Diseases

edited by

Y. TAKEDA

The Institute of Medical Science
The University of Tokyo
Tokyo, Japan

T. MIWATANI

Research Institute for Microbial Diseases
Osaka University
Osaka, Japan

1985 **MARTINUS NIJHOFF PUBLISHERS**
a member of the KLUWER ACADEMIC PUBLISHERS GROUP
BOSTON / THE HAGUE / DORDRECHT / LANCASTER

Distributors

for the United States and Canada: Kluwer Boston, Inc., 190 Old Derby Street, Hingham, MA 02043, USA
for Japan: KTK Scientific Publishers, 307 Shibuyadai-haim, 4-17 Sakuragaoka-cho, Shibuya-ku, Tokyo 150, Japan
for all other countries: Kluwer Academic Publishers Group, Distribution Center, P.O. Box 322, 3300 AH Dordrecht, The Netherlands

Library of Congress Cataloging in Publication Data

Main entry under title: CIP

Bacterial diarrheal diseases.

   (New perspectives in clinical microbiology)
   1. Diarrhea. 2. Bacterial diseases. 3. Epidemiology.
I. Takeda, Yoshifumi, 1935–   . II. Miwatani,
Toshio, 1928–   . III. Series. [DNLM: 1. Diarrhea.
2. Diarrhea--occurence. 3. Bacterial Infections.
4. Bacterial Infections--occurence. WI 407 B131]
QR201.D4B33   1984   616.9'2   84–1186

ISBN-13: 978-94-010-8709-4   e-ISBN-13: 978-94-009-4990-4
DOI: 10.1007/978-94-009-4990-4

Book Information

Joint edition published by: KTK Scientific Publishers, Tokyo, Japan and Martinus Nijhoff Publishers, Boston, USA

Copyright

PREFACE

Bacterial diarrheal diseases are a very important problem for human health, and many people, especially infants and children, die every year from diarrheal diseases, particularly in developing countries. Thus, in 1978 the World Health Organization initiated a Diarrhoeal Diseases Control Programme and is now working actively to control diarrheal diseases. The "International Symposium on Bacterial Diarrheal Diseases" which took place in Osaka from March 23rd to 25th, 1982, was organized by Osaka University with the support of the Ministry of Education, Science and Culture of the Japanese Government. The aim of this Symposium was to promote exchange of scientific information on bacterial diarrheal diseases, since studies in this field have progressed rapidly during the last few years due to work in many laboratories throughout the world.

It seems appropriate that this Symposium was held in Osaka, since during the past century Japanese bacteriologists have made a number of important contributions in the field of bacterial diarrheal diseases. Outstanding among these contributions are the recognition of *Shigella* as a causative agent of bacillary dysentery by Dr. Kiyoshi Shiga and the serotyping of *Vibrio cholerae* into the Ogawa, Inaba and Hikojima serotypes by Drs. Kabeshima and Nobechi. Moreover more recently, Dr. Tsunesaburo Fujino of Osaka University discovered *Vibrio parahaemolyticus* as the causative agent of an important diarrheal disease. Since geographically, Japan is situated near the developing countries of South East Asia, great efforts have been made by the Japanese scientific community to help in control of diarrheal diseases. It is certain that the Symposium stimulated and encouraged Japanese medical scientists and microbiologists to participate even more in research aimed at controlling diarrheal diseases.

We hope that publication of the Proceedings of this Symposium will be useful by making the contents of the Symposium fully available to scientists who are interested in this field, and that it will stimulate and encourage them to make further progress in the control of diarrheal diseases.

Yoshifumi Takeda
Toshio Miwatani

Contents

Bacterial Diarrheal Diseases, eds., Y. Takeda, T. Miwatani, 1-10.
Copyright © 1985 by KTK Scientific Publishers, Tokyo.

THE GLOBAL PROBLEM OF ACUTE DIARRHEAL DISEASES AND THE WHO DIARRHEAL DISEASES CONTROL PROGRAMME

M. H. Merson

Diarrhoeal Diseases Control Programme, World Health Organization, 1211 Geneva 27, Switzerland

The acute diarrheal diseases have long been recognized as a major cause of mortality and morbidity in infants and young children in the developing world. This paper will summarize (a) the magnitude of the problem; (b) the major bacterial agents of acute diarrhea; and (c) the global WHO programme for control of all acute diarrheal diseases.

The global problem

Past attempts to determine the magnitude of the diarrheal disease problem globally have resulted in a wide range of estimates(1). To try and obtain a more precise picture of the problem, WHO recently undertook a review of diarrhea surveillance data from articles published in the last three decades in English or French which described longitudinal, prospective, community-based studies of at least one year's duration in which no specific intervention was undertaken(2). In all the studies morbidity surveillance was carried out at least once every two weeks and mortality surveillance at least once a month. Two multi-country mortality studies in which death certificates were the basis for investigating the cause of death were also included. In all, 24 studies carried out in 18 countries in Asia, Africa, and Latin America were included in the analysis.

In the first five years of life the morbidity rate was highest for children 6-11 months of age (Fig. 1). The median incidence of diarrhea was 2.2 episodes per child per year in the under-five year age group and less than one episode per person per year in those above the age of five. In populations that were more frequently surveyed and were of comparatively smaller size, the median incidence in the under-five year age group was 3.0 episodes per child per year.

The highest mortality rates were in children below two years of age, with a median mortality rate of about 20 deaths per 1000 population (Fig. 2). The estimated case-fatality ratio in children below the age of five was 0.6 deaths per 1000 illnesses.

Based on 1980 population figures and the above calculated global median

2

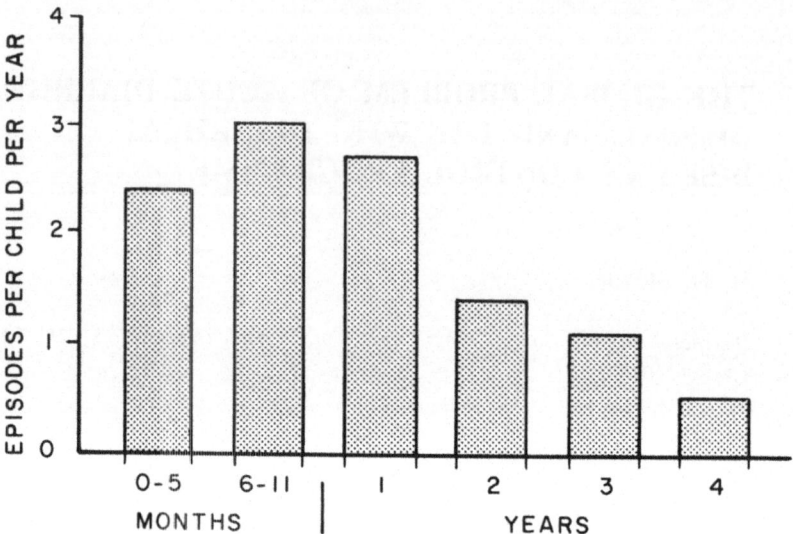

Fig. 1. Estimated median diarrheal morbidity rates in children less than 5 years old in developing countries, by age. (Based on: Snyder, J.D. & Merson, M.H., *Bull. Wld Hlth Org.*, **60**: 605–613 (1982). Reproduced by permission of WHO, Geneva, Switzerland.)

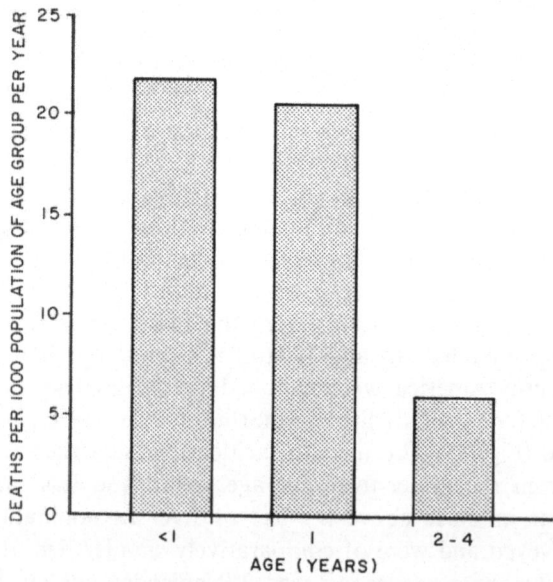

Fig. 2. Estimated median diarrheal mortality rates from active surveillance studies in Asia* and Latin America in children less than 5 years old, by age.
*Excluding China. (Based on: Snyder, J.D. & Merson, M.H., *Bull. Wld Hlth Org.*, **60**: 605–613 (1982). Reproduced by permission of WHO, Geneva, Switzerland.)

morbidity rate, the number of acute diarrheal episodes in 1980 in children less than five years of age in Africa, Asia (excluding China), and Latin America was estimated to be 744 million; when the median morbidity rates obtained in studies with the smallest populations and most frequent surveillance were used, the annual estimated number of cases came to a little over 1 billion. The annual number of deaths from acute diarrheal illness in children under five years of age was estimated to be 4.6 million for 1980; 80% of these deaths were in children under the age of two.

Despite the limitations inherent in these data obtained from different investigations carried out in widely varying cultural and geographic settings, it is clear that the problem of acute diarrhea is a staggering one. Besides causing high childhood mortality and morbidity, the diarrheal diseases are also a major contributor to malnutrition and represent a heavy load for national health budgets as they account for a large proportion of hospital attendances and admissions.

Bacterial diarrhoeal pathogens

In contrast to the situation existing a mere decade ago, when an etiologic agent could be identified in only 20% of acute diarrhea cases and the remainder were classified as "undifferentiated", it is now possible under ideal laboratory conditions to make a laboratory diagnosis in 70 - 80% of cases visiting treatment facilities. Among the known etiologic agents at least 13 bacteria have been clearly identified as diarrheal pathogens and there is increasing evidence that other Gram-negative organisms (e.g., Aeromonas) may occasionally cause diarrhea (Table 1). Some of these agents have been known for decades, but others have only recently been identified as etiologic agents of diarrhea. Among the newly identified agents, enterotoxigenic *Escherichia coli* (ETEC) and *Campylobacter jejuni* are known, along with rotavirus, to be important causes of infantile diarrhea in developing countries.

Enterotoxigenic *E. coli* have been found, when searched for, to be responsible, on the average, for about 25% of diarrhea cases in children and also to be an important cause of adult diarrhea(3). Studies in Bangladesh suggest that these organisms are most commonly spread through contaminated food or water(4). The major obstacle in estimating the importance of these organisms in developing countries has been the difficulty in differentiating them in the laboratory from

Table 1. Agents of acute diarrhoea

Bacteria	
Campylobacter jejuni	Yersinia enterocolitica
Enterotoxigenic Escherichia coli	Foodborne pathogens
Enteropathogenic Escherichia coli	- Staphylococcus aureus
Enteroinvasive Escherichia coli	- Clostridium perfringens
Salmonella	- Bacillus cereus
Shigella	Other Gram-negative organisms
Vibrio cholerae 01 (cholera)	- Klebsiella
Vibrio cholerae non-01 (NAG)	- Citrobacter
Vibrio parahaemolyticus	- Aeromonas

non-enterotoxin-producing *E. coli*. Recently an assay has been devised in Japan(5) which holds great promise as a simple diagnostic test for identifying strains producing heat-labile (LT) enterotoxin.

Campylobacter jejuni, originally known as *Vibrio fetus*, have consistently been found to be responsible for 10 - 15% of diarrhea cases in children in developing countries (Table 2) (6-10). Illness caused by these organisms is characterized especially by abdominal pain with diarrhea, or sometimes dysentery, and fever. The precise epidemiology of Campylobacter diarrhea has not yet been established, though there is increasing evidence from the developed countries, where the organism is also encountered as a frequent cause of diarrhea, that it may be a zoonosis similar to salmonellosis.

Of the "traditional" diarrheal pathogens, *Vibrio cholerae* O1 continues to cause special concern as the seventh pandemic of cholera, which began in 1961, has now spread to 92 countries, 12 of which have become infected since 1978. In a number of these cholera has become endemic, so that there is an increased risk of further spread to new areas. An important new finding has been that the *V. cholerae* O1 organism may have a free-living cycle that enables it to persist and multiply in the environment, particularly in estuarine and brackish waters, over long periods of time independent of human infections.

Concern about cholera and the need for accurate identification of *V. cholerae* O1 have led to the discovery of a number of other vibrios which are confirmed or suspected causes of diarrhea or wound infections (Table 3). Of those known to cause diarrhea there is one - *Vibrio parahaemolyticus* - whose importance as a diarrheal pathogen in adults, especially in Asian countries where shellfish are commonly consumed, has not been fully appreciated. For example, between 1969 and 1980, of 57,445 diarrhea cases seen at Bamrasnaradura Hospital in Bangkok, 5077 (9%) had *V. parahaemolyticus* isolated from their stools (11).

Another traditional bacterial pathogen which continues to be a major cause of acute diarrhea and dysentery, especially in young children, is *Shigella*, particularly *S. dysenteriae* type 1. This organism, which can cause a very severe illness characterized by a hemolytic-uremic syndrome, and often death, has given rise during the last decade to large epidemics in Central America, Asia (Bangladesh, India, Sri Lanka), and Africa (Zaire), where the responsible strains were resistant to many antibiotics. In this connexion, it is of interest to note that different plasmid compatibility groups have been found to be responsible for transmitting resistance (12).

Table 2. Campylobacter jejuni as a cause of acute diarrhoea

Country	Year	Age group	Number studied	% Campylobacter
Rwanda	1977	Children	204	11
Gambia	1979	< 5 y	246	15
Indonesia	1979	<10 y	144	10
Peru	1980	< 3 y	151	14
Bangladesh	1980	<10 y	199	12

Table 3. Vibrios causing infections in man

	Diarrhea	Wound infection
V. cholerae O1	+	–
V. cholerae non O1 (NAG)	+	–
V. parahaemolyticus	+	+
V. fluvialis (group F vibrios)	?	–
V. vulnificus	–	+
V. mimicus	+	?
V. alginolyticus	–	+
V. metschnikovii (enteric group 16)	?	–

There is some evidence that other bacteria besides those listed in Table 1, and as yet unidentified, may cause diarrhea. In studies carried out recently in Kenya (13) and Morocco (14) to evaluate the effect of doxycycline as a prophylactic for travelers' diarrhea, doxycycline had an overall efficacy of about 85% though no etiologic agent could be identified in 40% of the cases receiving placebo. This strongly suggests that unknown bacterial pathogens also play a role in travelers' diarrhea. The identification of these organisms and the elucidation of their role as agents of acute diarrhea in the developing countries are important areas for future research.

The WHO Diarrhoeal Diseases Control Programme

A number of significant advances in knowledge in the past decade in the areas of diagnosis, treatment, and prevention of acute diarrheas have provided a solid basis for a major attack on this vast global problem. These included, among others: (i) as mentioned above, the recognition of the role of new viral and bacterial agents as a cause of diarrhea; (ii) the finding that, except in extremely severe cases, dehydration in all diarrheas and in all age groups can be safely and effectively treated and prevented with a solution of Oral Rehydration Salts (ORS); and (iii) better understanding of the pathogenesis of many of the acute diarrheas and of the intestinal immune response, which offers new possibilities for developing better methods of treatment and prevention, including drugs and vaccines.

Recognizing the significance of these new developments, and as part of its overall commitment to primary health care as the key to Health for All by the Year 2000, the World Health Assembly in May 1978 established a global Diarrhoeal Disease Control (CDD) Programme. This Programme has as its immediate objective a reduction of the mortality caused by acute diarrheal diseases. Its longer-term objectives are to reduce the morbidity caused by these diseases and their associated ill effects, particularly malnutrition, in infants and young children, and to promote the self-reliance of countries in the delivery of health and social services for their control.

In order to attain its objectives, the Programme has been built up on two main components:

- a *health services (or control) component*, through which WHO is actively cooperating with Member States in the development of national CDD programmes as a part of primary health care, and

- a *research component*, through which support is being given to applied research to determine the best ways of applying available knowledge in national control programmes, and to biomedical research to find new tools for control, especially vaccines and drugs.

Health services component

The Programme is collaborating with Member States in the development of national CDD programmes applying a package of four major control strategies:

(a) To reduce diarrhea *mortality*:

○ the *treatment* of acute diarrhea, as early as possible in the course of illness, with emphasis on oral rehydration therapy using a balanced glucose-salt solution (ORS)°, accompanied by education of mothers on appropriate feeding of children during diarrhea and in convalescence.

(b) To decrease diarrhea *morbidity*:

○ the encouragement of *maternal and child care practices* that are important for the prevention of diarrhea, especially uninterrupted breast-feeding, preparation of safe weaning foods from local products, and good domestic and personal hygiene; and

○ the improvement of *environmental health practices*, especially by encouraging the proper use and maintenance of drinking water and sanitation facilities, and good food hygiene.

(c) To reduce diarrhea *mortality and morbidity*:

○ the *detection and control of epidemics*, especially of cholera.

The case management strategy is at present being given the highest priority, since the majority of deaths in acute diarrhea are due to dehydration and can be prevented through early oral rehydration therapy (15). Moreover, oral rehydration therapy has also been shown to have a beneficial long-term nutritional effect, resulting in better weight gain, when a nutritional message is given along with it (16).

At the country level WHO is working to promote this package of four strategies in three main areas: planning, training and evaluation (17). First, the CDD Programme is working closely with individual countries in the development of plans of operation for national diarrheal diseases control programmes. Second, it is very much involved in the training, especially management training, of senior-level and mid-level national staff. Technical training courses are also being organized, especially on the clinical and laboratory aspects of diarrheal diseases, and the Programme has produced several training manuals dealing with the treatment of diarrhea, ORS production, and laboratory diagnosis. Information is also widely

---

°ORS solution contains, in one litre of drinking water: 3.5 g sodium chloride, 2.5 g sodium bicarbonate, 1.5 g potassium chloride, and 20 g glucose.

disseminated through the global newsletter "Diarrhoea Dialogue", produced under contract by the Appropriate Health Resources and Technologies Action Group (AHRTAG) Limited, United Kingdom, as well as through special publications such as a half-yearly Bibliography on Acute Diarrhoeal Diseases to be produced shortly in collaboration with the National Library of Medicine, USA. Third, the Programme places great importance on the development of approaches to evaluation. A cluster sample survey approach has been developed for estimating diarrheal disease morbidity and mortality in an area or country, and an outline for comprehensive country programme reviews has been prepared (18).

Global targets have been set for these various activities for 1983 and 1989, as well as projected achievements assuming that these targets are met (Table 4). As of 1 February 1982, 31 countries had formulated plans of operation for national CDD programmes and in two-thirds of these programmes were operational, 20 countries were undertaking local production of ORS, and 55 countries had participated in management training courses.

Research component

The Programme's research component is regarded as an integral part of the control programme and has been designed to respond to the needs of national CDD programmes, which in turn can ensure that new research developments are rapidly applied. The research activities are managed, according the principle of peer review, by regional and global Scientific Working Groups which are responsible, respectively, for health services and biomedical research. Table 5 indicates the number of projects supported by the Programme to date in each area. Of these, 55% are in developing countries.

The Programme's research priorities in *health services (or applied) research* include:

   o studies of different methods for preparation and packaging of ORS;

Table 4. WHO CDD Programme : Services component

Projected targets	1983	1989
Countries with operational programmes	35	80
ORS production centres	20	30
Senior-level staff trained	300	720
Mid-level staff trained	320	980
Country programme evaluations	20	125
Projected achievements	**1983**	**1989**
Diarrhea cases under 5 years with access to oral rehydration therapy (percent)	25	50
Diarrhea cases under 5 years receiving oral rehydration therapy (percent)	12.5	37.5
Diarrhea deaths prevented annually in children under 5 years (million)	0.5	1.5

Table 5. Research component – current status
(at 28 February 1982)

Area	No of projects
Health services research	27
Biomedical research	
– Bacterial enteric infections	26
– Viral diarrheas	18
– Parasitic diarrheas	2
– Clinical management	10
Total	83

○ investigations of different approaches for delivery of oral rehydration therapy at village and family level;
○ etiological studies of acute diarrhea under different ecological and cultural conditions;
○ studies to determine optimal ways of promoting breast-feeding and preparation of safe, locally available weaning foods;
○ studies of traditional beliefs and practices regarding diarrheal disease, and evaluation of health education approaches to modify those that are harmful;
○ investigations of the most effective methods of environmental intervention to reduce the transmission of diarrheal disease agents, including methods of enlisting community participation.

In *biomedical research*, three Scientific Working Groups are coordinating research in (i) bacterial enteric infections, (ii) viral diarrheas, and (iii) drug development and clinical management of acute diarrheas. The priority areas in which research is being supported are listed below:
○ development of improved and simplified techniques for the laboratory diagnosis of the newer pathogens (e.g., rotavirus, enterotoxigenic *Escherichia coli*, and *Campylobacter*);
○ better characterization of the virulence factors in enterotoxigenic *E. coli*, *Vibrio cholerae* O1, and *Shigella*;
○ testing and development of new vaccines against typhoid fever, cholera, rotavirus, and enterotoxigenic *E. coli*;
○ studies on the mode of transmission of specific pathogens (especially rotavirus and *E. coli*);
○ studies on the interrelationship of nutrition and diarrhea (including optimal dietary therapy for children with diarrhea);
○ evaluation of new pharmaceutical approaches for the treatment of diarrhea; and
○ development of alternative means of presentation of ORS.

In the important areas of vaccine and drug development the following new approaches deserve special mention. A new live oral typhoid vaccine (strain Ty21a) is shortly to be field-tested. This vaccine has been shown to be highly effective for three years in an initial evaluation in a field trial in Egypt (19). An attempt is now being made to simplify the administration of the vaccine as a single dose in an enteric coated capsule, so that it will be more suitable for general public health use. Should this be successful, it is likely that an important new tool will be available for the control of typhoid fever. As regards rotavirus vaccine, three candidates are at present under development: two are live attenuated mutants of human rotavirus and the third is a bovine rotavirus vaccine. Various studies are attempting to develop antisecretory agents for diarrhea and the Programme is actively collaborating with several pharmaceutical companies in the study of compounds such as serotonin-antagonists, calcium/calmodulin inhibitors, and alpha agonists.

Another important research activity that the Programme is planning to initiate shortly is a multicentre etiology study to determine the relative importance of the various bacterial and viral agents as a cause of diarrhea in developing countries. This will be carried out conjointly with a hospital-based, case-control study of the etiology of diarrhea and will use a standard clinical and laboratory protocol to ensure the comparability of results.

Programme support

The Diarrhoeal Diseases Control Programme is being carried out with active support from the United Nations Children's Fund (UNICEF), the United Nations Development Programme (UNDP), and the World Bank, and has also received financial support from 14 governments and bilateral agencies. It is clear, however, that these resources constitute only a fraction of the total required to achieve the objectives of reduced mortality and morbidity, and to this end a vast and concerted effort will be needed on the part of national administrators and scientists in both developing and developed countries worldwide.

REFERENCES

1. Barua, D. 1981. Diarrhea as a global problem and the WHO programme for its control, p. 1-6. *In* T. Holme, J. Holmgren, M. H. Merson, and R. Möllby (eds), Acute enteric infections in children. New prospects for treatment and prevention. Elsevier/North-Holland Biomedical Press, Amsterdam.
2. Snyder, J. D., and M. H. Merson. 1982. The magnitude of the global problem of acute diarrhoeal disease: a review of active surveillance data. Bull. Wld Hlth Org. **60**: 605–613.
3. Möllby, R., and E. Bäck. 1981. Bacterial and parasitic agents in acute diarrheal disease in Sweden, p. 159–166. *In* T. Holme, J. Holmgren, M. H. Merson, and R. Möllby (eds.), Acute enteric infections in children. New prospects for treatment and prevention. Elsevier/North-Holland Biomedical Press, Amsterdam.
4. Black, R. E., M. H. Merson, B. Rowe, P. R. Taylor, A. R. M. Abdul Alim, R. J. Gross, and D. A. Sack. 1981. Enterotoxigenic *Escherichia coli* diarrhoea: acquired immunity and transmission in an endemic area. Bull. Wld Hlth Org. **59**: 263–268.
5. Honda, T., Q. Akhtar, R. I. Glass, and A. K. M. Golam Kibriya. 1981. A simple assay to detect *Escherichia coli* producing heat labile enterotoxin: results of a field study of the Biken test in Bangladesh. Lancet, **ii**: 609–610.
6. de Mol, P., and E. Bosmans. 1978. Campylobacter enteritis in Central Africa. Lancet **i**: 604.
7. Billingham, J. D. 1981. Campylobacter enteritis in The Gambia. Trans. roy. Soc. trop. Med. Hyg. **75**: 641–644.

8.   Ringertz, S., R. C. Rickhill, O. Ringertz, and A. Sutomo. 1980. *Campylobacter fetus* subsp. *jejuni* as a cause of gastroenteritis in Jakarta, Indonesia. J. clin. Microbiol. **12**: 538–540.

9.   Salazar, E. Unpublished data.

10.   Blaser, M. J., R. I. Glass, M. Imdadul Huq, B. Stoll, G. M. Kibriya, and A. R. M. A. Alim. 1980. Isolation of *Campylobacter fetus* subsp. *jejuni* from Bangladeshi children. J. clin. Microbiol. **12**: 744–747.

11.   Boonthai, P. 1981. Personal communication.

12.   Frost, J. A., B. Rowe, J. Vandepitte, and E. J. Threlfall. 1981. Plasmid characterisation in the investigation of an epidemic caused by multiply resistant *Shigella dysenteriae* type 1 in Central Africa. Lancet ii: 1074–1076.

13.   Sack, D. A., D. C. Kaminsky, R. B. Sack, J. N. Itotia, R. R. Arthur, A. Z. Kapikian, F. Ørskov, and I. Ørskov. 1978. Prophylactic doxycycline for travelers' diarrhea: results of a prospective double-blind study of Peace Corps volunteers in Kenya. New Engl. J. Med. **298**: 758–763.

14.   Sack, R. B., J. L. Froehlich, A. W. Zulich, D. Sidi Hidi, A. Z. Kapikian, F. Ørskov, I. Ørskov, and H. B. Greenberg. 1979. Prophylactic doxycycline for travelers' diarrhea. Gastroenterology **76**: 1368–1373.

15.   Baumslag, N., R. Davis, L. G. Mason, M. McQuestion, E. Sabin, J. Snyder, and A. Wiesenthal (eds.). 1980. Oral rehydration therapy: an annotated Bibliography. Pan American Health Organization, Washington, D. C.

16.   International Study Group. 1977. A positive effect on the nutrition of Philippine children of an oral glucose-electrolyte solution given at home for the treatment of diarrhoea. Bull. Wld Hlth Org. **55**: 87–94.

17.   Summary of Programme activities, January 1980 - April 1981. 1981. Unpublished document WHO/CDD/81.3. World Health Organization, Geneva.

18.   Manual for the planning and evaluation of national diarrhoeal diseases control programmes. 1981. Unpublished document WHO/CDD/SER/81.5. World Health Organization, Geneva.

19.   Wahdan, M. H., Ch. Sérié, R. Germanier, A. Lakany, Y. Cerisier, N. Guerin, S. Sallam, P. Geoffroy, A. Sadek El Tantawi, and P. Guesry. 1980. A controlled field trial of live oral typhoid vaccine Ty21a. Bull. Wld Hlth Org. **58**: 469–474.

Bacterial Diarrheal Diseases, eds., Y. Takeda, T. Miwatani, 11-23.
Copyright © 1985 by KTK Scientific Publishers, Tokyo.

THE VIBRIO DISEASES IN 1982: AN OVERVIEW

John P. Craig

Department of Microbiology and Immunology, Downstate Medical Center, State University of New York, Brooklyn, New York, U. S. A.

Members of the genus *Vibrio* are the causative agents of a major component of the diarrheal diseases of man, and of a small but intriguing number of systemic infections. In this brief overview I will outline my present perception of the nature and importance of diseases caused by vibrios, and then discuss a few of our own observations about toxin production by cholera vibrios. In other papers presented in this symposium, many of the participants will provide more detailed discussions of some of the topics which I can only introduce in this review.

Table 1 presents a very simplified summary of some of the important features of the six species of pathogenic vibrios which are now generally recognized. Cholera, in all of its epidemiologic forms, and food poisoning due to *Vibrio parahaemolyticus* continue to be responsible for the vast majority of morbidity caused by vibrios, and *Vibrio cholerae* cases, almost all of the mortality, in spite of the fact that case fatality ratios are very much higher for the rare cases of *Vibrio vulnificus* septicemia in compromised hosts (1).

In view of a number of recent findings, I think it is appropriate that henceforth all disease caused by *Vibrio cholerae*, including the non-O1 serotypes (or serovars) should be called cholera, fully recognizing that this disease appears in a number of epidemiologic forms. This view is supported by the fact that all heat-labile enterotoxins produced by this species appear to be very similar, and that, if minor differences occur, these differences are probably not associated with serotype (2). Rather, it seems more reasonable to take the view that all toxinogenic strains of all serotypes and both biotypes of the O1 serotype have the potential for producing essentially the same spectrum of clinical illness in which enterotoxin-mediated dehydrating diarrhea represents the severe extreme, and that the main feature distinguishing non-O1 serotypes is their epidemiologic pattern. There is thus far no documented instance of non-O1 serotypes being involved in true epidemic spread, or appearing simultaneously or sequentially in several geographic areas. Thus, most non-O1 disease has been sporadic, or has occurred in non-dispersing localized epidemics. (3, 4, 5). This is also true so far of *Vibrio mimicus* and *Vibrio fluvialis*, although it is impossible to be certain that epidemic or even pandemic cholera in the nineteenth and early twentieth century was not caused at times by non-O1 serotypes or by these newly recognized species. The el tor biotype of the O1 serotype

Table 1. Pathogenic vibrios and some of their properties

Organism	Disease	Gut Mucosal Colonization	Tissue Invasion	Bacteremia	Enterotoxin LT	Enterotoxin ST	Salt Required
Vibrio cholerae Serotype 0:1 classical and eltor biotypes	Cholera (sporadic, endemic, epidemic &	+	0	0	+	0	0
Non-0:1 Serotypes	pandemic)	+	0	0	+	+	0
V. mimicus (Suc⁻)	Cholera-like diarrhea	+	0	0	(+)[1]	+	0
V. fluvialis (Group F, EF6)	Cholera-like diarrhea	+	0	0	(+)	+	+
V. parahaemolyticus	Sea food gastro-enteritis	+	0	0	(+)	0	+
V. alginolyticus	Wound Infections	0	+	0	0	0	+
V. vulnificus (Lac⁺)	Cellulitis & septicemia	0	+	+	0	0	+

[1] (+) Enterotoxic activity not demonstrated but filtrates exhibit properties suggesting enterotoxin.

has been clearly associated with both smoldering endemicity and pandemic spread (6) and the classical biotype with endemic cholera in the Indian subcontinent and presumably pandemic spread in ages past (7).

Thus the property which confers the ability to engage in pandemic spread, which might best be called "dispersiveness", a term introduced by the German epidemiologist Sticker over 70 years ago (8), is a property to be reckoned with, but one which we can measure only in retrospect, and for which no laboratory tests have been devised.

Vibrio mimicus, which until recently was merely a cholera vibrio which could not ferment sucrose (9), as well as *Vibrio fluvialis* (10), should tentatively be viewed as members of a cholera vibrio cluster, since they appear to produce disease in the same clinical spectrum as *Vibrio cholerae*, and both have been shown to produce exotoxins in vitro which exhibit some of the properties of cholera enterotoxin (11, 12, 13, 14). The recent outbreaks of *V. fluvialis* diarrhea suggest that they could have been accepted as cholera both clinically and epidemiologically in earlier times before the more recent laboratory tests were available (15). Heat-stable enterotoxins, biologically similar to *E. coli* ST, have been demonstrated in some strains of non-O1 *V. cholerae*, *V. mimicus* and *V. fluvialis* (5, 11, 14). Their role in pathogenesis is not yet known. The greater salt requirement of *V. fluvialis* places it in the broad group of halophilic vibrios, and this may play an important role in determining its epidemiologic pattern (10).

The other halophilic vibrios are pathogenetically really quite different from the cholera group. *V. parahaemolyticus* appears at first to resemble the cholera group because of its marked susceptibility to serum killing and phagocytosis so that it colonizes the human host mainly as a mucosal surface infection (16). There is evidence, however, that penetration of intestinal epithelial cells (17) and ulceration of the bowel do occur (18). Although intensive efforts have been made to determine how this organism stimulates fluid secretion, this mechanism is still unknown (3). Although the thermostable hemolysin may be capable of doing some damage to intestinal cell membranes, other factors are clearly responsible for the diarrhea seen in disease. Honda has shown that anti-hemolysin antibody is incapable of preventing the fluid accumulation evoked by living cells in the rabbit ligated ileal loop assay (19).

V. parahaemolyticus is reported to produce a substance which causes elongation of Chinese hamster ovary cells (20), hence the plus sign in parentheses in Table 1, but enterotoxic activity of cell-free preparations has not yet been demonstrated (3). The thermostable hemolysin causes increase in vascular permeability in cutaneous blood vessels with peak activity at one to two hours after infection (19). This is reminiscent of the permeability factor (PF) activity of *Clostridium perfringens* alpha toxin (phospholipase C) and *E. coli* ST (21, 22) but it must be emphasized that relatively few molecules which have PF activity are also enterotoxins. When the diarrheagenic principle of *V. parahaemolyticus* is finally revealed, it is likely that it will represent a previously unrecognized hypersecretory mechanism. An understanding of this mechanism is an important goal, because it may explain not only *V. parahaemolyticus* diarrhea, but may help to explain the enteropathogenicity of non-toxinogenic strains of *V. cholerae* as well.

The invasive vibrios, *Vibrio alginolyticus* and *V. vulnificus* closely resemble *V. parahaemolyticus* in their salt requirements, their bacteriological properties and their ecology (23, 24). All are normal inhabitants of marine environments, and infection is acquired exclusively by consumption of contaminated seafood or injection of contaminated seawater (3). However, they differ strikingly from *V. parahaemolyticus* in their invasive tendency. Not only do they penetrate the gut wall readily, but they possess surface antigens which resist phagocytosis (25, 26) and they are much less susceptible to the bactericidal activity of normal human serum than is *V. parahaemolyticus* (16). Most of the septicemic cases of *V. vulnificus* infection have been in patients which chronic liver disease, often with hemochromatosis (1). There is experimental evidence to suggest that increased available iron along with poor complement-mediated serum killing may account for the high susceptibility in these patients (27). Nevertheless, it is striking that tissue invasion and septicemia do not occur with the cholera group of vibrios, even in the most debilitated patients or in patients with chronic liver disease. So marked is this difference that in experimental animals orally or intestinally administered *V. vulnificus* fails to colonize the intestinal mucosa, but passes directly into the tissues to establish fatal septicemia (26). Experimental findings differ concerning the presence of exotoxins in cell-free filtrates. Some investigators have shown that only viable cells cause the marked increase in vascular permeability leading to protein and water loss into the extravascular tissues, edema, hemoconcentration, hypovolemic shock and death (26). Others have demonstrated lethal, heat-labile, antigenic cytolysins in cell-free filtrates (28). Therefore, the mechanism(s) of pathogenesis for this species is certainly not yet explained, but the facts that are known emphasize the extreme diversity of pathogenetic potential within one genus of organisms which appear to be genetically closely related.

I would now like to return to further discussion of the cholera group of vibrios. Historians have described seven major pandemics of cholera between 1817 and 1982 (6, 7). These are summarized in Fig. 1. The roman numerals indicate the numbers which have been assigned to these periods of wide-spread dissemination. It is obvious that during the past century and a half, the world has been in the throes of what have been called pandemics of cholera much more often than not. In the interpandemic periods, many of which were very short, indeed, it was usually assumed that the organisms disappeared from the unaffected regions, and that cholera has been permanently endemic only in the Indian subcontinent, and perhaps other parts of southeast Asia, and the adjacent islands. It is from these endemic foci that cholera has been thought to sally forth repeatedly over the same trade and travel routes. Even during the seventh pandemic, the path of "advancing" cholera was strikingly similar to and in many cases identical to previous paths followed in the 19th century (6). Moreover, it has been assumed that all pandemics from I through VI were caused by the classical biotype of serotype O1 of *V. cholerae*. I wonder whether either of these assumptions is warranted. In view of newer knowledge of the ecology of cholera vibrios, it appears likely that all biotypes

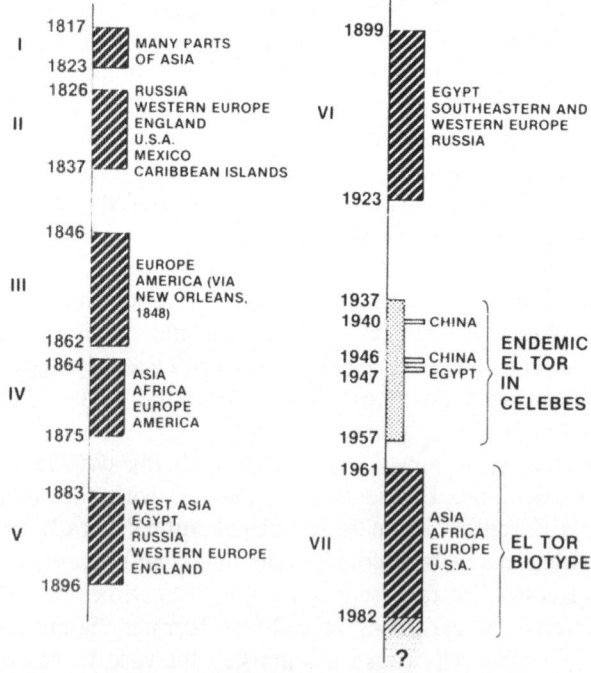

Fig. 1. Pandemic and Epidemic Cholera, 1817–1982.

and serotypes can be autochthonous members of certain bodies of water, especially brackish estuaries, where they can lead an existence independent of man (29, 30). Should we not leave open the possibility that some or all of the apparent pandemics may have been due, at least in part, to local recrudescenses of disease caused by vibrios which had persisted in the local environment over long periods of time, giving rise to periodic marked fluctuations in the incidence of clinically apparent disease owing to local factors which are still not understood? Recent experience with el tor strains in the southern United States between 1973 and 1981 demonstrates that a single strain may have persisted over a very wide band stretching several hundred kilometers along the U.S. coast of the Gulf of Mexico without recognizable person-to-person spread (31). Recently introduced laboratory methods, especially improved phage typing systems, should enable us to differentiate between persistance in the environment and introduction of strains from other areas by human intervention.

Even with earlier laboratory methods, the observations of Dutch investigators in the Celebes during the two decades before the Seventh Pandemic demonstrated endemic persistence without high clinical disease incidence (32, 6). It has been assumed that those Indonesian strains actually were transported by human agency throughout the six continents to produce the Seventh Pandemic. However, hemolysin, polymyxin B and bacteriophage markers have clearly shown that several different sub-biotypes have appeared within the broader el tor biotype during this pandemic (33). Is it possible that these subtypes did not all originate by mutation from a single parent "pandemic strain", but that they had been living in the environments of several continents all along, and that multiple local epidemics due to ecologic changes which we still do not understand could have created the appearance of pandemic contiguous spread? I think that these possibilities should be considered as new methods are developed for labeling and tracing these organisms more precisely through time and space.

One of the biotypical variables in *V. cholerae* which have interested us for some time is the variation in amount of enterotoxin produced under different growth conditions. Using the rabbit skin PF assay, we can detect as little as 100 pg cholera enterotoxin per ml of crude culture filtrate, making it possible to screen large numbers of strains to determine their in vitro yield. One of the problems which arises with this assay, as with all assays of biologic activity in crude filtrates, is the differentiation between very small amounts of holotoxin and the non-specific blueing caused by as yet unknown factors. To overcome this problem we have developed a simple permeability factor neutralization assay (PFNA) utilizing heat, G_{MI} ganglioside, and cholera antitoxin, to determine whether the PF effect is abolished by these three treatments. Table 2 illustrates the results of such a test on a few strains of *V. cholerae*. Organisms were grown in shallow cultures of casamino acids-yeast extract-glucose medium at 30°C under both resting and shaken conditions. The amount of PF activity in cell-free 24 hr culture filtrates is expressed by a blueing score which incorporates lesion size and intensity. Reduction of this blueing score 4-fold or more by all three treatments has been arbitrarily accepted as indication of the production of specific cholera-like enterotoxin. The scores for strain 569B and for resting culture of 7946 were reduced more than 4-fold

Table 2. PF blueing scores of some representative strains of V. cholerae

Strain	Type/Subtype (Biotype)	Culture Condition	Final Dilution	Blueing Score[a]				
				Control	Heated	C_{M1}[b]	CAT[c]	CT[d]
569B	O:1/Inaba	R[e]	1:2	36	0	0	0	+
	(Classical)	S[e]	1:3200	64	1	1	0	+
7946	O:1/Ogawa	R	1:2	50	10	9	9	+
	(El Tor)	S	1:2	47	12	19	20	±
1196-78	O:1/Ogawa	R	1:2	4	2	4	6	-
	(El Tor)	S	1:2	0	1	1	3	-
2633-78	O:1/Ogawa	R	1:2	17	19	20	17	-
	(El Tor)	S	1:2	4	1	4	2	-
5163	O:25	R	1:2	43	0	43	47	-
		S	1:2	0	0	0	0	-
MS-063	O:42	R	1:4	7	10	7	10	-
		S	1:4	22	14	23	23	-
E8498	O:344	R	1:2	51	3	12	10	+
		S	1:2	44	13	21	18	±

[a] Product of mean lesion diameter (mm) and intensity

[b] With G_{M1} ganglioside, 25 µg/ml

[c] With cholera antitoxin, NIH Lot 001, 40 AU/ml

[d] Cholera toxin present, +; absent -; indeterminate ±

[e] R: resting cultures; S: shaken

by all three treatments. The shaken culture of 7946 contained PF which was only partly neutralized, indicating that, in addition to enterotoxin, this strain produced non-specific PF under this growth condition. Strains 1196-78 and 2633-78 represent two kinds of non-toxinogenic O1 strains. 1196-78 produced almost no PF in either resting or shaken cultures, but 2633-78 produced moderate amounts of heat-stable, non-specific PF in resting cultures, which might be confused with enterotoxin if the PFNA had not been used. Strains 5163 and MS-063 are non-toxinogenic non-O1 strains with different patterns of non-specific PF production. E8498, a non-O1 strain isolated from the environment, produced a great deal of non-specific PF in shaken culture, but the resting filtrate contained PF activity which was reduced more than 4-fold by all three treatments. On this basis, E8498 was considered to be toxinogenic, and this was later confirmed by purifying the toxin and demonstrating that it was indistinguishable biologically and immunologically from cholera enterotoxin (34, 35).

Twenty-four strains (10 non-toxinogenic and 14 toxinogenic) were tested for biologically active holotoxin production by the PFNA and for the presence of sequences coding for the toxin gene by the DNA probe technique using both cholera toxin and Escherichia coli heat-labile toxin (LT) probes by Dr. James Kaper (36). There was complete agreement between the two assays in this series. Similarly, 23 strains were examined by PFNA and for specific cholera antitoxin-binding material by G_{M1}ELISA by Dr. Jan Holmgren (37). There was excellent correlation in all but one strain. In that case, the strain produced very little PF-active holotoxin, but a high ELISA reading. Further testing in a subunit-specific ELISA showed that this strain produced excess B subunit. It therefore appears that PFNA is capable in most instances of differentiating between cholera entertoxin and non-specific PF in crude culture filtrates.

We have now examined over 300 strains of *V. cholerae* using the PFNA, and the results are summarized here. There was marked variation in in vitro toxin production even among strains freshly isolated from purging cholera patients and subjected to only minimal serial passage. Fig. 2 shows the distribution of PF content for the three groups of cholera vibrios. Since holotoxin production is dependent on growth conditions (see below), the data in Fig. 2 show the maximal output observed for each strain. Toxin content of culture filtrates is expressed on the abscissa as the $\log_{10}$ of 4 mm blueing doses (BD_4) per ml. Thus, since classical strains nearly always produce more toxin in shaken than in resting cultures, only shaken culture data are presented here. The reverse is true for el tor strains. Non-O1 strains tend to be more like el tor strains. All 32 classical strains were toxinogenic. They varied in toxin output over a range of approximately 300,000-fold. Twenty four of the 139 el tor strains, including isolates from both patients and the environment, proved to be non-toxinogenic based on the PFNA. The amount of non-specific blueing produced by non-toxinogenic strains never exceeded 1000

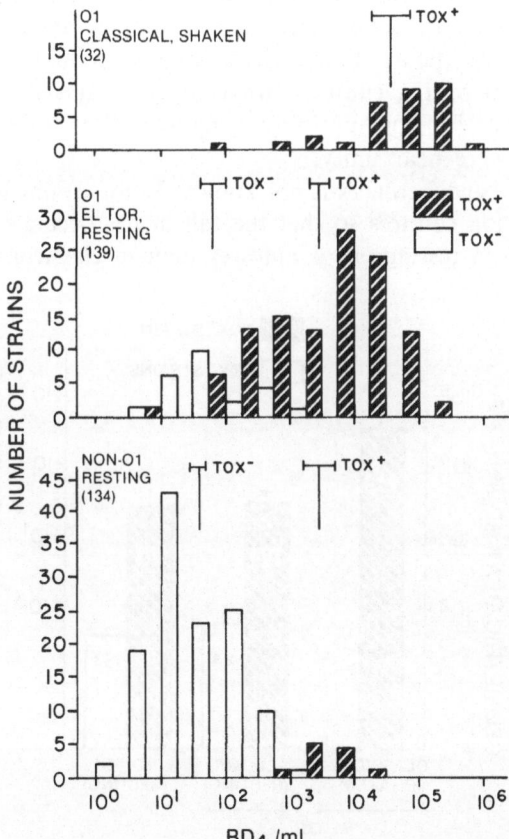

Fig. 2. *In Vitro* Production of Vascular Permeability Factor by Strains of *Vibrio cholerae*.

blueing doses per ml, however, so that strains producing more than this can usually be presumed to be toxinogenic. Toxin production in toxinogenic el tor strains varied over a 300,000-fold range, but at a 10-fold lower mean than for classical strains. It is clear that many toxinogenic strains produce very low levels of toxin in vitro. The non-O1 strains which we have examined were predominantly non-toxinogenic, but the mean for strains which were toxinogenic was essentially identical to that of toxinogenic el tor strains.

These results are summarized in Fig. 3. In terms of biological equivalence with the purified enterotoxin prepared from the classical strain 569B, classical strains produced an average of about 300 ng/ml, and toxinogenic el tor and non-O1 strain about 30 ng/ml. It seems clear therefore that any difference in pathogenicity between el tor and non-O1 strains is not based on differences in enterotoxin production potential, but rather on other less well-defind virulence factors.

Finally, there appears to be a consistent difference in the ratios of toxin produced in shaken and resting cultures by classical and el tor strains. The distribution of these ratios is shown in Fig. 4. The zero point on the abscissa represents equal toxin production in both growth conditions, that is, a ratio of 1.0. Classical strains all had ratios above 1.0, while el tor strains were predominantly less than 1.0, signifying that more toxin was produced in resting than in shaken cultures. Non-O1 strains clustered around unity. These findings are summarized in Fig. 5, which shows that, on the average, classical strains produced 100 times as much toxin in shaken as in resting cultures, while el tor strains produced only about 1/7th as much. Ratios for non-specific blueing as well as for the toxin produced by non-O1 strains were near unity.

The basis for these differences is not known. El tor strains metabolize glucose more rapidly in resting cultures so that the fall in pH occurs earlier and returns to neutrality sooner in resting el tor cultures than in classical cultures, but it is

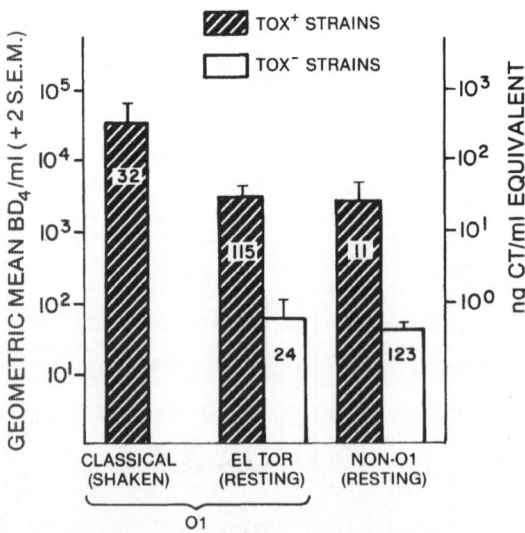

Fig. 3. *In Vitro* Production of Vascular Permeability Factor by Strains of *Vibrio cholerae* O1 and NonO1.

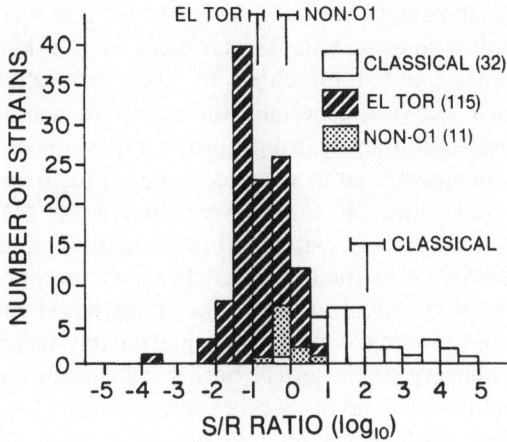

Fig. 4. Distribution of Ratios of PF Content of Shaken/Resting Cultures of Tox$^+$ Strains of *Vibrio cholerae*.

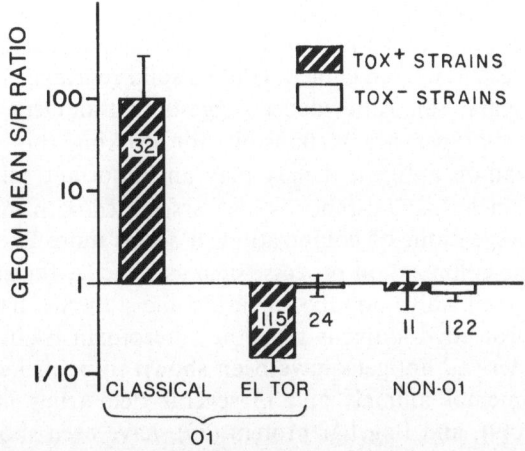

Fig. 5. Ratios of PF Content of Shaken/Resting Cultures of Tox$^+$ and Tox$^-$ Strains of *Vibrio cholerae* O1 and Non-O1.

not certain that this is the critical factor. There is no evidence that these ratios are based on excessive production of B subunit, or on more rapid dissociation of subunits by one or the other biotype. The difference in S/R ratio appears to be consistent, and for the strains examined thus far, about as reliable as any of the conventional labels used to distinguish the two biotypes. One may speculate about whether this difference may reflect a property which is correlated with differences in capacity to survive in the environment.

It is well-recognized that hemolysin production varies among O1 strains of *V. cholerae*, but the distribution of hemolysin-producing capacity among non-O1 strains has not been described in detail. Hemorrhagic factor demonstrable by intracutaneous injection in rabbits has been described for a few non-O1 strains (38, 39), but its distribution among non-O1 serotypes is not known. No role in pathogenesis has been suggested for either of these extracellular products, but their marked biological activity, especially the action of hemorrhagic factor on blood vessels, suggests that they warrant further study.

It has now been demonstrated in volunteers that el tor strains which produce very low levels of toxin in vitro can cause severe cholera (40, 41). Moreover, since diarrhea has now been clearly associated with non-toxinogenic el tor and non-O1 strains (42, 5), the search is on for other diarrheagenic mechanisms. It has been known for some time that colonization of the small bowel mucosa is essential for disease production in animal models (43), presumably in order to assure the most efficient toxin delivery to the brush border cell membrane. However, it is possible that colonization itself involves other mechanisms which induce net fluid hypersecretion. In their early work on toxinogenic *E. coli*, Smith and his colleagues showed that non-toxinogenic strains possessing the adherence factor K-88 were capable of producing mild diarrhea in piglets (44). Recognition of the complexity of these relationships has led to greater attention recently to the roles of chemotaxis, directed motility and adherence in the pathogenesis of vibrio diarrheas (45).

One of the most important findings during the past decade has been the clear demonstration that recovery from cholera confers solid resistance to live rechallenge lasting up to three years (46). All evidence suggests that antigens common to both Ogawa and Inaba subtypes are responsible for evoking this immunity. Since enterotoxin is a common antigen, it may play an important role as a protective antigen. However, since this resistance is also associated with marked inhibition, and perhaps total prevention, of colonization, it seems more likely that other antigens involved in the colonization process, such as flagella, flagellar sheath, outer membrane proteins, cell wall lipopolysaccharide and adhesins have an even more important role as protective antigens than the enterotoxin itself. Whole cell vaccines free of toxin-derived antigens have been shown to be protective against live challenge in experimental animals and in several field trials (47, 48). Purified lipopolysaccharide (49), and flagellar protein (50), have been shown to be protective in experimental animal models, but their relative contribution to the immunity acquired during disease is not at all clear. The possible protective roles of outer membrane protein (endotoxin protein), flagellar sheath antigen, adhesin (lectin) and extracellular enzymes have not been individually assessed, so that at present it is not possible to say which, if any, of these factors contributed to the protective effect of whole-cell vaccine. In enterotoxinogenic *E. coli*, surface pili have been shown to mediate attachment and there is evidence from animal models that local anti-pili antibody can be protective (51). No such clear cut colonization factors have yet been demonstrated in cholera, although the adhesin associated with hemagglutination may prove to play some role in this process (52).

In summary, the important role of enterotoxin has now been well established for at least some strains of cholera vibrios. In order to explain cholera pathogenesis and immunity as well as the mechanisms by which hypotoxinogenic and non-toxinogenic strains cause disease and confer acquired resistance, future investigation will of necessity focus on other properties of these organisms, especially those which determine their successful colonization of the intestinal mucosa.

REFERENCES

1. Blake, P. A., M. H. Merson, R. E. Weaver, D. G. Hollis, and P. C. Heublein. 1979. Disease caused by a marine vibrio. N. Engl. J. Med. **300**: 1–5.
2. Yamamoto, K., Y. Takeda, T. Miwatani, and J. P. Craig. 1982. Molecular heterogeneity of *Vibrio cholerae* non-O1 enterotoxin. This symposium.
3. Blake, P. A., R. E. Weaver, and D. G. Hollis. 1980. Diseases of humans (other than cholera) caused by vibrios. Ann. Rev. Microbiol. **34**: 341–367.
4. Hughes, J. M., D. G. Hollis, E. J. Gangarosa, and R. E. Weiner. 1978. Non-cholera vibrio infections in the United States. Ann. Int. Med. **88**: 602–606.
5. Spira, W. M., and R. R. Daniel. 1979. Biotype clusters formed on the basis of virulence characters in non-O Group 1 *Vibrio cholerae*, In Proceedings of the 15th Joint Cholera Conference, U.S.-Japan Coop. Med. Sci. Program, Bethesda, July 23–25, 1979, U.S. Dept. of Health, Education and Welfare, National institutes of Health, NIH Publication No. 80–2003, February, 1980, pp. 440–457.
6. Kamal, A. M. 1974. The Seventh Pandemic of Cholera, P. 1–14, In D. Barua and W. Burrows (ed.), Cholera, W. B. Saunders, Co., Philadelphia.
7. Pollitzer, R. 1959. Cholera. World Health Organization Monograph Series No. 43, World Health Organization, Geneva.
8. Sticker, G. 1912. Abh. a. d. Seuchengeschichte, II Bd., Die Cholera, Giessen, as quoted by Greenwood, M., 1935, Cholera, pp. 165–172 In Epidemics and Crowd Diseases, Williams and Norgate, Ltd., London.
9. Davis, B. R., G. R. Fanning, J. M. Madden, A. G. Steigerwalt, H. B. Bradford, Jr., H. L. Smith, Jr., and D. J. Brenner. 1981. Characterization of biochemically atypical *Vibrio cholerae* strains and designation of a new pathogenic species, *Vibrio mimicus*. J. Clin. Microbiol. **14**: 631–639.
10. Lee, J. V., P. Shread, A. L. Furniss, and T. Bryant. 1981. Taxonomy, and description of *Vibrio fluvialis*, sp. nov. (Synonym Group F vibrios, Group EF6). J. Appl. Bact. **50**: 73–95.
11. Brenner, D. J., S. Moseley, B. R. Davis, G. R. Fanning, and A. G. Steigerwalt. 1981. Choleratoxin and heat-stable enterotoxin production by *Vibrio mimicus*. Abstr. In Proceedings of the 17th Joint Cholera Conference, U.S.-Japan Coop. Med. Sci. Program, Baltimore, October 25–28, 1981, p. 20.
12. Sanyal, S. C., R. K. Agarwal, E. Annapurna, and J. V. Lee. 1980. Enterotoxicity of Group F vibrios. Jpn. J. Med. Sci. and Biol. **33**: 217–222.
13. Lockwood, D. E., A. S. Kreger, and S. H. Richardson. 1982. Detection of toxins produced by *Vibrio fluvialis*. Infect. Immun. **35**: 702–708.
14. Kudoh, Y., M. Tsuno, S. Matsushita, S. Yamada, K. Ohta, S. Sakai, and M. Ohashi. 1981. Enteropathogenicity and some biological features of Group F (EF6) vibrio isolates. Abstr. In Proceedings of the 17th Joint Cholera Conference, U.S.-Japan Coop. Med. Sci. Program, Baltimore, October, 25–28, 1981, p. 54.
15. Furniss, A. L., J. V. Lee, and T. J. Donovan. 1977. Group F, a new vibrio? Lancet, **2**: 565.
16. Carruthers, M., and M. J. Kabat. 1981. *Vibrio vulnificus* (lactose-positive vibrio) and *Vibrio parahaemolyticus* differ in their susceptibilities to human serum. Infect. Immun. **32**: 964–966.
17. Calia, F. M., and D. E. Johnson. 1975. Bacteremia in suckling rabbits after oral challenge with *Vibrio parahaemolyticus*. Infect. Immun. **11**: 1222–1225.
18. Bolen, J. L., S. A. Zamiska, and W. B. Greenough, III. 1974. Clinical features in enteritis due to *Vibrio parahaemolyticus*. Am. J. Med. **57**: 638–641.
19. Honda, T. 1982. Pathogenesis of *Vibrio parahaemolyticus*. This symposium.
20. Honda, T., M. Shimizu, Y. Takeda, and T. Miwatani. 1976. Isolation of a factor causing morphological changes of Chinese hamster ovary cells from the culture filtrate of *Vibrio parahaemolyticus*. Infect. Immun. **14**: 1028–1033.

21. Elder, J. M., and A. A. Miles. 1957. The action of the lethal toxins of gas-gangrene clostridia on capillary permeability. J. Path. & Bact. **74**: 133–145.

22. Craig, J. P., Y. Yamamoto, T. Takeda, Y. Takeda, and T. Miwatani. 1981. Vascular permeability activity of *Escherichia coli* heat-stable enterotoxin. Infect. Immun. **33**: 473–476.

23. Zen-Yoji, H., R. A. LeClair, K. Ohta, and T. S. Montague. 1973. Comparison of *Vibrio parahaemolyticus* cultures isolated in the United States with those isolated in Japan. J. Infect. Dis. **127**: 237–241.

24. Farmer, J. J., III. 1979. *Vibrio ("Beneckea") vulnificus*, the bacterium associated with sepsis, septicaemia and the sea. Lancet **2**: 903.

25. Poole, M. D., and J. D. Oliver. 1978. Experimental pathogenicity and mortality in ligated ileal loop studies of the newly reported halophilic lactose-positive *Vibrio* sp. Infect. Immun. **20**: 126–129.

26. Bowdre, J. H., M. D. Poole, and J. D. Oliver. 1981. Edema and hemoconcentration in mice experimentally infected with *Vibrio vulnificus*. Infect. Immun. **32**: 1193–1199.

27. Wright, A. C., L. M. Simpson, and J. D. Oliver. 1981. Role of iron in the pathogenesis of *Vibrio vulnificus*. Infect. Immun. **34**: 503–507.

28. Kreger, A., and D. Lockwood, 1981. Detection of extracellular toxin(s) produced by *Vibrio vulnificus*. Infect. Immun. **33**: 583–590.

29. Colwell, R. R., R. J. Seidler, J. Kaper, S. W. Joseph, S. Garges, H. Lockman, D. Maneval, H. Bradford, N. Roberts, E. Remmers, I. Huq, and A. Huq. 1981. Occurrence of *Vibrio cholerae* serotype O1 in Maryland and Louisiana estuaries. Appl. Environ. Microbiol. **44**: 555–558.

30. Colwell, R. R. 1982. Ecology of *Vibrio cholerae* and *Vibrio parahaemolyticus* and related vibrios in the natural environment. This symposium.

31. Blake, P. A., D. T. Allegra, J. D. Snyder, T. J. Barrett, L. McFarland, C. T. Caraway, J. C. Feeley, J. P. Craig, J. V. Lee, N. D. Puhr, and R. A. Feldman. 1980. Cholera–a possible endemic focus in the United States. N. Engl. J. Med. **302**: 305–309.

32. de Moor, C. E. 1965. The New Guinea Epidemic and the El Tor Problem, p. 17–18, *In* Proceedings of the Cholera Research Symposium, Honolulu, January 24–29, 1965. U.S. Govt. Printing Office, Washington, D. C.

33. Gallut, J. 1974. The Cholera Vibrios, p. 17–40 *In* D. Barua and W. Burrows (ed.) Cholera. W. B. Saunders, Co., Philadelphia.

34. Craig, J. P., K. Yamamoto, Y. Takeda, and T. Miwatani. 1981. Production of cholera-like enterotoxin by a *Vibrio cholerae* non-O1 strain isolated from the environment. Infect. Immun. **34**: 90–97.

35. Yamamoto, K., Y. Takeda, T. Miwatani, and J. P. Craig. 1982. Purification and some properties of an enterotoxin from *Vibrio cholerae* non-O1 that is identical to cholera enterotoxin. Abstr *In* Proceedings of the 17th Joint Conference on Cholera, U.S.-Japan Coop. Med. Sci. Prog., Baltimore, October 25–28, 1981. pp.85–86.

36. Kaper, J. B., S. L. Moseley, and S. Falkow. 1981. Molecular characterization of environmental and non-toxinogenic strains of *Vibrio cholerae*. Infect. Immun. **32**: 661–667.

37. Svennerholm. A.-M., and J. Holmgren. 1978. Identification of *Escherichia coli* heat-labile enterotoxin by means of a ganglioside immunosorbent assay (G_{MI}-ELISA) procedure. Curr. Microbiol. **1**: 19–27.

38. Ohashi, M., T. Shimada, and H. Fukumi. 1972. *In vitro* production of enterotoxin and hemorrhagic principle by *Vibrio cholerae*, NAG. Jpn. J. Med. Sci. Biol. **25**: 179–194.

39. Zinnaka, Y., S. Fukuyoshi, and Y. Okamura. 1973. Some observations on the NAG vibrio toxin. pp. 116–123 *In* H. Fukumi and M. Ohashi (ed.) Proceedings of the 8th Joint Conference on Cholera, U.S.-Japan Coop. Med. Sci. Prog., Tokyo, Japan, August, 1972. The Japanese Cholera Panel, National Institute of Health, Tokyo.

40. Levine, M. M., R. E. Black, M. L. Clements, D. R. Nalin, L. Cisneros, and R. A. Finkelstein. 1981. Volunteer studies in development of vaccines against cholera and enterotoxigenic *Escherichia coli*: a review. pp. 443–459, *In* T. Holme, J. Holmgren, M. H. Merson and R. Mollby (ed.), Acute Enteric Infections of Children. New Prospects for Treatment and Prevention. Elsevier/North-Holland Biomedical Press, Amsterdam.

41. Unpublished observations by the author.
42. Morbidity and Mortality Weekly Report, 1980. **50**: 601. U.S. Dept. of Health and Human Services, Public Health Service, U.S.A.
43. Freter, R. 1969. Studies of the mechanism of action of intestinal antibody in experimental cholera. Tex. Rep. Biol. Med. **27**: suppl. 1, pp. 299–316.
44. Smith, H. W., and M. A. Linggood. 1971. Observations on the pathogenic properties of K88, HlY and ENT plasmids of *Escherichia coli* with particular reference to porcine diarrhea. J. Med. Microbiol. **4**: 467–485.
45. Freter, R. 1980. Association of enterotoxigenic bacteria with the mucosa of the small intestine: mechanisms and pathogenic implications, p. 155–170 *In* Ö. Ouchterlony and J. Holmgren (ed.), Cholera and Related Diarrheas, 43rd Nobel Symp., Stockholm, 1978, S. Karger, Basel.
46. Levine, M. M. 1980. Immunity to cholera as evaluated in volunteers. pp. 195–203 *In* Ö. Ouchterlony and J. Holmgren (ed.) Cholera and Related Diarrheas, 43rd Nobel Symp., Stockholm, 1978. S. Karger, Basel.
47. Peterson, J. W. 1979. Synergistic protection against experimental cholera by immunization with cholera toxoid and vaccine. Infect. Immun. **26**: 528–533.
48. Feeley, J. C., and Gangarosa, E. J. 1980. Field trials of cholera vaccine, pp. 204–210 *In* Ö. Ouchterlony and J. Holmgren (ed.), Cholera and Related Diarrheas. 43rd Nobel Symp., Stockholm, 1978. S. Karger, Basel.
49. Svennerholm, A.-M., and J. Holmgren. 1976. Synergistic protective effect in rabbits of immunization with *Vibrio cholerae* lipopolysaccharide and toxin/toxoid. Infect. Immun. **13**: 735–740.
50. Yancey, P. J., D. L. Willis, and L. J. Berry. 1979. Flagella-induced immunity against experimental cholera in adult rabbits. Infect. Immun. **25**: 220–228.
51. Moon, H. W., and R. E. Isaacson. 1980. Pili of enterotoxigenic *Escherichia coli* as protective antigens in live oral vaccines, Abstr *In* Proceedings of the 16th Joint Cholera Conference, U.S.-Japan Coop. Med. Sci. Prog., October 1980, Gifu, Japan.
52. Finkelstein, R. A., and L. F. Hanne. 1982. Hemagglutinins (colonization factors?) produced by *Vibrio cholerae*, Abstr *In* Proceedings of the 17th Joint Cholera Conference, U.S.-Japan Coop. Med. Sci. Prog., Baltimore, October 25–28, 1981.

This work was supported by Public Health Service Conract AI 92602 from the National Institute of Allergy and Infectious Diseases and by grant C6/181/49 from the Diarrheal Diseases Control Program of the World Health Organization, United Nations.

*This work has subsequently been published as follows: Yamamoto, K., Y. Takeda, T. Miwatani and J. P. Craig. Purification and Some Properties of a Non-O1 *Vibrio cholerae* Enterotoxin that is Identical to Cholera Enterotoxin. Infect. Immun. **39**: 1128–1125, 1983.

Bacterial Diarrheal Diseases, eds., Y. Takeda, T. Miwatani, 25-36.
Copyright © 1985 by KTK Scientific Publishers, Tokyo.

EPIDEMIOLOGY OF INFANTILE BACTERIAL DIARRHEAL DISEASE IN BRAZIL

L. R. Trabulsi[1], M. R. F. Toledo[1], J. Murahovschi[2], U. F. Neto[1], and J. A. N. Candeias[3]

Department of Microbiology, Immunology and Parasitology, Escola Paulista de Medicina, São Paulo[1]
Clinica Infantil do Ipiranga, São Paulo[2]
Department of Microbiology and Immunology, Instituto de Ciências Biomédicas, USP, São Paulo[3]

Although we are supposed to present a paper on the epidemiology of infantile diarrhea in Brazil, we will not attempt to cover the whole subject. On the contrary, this paper will deal basically with the prevalence of the principal enteropathogenic bacteria and viruses in the feces of infants with endemic diarrhea and control groups. We should also initially say that we are not going to present data from all over Brazil. First of all, no data are available for many areas of the country and second, most of the available data concern infants of low socio-economic level.

Just to show the importance of infantile diarrhea in Brazil, two examples were selected from studies conducted in São Paulo:
1) Approximately 1/3 of the pediatric emergency visits to public hospitals were due to acute diarrhea in the last three years (data not published);
2) in the report of the Inter-American Investigation of Mortality in Childhood, published in 1973 (18) it was shown that the infant mortality rate determined by infectious diseases was 24.3 per thousand live births and that about 80% of the infections were represented by diarrheal disease.

However, according to the State Department of Statistic the number of infantile deaths due to "enteritis and other diarrheal diseases" fell about 40% from 1977 to 1979 in São Paulo. Data for the last two years were not available.

Prevalence of the individual enteropathogens

Escherichia coli

At present, we know at least 3 categories of *E. coli* which cause infantile diarrhea. The oldest one is the traditional enteropathogenic *E. coli* serotypes associated with infantile diarrhea, or EPEC. In this category we may include around 14-18 O serogroups, but in our studies we have been looking for only serogroups

O26, O55, O86, O111, O119, O125, O126 and O127. *E. coli* serogroups O128ac and O124 are not considered as EPEC in our laboratory because the first is an enterotoxin ST producer (19) and the second is invasive (28).

The EPEC serogroups mentioned are very important cause of infantile diarrhea in Brazil and this has been so for at least 20 years. In studies carried out in different periods during the 1960s and the 1970s in São Paulo, EPEC was found in about 25 – 34% of infants with diarrhea, an isolation frequency higher than the joint isolation frequency of *Shigella* and *Salmonella* in the same studies (11, 12). However, EPEC has its greatest importance in the first 6 months of life. In the study summarized in table 1, involving 558 children with acute diarrhea and carried out in the last 5 years in São Paulo, EPEC was found in 35% of the children less than 6 months old, in 16% of those aged 6 to 11 months, but only in about 3% of those with or over 12 months of age. In the same table, it is shown that the isolation rate of EPEC for 181 control children matched by age, socio-economic level and study period was about 5% only. As shown in table 2, *E. coli* O111ab and *E. coli* O119 represented about 81% of all EPEC isolates in the preceding study. Table 3 shows the O:H types within each O serogroup. If we consider that the large majority of *E. coli* O111ab isolates was non-motile

Table 1. Frequency of EPEC in feces of 558 children with acute diarrhea and in 181 controls studied in São Paulo between 1977 and 1982

Age (months)	Children with diarrhea		Controls	
	Nọ	Nọ with EPEC	Nọ	Nọ with EPEC
0-5	359	126 (35.1%)	95	5 (5.3%)
6-11	95	15 (15.8%)	32	2 (6.2%)
≥12	104	3 (2.9%)	54	2 (3.7%)
Total	558	144 (25.8%)	181	9 (5.0%)

Table 2. Frequency of isolation of EPEC O serogroups in São Paulo between 1977 and 1978

O Serogroups	Nọ of isolates	
26	8 (5.9%)	
55	9 (6.7%)	
86	4 (3.0%)	
111ab	69 (51.5%)	81.3%
119	40 (29.8%)	
125	1 (0.7%)	
126	3 (2.2%)	
Total	134 (100%)	

Table 3. Serotypes (O:H) of EPEC
          isolated from children in
          São Paulo between 1977
          and 1978

Serotypes	Nọ of isolates
O26:H⁻	6
O26:H11	1
O26:H32	1
O55:H⁻	4
O55:H6	3
O55:H7	2
O86:H34	4
O111ab:H⁻	37
O111ab:H2	29
O111:H?	3
O119:H⁻	2
O119:H6	38
O125:H21	1
O126:H21	2
O126:H27	1

or had H2 antigen, and that out of the 40 *E. coli* O119 strains 2 were non-motile and 38 had H6 antigen, we came to the pratical conclusion that in São Paulo we can make a complete identification of most EPEC using just two O and two H sera. It is interesting to note that the occurrence of these O:H types has been stable in the last 20 years and that the majority of them correspond to the same O:H types reported by Ewing et al. (5) as basically isolated from children with diarrhea.

We are emphasizing these aspects of EPEC because several workers are not including the search for these bacteria in their studies on infantile diarrhea and it seems to us that they are very important etiological agents and can be easily and accuratly identified.

Infantile diarrhea caused by EPEC in developed countries has been described most of the times in association with hospital outbreaks. The following evidence strongly suggest that hospitals have been the direct or indirect source of EPEC infections in a large part of our cases. 1) *E. coli* O111 and O119 have been isolated from the environment in several hospital nurseries (17); 2) the larger the number of hospital admissions of an infant the more it has EPEC infections (data not published); and 3) most EPEC strains isolated from infants with endemic diarrhea are typical hospital strains in its pattern of drug resistance (14, 29). So, it is probable that endemic EPEC infections in São Paulo are nosocomial infections basically. This permanent source of infection would be a satisfactory explanation for the persistently high isolation rate for EPEC in infants in the first months of life.

The other category of *E. coli* that cause infantile diarrhea is enterotoxigenic *E. coli*, or ETEC. The first study in Brazil on the role played by these bacteria in infantile diarrhea was conducted by Guerrant et al. (8) in 1975. These authors found that among 38 children with diarrhea 21 were carriers of ETEC. Most isolates were LT-only strains. From 18 controls without diarrhea, only one ETEC strain was isolated. More recently, Magalhães et al. (9) found that 7 or 12% of 60 children with diarrhea in Recife, a northeastern city of Brazil, were carriers of ETEC strains of the three toxigenic phenotypes. No ETEC strains were isolated from 21 children without diarrhea. Now we would like to present the results of a study that we conducted in São Paulo in the years 1978 and 1979, involving 245 children with diarrhea and 96 without symptoms of gastrointestinal disorders.

Table 4 shows that ETEC was isolated from 13.0% of the children with diarrhea and from 11.4% of the control group. However, if we consider these children according to their age groups, we will see that in the control group only the children with or over 12 months of age were carriers of ETEC. Furthermore, these ETEC strains were LT-only without exception. Table 5 shows the distribution of strains LT/ST, ST-only and LT-only in the three age groups of the children with diarrhea. Most of the LT/ST and ST-only strains were isolated from those children 5 months of age or less. Table 6 shows the ETEC serotypes and, in general, they correspond to those referred by other authors (9, 13). It is noteworthy the absence

Table 4. Frequency of ETEC in feces of 245 children with acute diarrhea and in 96 controls studied in São Paulo between 1977 and 1978

Age (months)	Children with diarrhea		Controls	
	NQ	NQ with ETEC	NQ	NQ with ETEC
0-5	161	21 (13.0%)	39	0 (0.0%)
6-11	27	2 (7.4%)	18	0 (0.0%)
≥12	57	9 (15.8%)	39	11*(28.2%)
Total	245	32 (13.0%)	96	11 (11.4%)

* These strains are LT-only.

Table 5. Frequency of LT, ST and LT/ST *E coli* strains in the feces of 245 children with acute diarrhea studied in São Paulo between 1977 and 1978

Age (months)	NQ of cases	NQ of cases with			
		LT	ST	LT/ST	Total
0-5	161	1 (0.6%)	10 (6.2%)	10 (6.2%)	21 (13.0%)
6-11	27	0 (0.0%)	1 (3.7%)	1 (3.7%)	2 (7.4%)
≥12	57	7 (12.2%)	1 (1.7%)	1 (1.7%)	9 (15.8%)
Total	245	8 (3.3%)	12 (4.9%)	12 (4.9%)	32 (13.0%)

Table 6. Serotypes (O:H) of ETEC isolated from children
in São Paulo between 1977 and 1978

Enterotoxigenic phenotype	Serotype	Nọ of isolates
LT/ST	O6:H16	7
	O63:H‾	5
	O139:H28	3
	O25:H42, O6_2:H‾,	5 (one
	NT:H4, NT:H‾, R:H‾	of each)
ST	O128ac:H21	4
	O128ac:H12	3
	O128ac:H7	2
	O128ac:H‾	2
	NT	4
LT	O139:H28	2
	O60:H2	2
	O78:H10	2
	O8:H4, o8:H5, O8:H8,	6 (one
	O8:H9, O25:H‾, O114:H21	of each)

NT, negative with O1-O157 sera.

Table 7. Distribution of ETEC phenotypes in human
feces, food and water

Phenotype	Human		Food[a]	Water[b]
	Diarrhea	No diarrhea		
LT[c]	+	+	+	+
ST	+	-	-	-
LT/ST	+	-	-	-

[a] From animals.
[b] From rivers and drinking water.
[c] Serotypes are not the same in the three sources.

in São Paulo of serotypes O78:H11 and H12. With the objective of learning about the human sources of infection by ETEC we have investigated the presence of these bacteria in food and water (20). Table 7 shows that only LT strains have been isolated from the two sources. However, the serotypes of these strains were extensively different from those isolated from humans.

Finally, we have invasive *E. coli*, whose known O serogroups are the following: O28ac, O29, O112ac, O124, O136, O143, O144, O152, O164, and "*E. coli* São Paulo" (22). Table 8 shows that invasive *E. coli* was found in all age groups, but with low frequency rate. In a study carried out in the 1960s we detected in-

Table 8.   Frequency of EIEC in feces of 558 children with
           acute diarrhea and in 181 controls studied in
           São Paulo between 1977 and 1982

Age (months)	Children with diarrhea		Controls	
	No.	No. with EIEC	No.	No. with EIEC
0-5	359	2 (0.5%)	95	0 (0.0%)
6-11	95	2 (2.1%)	32	0 (0.0%)
≥12	104	3 (2.9%)	54	1 (1.8%)
Total	558	7 (1.2%)	181	1 (0.5%)

vasive *E. coli* in about 6% (9 of 154) of the children with diarrhea in São Paulo. In our experience, invasive *E. coli* seems to be more frequent in older children and in adults (28).

Shigella

Shigella is an well known agent of infantile diarrhea all over the world. The frequency of these bacteria in children with diarrhea and controls in São Paulo is shown in table 9. It is lower than those reported in the 1950s and 1960s by several authors (14). Around 70% of the children with shigellosis are infected with *Shigella flexneri*, 20% with *Shigella sonnei* and the remaining 10% with *Shigella dysenteriae* or *Shigella boydii*. It should be mentioned that practically all *Shigella dysenteriae* isolates are type 2 (14) and most *Shigella boydii* isolates are an aerogenic variant of *Shigella boydii* 14 (27).

Salmonella

Data obtained in the last 20 years indicate that the frequency of infantile diarrhea caused by *Salmonella* has doubled between 1969 and 1980 in São Paulo (16, 24). Furthermore, extraintestinal infections by these bacteria, including meningitis and septicemias, became relatively frequent in the same period. The explanation for these changes seems to be a large epidemic of *Salmonella typhimurium*

Table 9.   Frequency of Shigella in feces of 558 children
           with acute diarrhea and in 181 controls studied
           in São Paulo between 1977 and 1982

Age (months)	Children with diarrhea		Controls	
	No.	No. with Shigella	No.	No. with Shigella
0-5	359	15 (4.2%)	95	0 (0.0%)
6-11	95	7 (7.4%)	32	1 (3.1%)
≥12	104	11 (10.6%)	54	3 (5.5%)
Total	558	33 (5.9%)	181	4 (2.2%)

infections that broke out in the 1960s and persists until today. The epidemic was first recorded in 3 nurseries in 1969 (25) and since then it has spread to several other nurseries and to the community. At present, we may say that we have in São Paulo and probably in other cities of Brazil a kind of vicious circle in which the nurseries feed the community with *S. typhimurium* and the community feeds the nursery. According to this, we may say that endemic infantile diarrhea caused by *S. typhimurium* in São Paulo is to a large extent nourished by the hospital nurseries, in a manner similar to that mentioned for EPEC. Table 10 shows the frequency of *Salmonella* among 558 children with diarrhea and 181 controls, studied

Table 10. Frequency of Salmonella in feces of 558 children with acute diarrhea and in 181 controls studied in São Paulo between 1977 and 1982

Age (months)	Children with diarrhea		Controls	
	No.	No. with Salmonella	No.	No. with Salmonella
0-5	359	30 (8.3%)	95	6 (6.3%)
6-11	95	8 (8.4%)	32	0 (0.0%)
≥12	104	2 (1.9%)	54	2 (3.7%)
Total	558	40 (7.2%)	181	8 (4.4%)

Table 11. Some characteristics of the epidemic and non-epidemic strains of Salmonella typhimurium found in São Paulo

Characteristics	Strains	
	Epidemic	Non-epidemic
Beta-galactosidase	+ (plasmid mediated)	-
Antigens	1,4,12:i-1,2	1,4,5,12:i-1,2
Phage types (Felix-Callow)	non-typable	typable
Drug resistance	1) Usually resistant to trimethoprim-sulfa-methoxazole, nalidix acid, ampicillin, cephalosporin, te-tracycline, kanamy-cin, chloramphenicol	Usually sensitive to the same drugs
	2) Most isolates resistant to gentamycin	Never resistant to gentamycin
	3) Some isolates resistant to colistin	Never resistant to colistin
Mouse virulence	Reduced	Expected

between 1977 and 1982. About 80% of the *Salmonella* isolates were the epidemic strain of *S. typhimurium*. In table 11 are shown some characteristics of this *Salmonella* (1, 2, 7, 15, 26).

Yersinia enterocolitica

Y. enterocolitica seems to be a rare cause of infantile diarrhea in Brazil. In a survey conducted in our laboratory in the last 4 years we found the bacteria in only 3 children with diarrhea out of more than 500 studied. In Rio de Janeiro, in a study conducted by Stumpf et al. (23) in 1978, *Y. enterocolitica* was found in 4 (5.7%) of 70 children with diarrhea. In spite of the low frequency of infantile diarrhea caused by *Y. enterocolitica*, the bacteria have been found in several animal species and foods in Brazil (6).

Campylobacter fetus ssp. jejuni

The studies conducted in Brazil on the association of *Campylobacter fetus* ssp. *jejuni* with infantile diarrhea are three in number. Ricciardi et al. (21) found the bacteria in the feces of 14 (6.4%) of 271 children with diarrhea, in Rio de Janeiro. In Recife, a northeastern city of Brazil, Marcelo Magalhães (personal communication) found *Campylobacter fetus* ssp. *jejuni* in 17 (18.9%) of 90 infants with diarrhea and in 8 (17.8%) of 45 controls. In São Paulo, we are conducting a study that already involves 266 children with diarrhea and 78 controls. The frequency of *Campylobacter fetus* ssp. *jejuni* in the first group has been of 6.0% and in the second of 9.0% (Table 12).

Rotavirus

Rotavirus has been investigated in several areas of Brazil and has been found in 20 – 30% of the children with endemic diarrhea (3, 4). Prevalence has been high in the cold months of the year and in infants over 5 months of age.

Table 12. Frequency of Campylobacter fetus ssp. jejuni in feces of 266 children with diarrhea and in 78 controls studied in São Paulo between 1980-1982

Age (months)	Children with diarrhea		Controls	
	No.	No. with C. jejuni	No.	No. with C. jejuni
0-5	132	9 (6.8%)	35	2 (5.7%)
6-11	62	2 (3.2%)	14	2 (14.3%)
≥12	72	5 (6.9%)	29	3 (10.3%)
Total	266	16 (6.0%)	78	7 (9.0%)

Prevalence of enteropathogenic bacteria and Rotavirus. Mixed infections

Table 13 shows that results of a study on the etiology of acute diarrhea we have been carrying out in São Paulo since March 1981 and in which we looked for EPEC, ETEC, EIEC, *Shigella, Salmonella, Y. enterocolitica, Campylobacter fetus* ssp. *jejuni* and *Rotavirus* in the feces of each of the children included in the study. We would like to comment on two aspects of the results obtained. First, we did not succeed in finding an etiological agent for a large number of cases in the two age groups investigated. Of course we may think of several explanations for this finding, including the possibility that we still do not know all the bacteria and viruses that may cause diarrhea. The second point to which we would like to call your attention is the high number of cases with mixed infections. This is a largely unknown aspect of infantile diarrhea that involves pro-

Table 13. Frequency of enteropathogenic bacteria and Rotavirus in feces of 190 children with acute diarrhea studied in São Paulo in 1981

Enteropathogenic agent	Age (months)	
	0-5	≥6
	Diarrhea (118)	Diarrhea (72)
EPEC	30 (25.4%)	4 (5.5%)
ETEC	7 (5.9%)	2 (2.7%)
EIEC	0 (0.0%)	2 (2.7%)
Shigella	5 (4.2%)	3 (4.2%)
Salmonella	5 (4.2%)	3 (4.2%)
C. jejuni	2 (1.7%)	1 (1.4%)
Y. enterocolitica	0 (0.0%)	0 (0.0%)
Rotavirus	8 (6.7%)	7 (9.7%)
2 or more	18 (15.2%)	18 (25.0%)
Total	75 (63.5%)	40 (55.5%)

Table 14. Frequency of association among enteropathogenic agents in a study conducted in São Paulo in 1981

Enteropathogenic agent	No. of isolates	No. in association
EPEC	58	23 (39.6%)
ETEC	17	8 (47.0%)
EIEC	3	1 (33.3%)
Shigella	18	10 (55.5%)
Salmonella	23	10 (43.4%)
C. jejuni	10	6 (60.0%)
Rotavirus	30	13 (43.3%)
Total	159	71 (44.6%)

Table 15. Frequency of EPEC, Shigella and Salmonella in feces of children with acute diarrhea in the cities of Botucatu and São Paulo, in 1965-1969

City	No. of cases	No. with				
		EPEC	Shigella	Salmonella	Mixed	Total
Botucatu	805	37 (4.6%)	76 (9.4%)	29 (3.6%)	3 (0.4%)	145 (18.0%)
São Paulo	305	93 (30.5%)	14·(4.6%)	11 (3.6%)	12 (3.9%)	130 (42.6%)

blems of epidemiology, diagnoses, pathogenesis and even treatment. Surprisingly enough, table 14 shows that each of the etiological agent investigated came out with a companion with a high frequency rate.

Now I would like to mention some of the more pertinent characteristics of the children that have been most studied in Brazil in regard to diarrheal diseases.

They frequently live in over populated slums in the surroundings of large cities, where the hygiene standards are particularly poor. Also, these children are most often undernourished and make use of the generally over-crowded public hospitals where the nursing staff is not sufficiently skilled and the young doctors working without supervision are liable to make abusive use of antibiotics. Unfortunately, we do not have studies on infantile diarrhea in the other sectors of the Brasilian population, but the incidence of this illness and probably the prevalence of the different etiological agents are different from those here presented. Just to exemplify the latter possibility, we would like to compare in table 15 the results of two studies carried out in the state of São Paulo between 1965 and 1969, both with children belonging to low income families making use of Public Health Services. One study was conducted in the capital of São Paulo and the other in Botucatu, a small university city in the countryside of the state. As you can see, EPEC was found almost 7 times more frequently in the capital than in Botucatu. Shigella was found twice more often in Botucatu than in São Paulo. The positive cultures and mixed infections were more frequent in São Paulo than in Botucatu.

We thank Wanda M. Cintra de Camargo for revewing the English text.

REFERENCES

1. Affonso, M. H. T., M. R. F. Toledo, and L. R. Trabulsi. 1977. Natureza genética da fermentacão de lactose em amostras de *Salmonella typhimurium*. Rev. Microbiol. **8**: 110–116.
2. Almeida, P. C., and L. R. Trabulsi. 1974. Caracteristicas culturais, bioquimicas, sorológicas e virulência de amostras de *Salmonella typhimurium* fermentadora de lactose. Rev. Microbiol. **5**: 27–35.
3. Baldacci, E. R., J. A. N. Candeias, J. C. Breviglieri, and S. J. E. Grisi. 1979. Etiologia viral e bacteriana de casos de gastroenterite infantil: uma caracterizacão clinica. Rev. Saúde Públ. **13**: 47–53.
4. Candeias, J. A. N., C. P. Rosenburg, and M. L. Rácz. 1978. Identificacão por contraimunoelectroforese de rotavirus em casos de diarréia infantil. Rev. Saúde Públ. **12**: 99–103.
5. Ewing, W. H., B. R. Davis, and T. S. Montague. 1963. Studies on the occurrence of *Escherichia*

coli serotypes associated with diarrheal disease. CDC Publ. Center for Disease Control. Atlanta, Ga.

6. Falcão, D. P. 1981. Présence de *Yersinia enterocolitica* et *Yersinia pseudotuberculosis* en Amérique Latine. Rev. Microbiol. **21**: 5-10.

7. Falcão, D. P., L. R. Trabulsi, F. W. Hickman, and J. J. Farmer III. 1975. Unusual Enterobacteriaceae: lactose-positive *Salmonella typhimurium* which is endemic in São Paulo, Brazil. J. Clin. Microbiol. **2**: 349-353.

8. Guerrant, R. L., R. A. Roger, P. M. Kirschenfeld, and M. A. Sande. 1975. Role of toxigenic and invasive bacteria in acute diarrhea of childhood. N. Engl. J. Med. **293**: 567-573.

9. Magalhães, M., M. Andrade, and A. E. Carvalho. 1981. Pathogenic *Escherichia coli* associated with infantile diarrhea. Rev. Microbiol. **12**: 38-41.

10. Merson, M. H., F. Ørskov, I. Ørskow, R. B. Sack, I. Huq, and F. T. Koster. 1979. Relationship between enterotoxin production and serotype in enterotoxigenic *Escherichia coli*. Infect. Immun. **23**: 325-329.

11. Murahovschi, J., and D. Ciochetti. 1963. Estudo sobre a etiologia das diarréias agudas do lactente. J. Pediatr. **28**: 1-50.

12. Murahovschi, J., and L. R. Trabulsi. 1976. Sindrome diarréica aguda no lactente. Pediatr. Prat. **47**: 13-31.

13. Ørskov, I., and F. Ørskov. 1977. Special O:K:H serotypes among enterotoxigenic *E. coli* strains from diarrhea in adults and children. Occurrence of the CF (colonization factor) antigen and of hemagglutinating abilities. Med. Microbiol. Immunol. **163**: 99-110.

14. Pessôa, G. V. A., C. T. Calzada, E. S. Peixoto, C. E. A. Melles, E. Kano, M. Raskin, V. Simonsen, and K. Irino. 1978. Ocorrência de bactérias enteropatogênicas em São Paulo no septênio 1970-76. III-Sorotipos de *Shigella* e de *Escherichia coli* da gastrenterite infantil. Rev. Inst. Adolfo Lutz. **38**: 129-139.

15. Pessôa, G. V. A., K. Irino, C. E. A. Melles, C. T. Calzada, M. Raskin, and E. Kano. 1978. Ocorrência de bactérias enteropatogênicas em São Paulo no septênio 1970-76. II-O surto epidêmico de *Salmonella typhimurium* em São Paulo. Rev. Inst. Adolfo Lutz. **38**: 107-127.

16. Pessôa, G. V. A., K. Irino, C. T. Calzada, C. E. A. Melles, and E. Kano. 1978. Ocorrência de bactérias enteropatogênicas em São Paulo no septênio 1970-76 I-Sorotipos de *Salmonella* isolados e identificados. Rev. Inst. Adolfo Lutz, **38**: 87-105.

17. Pessôa, G. V. A., R. T. Suguimori, K. Irino, M. Raskin, and C. T. Calzada. 1980. Isolamento de enterobactérias patogênicas em bercários do municipio de São Paulo. Rev. Inst. Adolfo Lutz. **40**: 107-127.

18. Puffer, R. R., and C. V. Serrano. 1973. Patterns of mortality in childhood. Pan American Health Organization, Sc. Pub. 262.

19. Reis, M. H. L., A. F. P. Castro, M. R. F. Toledo, and L. R. Trabulsi. 1979. Production of heat-stable enterotoxin by the 0128 serogroup of *Escherichia coli*. Infect. Immun. **24**: 289-290.

20. Reis, M. H. L., J. C. Vasconcelos, and L. R. Trabulsi. 1980. Prevalence of enterotoxigenic *Escherichia coli* in some processed raw food from animal origin. Appl. Environ. Microbiol. **39**: 270-271.

21. Ricciardi, I. D., M. C. S. Ferreira, S. S. Otto, N. Oliveira, A. Sabrá, and C. F. Fontes. 1979. Thermophilic Campylobacter-associated diarrhoea in Rio de Janeiro. Rev. Bras. Pesq. Med. Biol. **12**: 189-191.

22. Silva, R. M., M. R. F. Toledo, and L. R. Trabulsi. 1980. Biochemical and cultural characteristics of invasive *Escherichia coli*. J. Clin. Microbiol. **11**: 441-444.

23. Stumpf, M., I. D. Ricciardi, N. Oliveira, A. Sabrá, and M. Bernhoeft. 1978. *Yersinia enterocolitica* as a cause of infantile diarrhoea in Rio de Janeiro, Brazil. Rev. Bras. Pesq. Med. Biol. **11**: 383-384.

24. Taunay, A. E. 1968. Diagnóstico bacteriológico das salmonelas de origem animal, sua importância e frequência no municipio de São Paulo. Rev. Inst. Adolfo Lutz. **28**: 43-69.

25. Taunay, A. E., J. R. C. Novaes, and G. V. A. Pessôa. 1971. Infeccões por enterobactérias no municipio de São Paulo. Provável disseminacão por via aérea. Rev. Inst. Adolfo Lutz. **31**: 113-116.

26. Toledo, M. R. F., M. H. L. Reis, J. Murahovschi, R. Cury, S. R. T. S. Ramos, E. S. Fiore, E. Y. Schussel, and L. R. Trabulsi. 1979. Ocorrência de uma variante de *Salmonella typhimurium* que fermenta a lactose tardiamente. Rev. Microbiol. **10**: 103–105.
27. Toledo, M. R. F., R. M. Silva, and L. R. Trabulsi. 1981. Sachś "Enterobacterium A12" is an aerogenic variant of *Shigella boydii* 14. Int. J. Syst. Bacteriol. **31**: 242–244.
28. Trabulsi, L. R., M. R. Fernandes, and M. E. Zuliani. 1967. Novas bactérias pathogênicas para o intestino do homem. Rev. Inst. Med. Trop. São Paulo. **9**: 31–39.
29. Zuliani, M. E., and L. R. Trabulsi. 1969. Estudos sobre a *E. coli* O111:B4. III-sensibilidade "in vitro à sulfadiazina e a 6 antibióticos. Rev. Inst. Med. Trop. São Paulo. **11**: 323–334.

Bacterial Diarrheal Diseases, eds., Y. Takeda, T. Miwatani, 37–52.
Copyright © 1985 by KTK Scientific Publishers, Tokyo.

EPIDEMIOLOGY OF DIARRHOEAL DISEASES IN BANGLADESH

M. U. Khan, and W. B. Greenough III

International Centre for Diarrhoeal Disease Research, Bangladesh Dacca, Bangladesh

Bangladesh is a small country of 55,598 square miles yet has nearly 100 million people. It lies on the Northeast portion of the Indian sub-continent (Fig. 1). The climate is sub-tropical with a dry and wet season (Fig. 2). It is situated on a delta formed by three great rivers–the Ganges, Brahmaputra and Meghna. At peak flow there is a flux of five million cubic feet per second which is twice that of the Mississippi River (1). Thus crowding and water have a great influence and determine the patterns of life and illness in this country. There are few accurate health data for Bangladesh. The International Centre for Diarrhoeal Diseases Research, Bangladesh (ICDDR,B) formerly the Cholera Research Laboratory (CRL) has kept careful records for nearly twenty years in a rural area in the centre of the country (Fig. 3). In addition, a Treatment Centre for diarrhoea has been in operation in Dacca, the largest city. The information presented in this paper is derived from these populations. Studies in Teknaf, another field area is different in many ways from other parts of Bangladesh started much later (Fig. 1).

Diarrhoea as a Cause of Death

Diarrhoea was the most important component contributing to the overall mortality by age during 1979-80 (Table 1). The preponderance of death due to dysentery reflects effective treatment of cholera and watery diarrhoea in Matlab area (2). In other areas higher death rates pertain. Death, however gives only a small indication of the scope of the problem. It is seen from a recent study on urban families in the lower economic bracket that every member of a family had over six episodes of diarrhoea each year (3). Another rural study shows that infants aged between 9-11 months had over 4 episodes and children less than 5 year old had approximately 4 episodes per year in Matlab (4). If a definition of "disabling diarrhoea" is used, the overall rate drops to less than 0.1 attack per person per year (5). Thus when discussing diarrhoea rates it is important to know the intensity of surveillance and definition of severity used by the field worker. Despite lack of firm data the problem is large and has given a sense of urgency to statements by politicians interested in health (6).

38

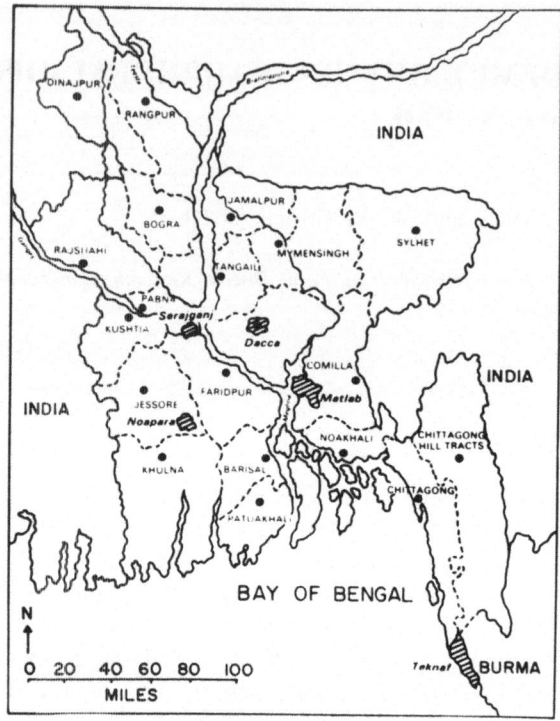

Fig. 1. Map of Bangladesh showing boundaries of districts. Hatched areas indicate study project areas of the International Centre for Diarrhoeal Disease Research.

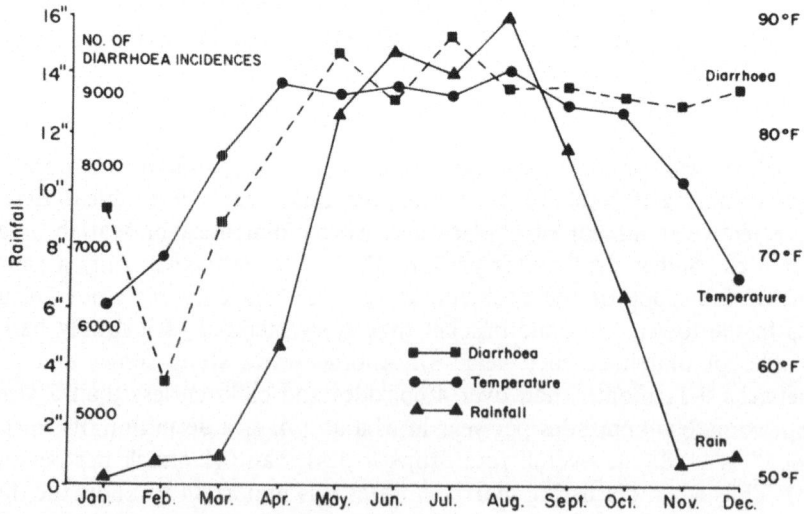

Fig. 2. Temperature, rainfall and incidence of diarrhoea by month: Dacca (Source Meteorological Department and ICDDR, B Hospital Dacca).

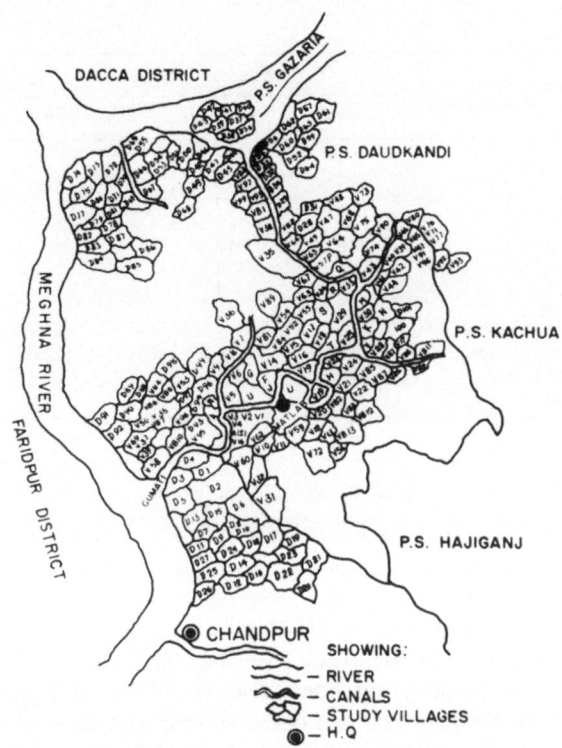

Fig. 3. ICDDR,B Surveillance area in Matlab, 1977.

Table 1. Death rates in 1979 and 1980 by age and sex in matlab

Age at death	1979: Rate per 1000 population			1980: Rate per 1000 population		
	Both Sexes	Males	Females	Both Sexes	Males	Females
All ages	13.8	13.4	14.2	13.1	12.0	14.1
Under 1 year	116.4*	118.7*	114.0*	105.1	91.0	120.1
1-4 years	21.6	16.1	27.6	21.7	16.1	27.8
5-9	4.8	4.5	5.2	3.1	2.8	3.5
10-14	0.9	0.8	1.1	.9	.7	1.1
15-19	1.6	0.7	2.5	1.4	1.0	1.8
20-24	2.5	1.9	3.0	1.5	1.2	1.9
25-29	2.3	1.5	3.1	3.0	2.4	3.6
30-34	3.2	2.4	3.9	2.1	1.1	3.0
35-39	4.1	3.2	4.8	4.4	4.5	4.3
40-44	4.4	5.4	3.6	4.5	7.1	2.2
45-49	10.4	13.1	7.5	8.0	8.9	7.0
50-54	11.3	13.1	9.3	12.7	14.0	10.3
55-59	21.5	24.6	18.1	15.9	14.8	17.0
60-64	30.0	32.6	27.0	26.3	26.4	26.2
65+	75.4	68.3	84.1	72.0	69.8	74.6

* Rate per 1000 live births: Source: Mr. M. K. Chowdhury
Statistics Branch, ICDDR,B

Table 2. Causes of diarrhoea in rural Bangladesh

% of pathgens: identified	Age of patients			All ages
	2 yrs.	2-9 yrs.	10 yrs.+	
ETEC: All	28	24	43	32
ST	17	15	22	19
ST/LT	7	7	19	11
LT	4	1	2	2
Rotavirus	46	12	9	24
Vibrio Cholerae	2	34	14	14
NAG/NCV	5	4	11	7
Shigella	5	10	5	6
E. Histolytica	1	13	8	4
EF-6 organism	1-4	1-2	1-2	<1
Salmonella	<1	<1	<1	<1
G. lamblia	1	1-4	1-4	<1-2
	89	98	91	90

Source: Ref. No. 2, 7

Etiology

In 1962 an etiology could be accurately assigned in only 20% of the cases. By 1980, an agent could be identified in nearly 90% of cases recognized (7). The important pathogens causing diarrhoeal diseases in Bangladesh are shown in Table 3 and 4 (2, 7, 8). Of the bacterial pathogens enterotoxigenic *E. coli*, *Vibrio cholerae*, other vibrios, *Shigellae*, Salmonella and *Campylobacter* are common. The two most important protozoae are *E. histolytica* and *G. lamblia*. Rotavirus is very common in young children in Bangladesh. It is likely that other viruses are also present and will by recognized by electron microscopy. In children under 2 years of age, rotavirus accounts for nearly 50% of all diarrhoea. Three strains of rotavirus have been isolated. The second most common pathogen is enterotoxigenic *E. coli* causing nearly 25% of all cases. *Vibrio cholerae* and non O1 vibrios are responsible for 5-10% of all diarrhoea. Shigella accounts for 5-10%. *Campylobacter* is a recently discovered agent and occurs in 12% of the hospitalized cases in Dacca (8) and 48% of the hospitalized cases in Matlab (9) among children less than 5 years old. Now *Shigella flexneri* alone constitutes about 70% of all shigella

Table 3. Population of various diarrhoeal cases hospitalised per 100 patients

cholera (Inaba + Ogawa)	12.0
NAG/NCV/F-6	9.0
Rotavirus	23.0
Shigella	5.0
ETEC	25.0
G. Lamblia	2.0
Salmonella	<1.0
E. Histolytica	3.0
Mixed infection	6.0
Total	86.0

Table 4. Enteric pathogens from diarrhoeal patients of ICDDR,B Dacca hospital (December 1979 – November 1980)

Pathogen		Percent detected
Enterotoxigenic E. coli total		20
ST	10	–
LT	3	–
ST+LT	7	–
Rotavirus total	–	19
Campylobacter spc. jejuni		14
Shigella total	–	12
Sh. flex	7	–
Sh. dyst.	3	–
Sh. sonn	1	–
Sh. Boyd.	1	–
Vibrios	–	7
O1	6	–
Non O1	1	–
Entameba histolytica	–	6
Giardia Iamblia	–	6
Pleisiomonas*	–	5
Aeromonas*	–	1
Total isolation		91

* Sanyal, S.C. T.C. cases only
  Source. Ref. no. 8

cases. Although *Sh. dysenteriae* was rare before 1970, an epidemic occurred after 1972. Of the ETEC, stable toxin (ST) producing ones are most common. Non O1 vibrios of Heiberg group III, V and VI are more common. A new bacteria, EF-6, (F group vibrios) associated with an epidemic of diarrhoea in 1976-77 (10) continues to be isolated sporadically. There are over 30 hospitalized cases of diarrhoea per year per 1000 population, where good treatment facilities exist (Table 5). There are however large seasonal and year to year variations as can most easily be seen for cholera (Fig. 4). At present *Vibrio cholerae* in Bangladesh are of the El Tor biotype. Ogawa and Inaba are equally common and shift periodically (Fig. 5).

Table 5. Rate of hospitalization with diarrhoea of different etiologies per year

Pathogens isolated	Hospitalized per 1000 population/yr.
Vibrio cholerae	3.7
NCV/NAG	3.1
Shigella	1.5
ETEC	3.1
Rotavirus	7.5
Others: (G. Lamblia, E. Hist. Salm, Campy, Staph, ETEC.)	6.4
Total	30.3

42

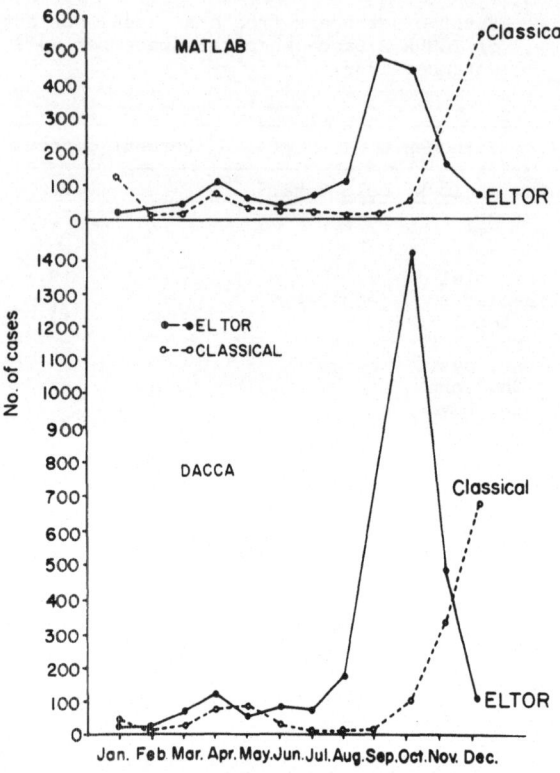

Fig. 4. Seasonality of cholera cases in Dacca and Matlab classical and eltor (3 years average).

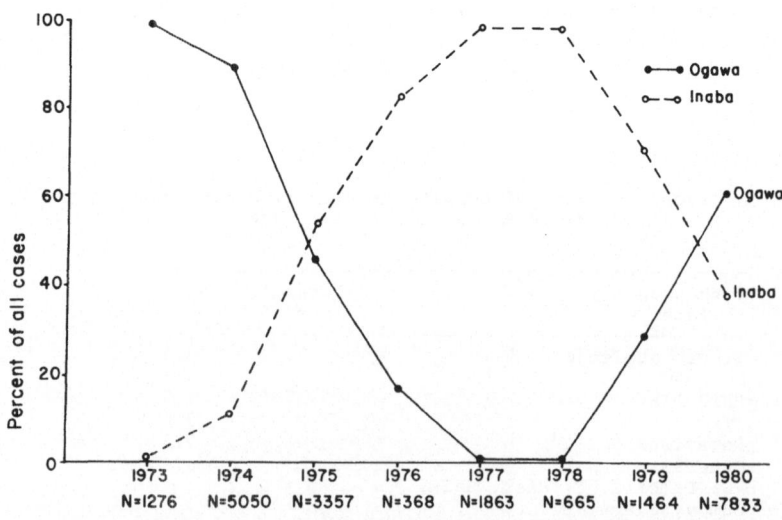

Fig. 5. Shift of serotypes of *V. cholerae* 1973 - 1980 Dacca city.

The rate of hospitalization varies by causes of diarrhoea (Table 5). Rotavirus and individuals infected with enterotoxigenic *E. coli* are more likely to be hospitalized.

Age

Incidence in hospitalized cases by age and sex for the etiological agents are shown in Figs. 6-10. Most diarrhoeal diseases are endemic in Bangladesh, but with seasonal variations and 10 year cycles of increase and decrease. The age distribution of diarrhoeal diseases in Bangladesh differs from developed countries. Almost all age groups are infected by pathogens which can cause diarrhoea in

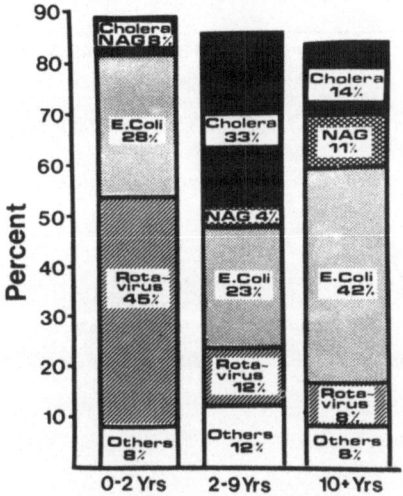

Fig. 6. Etiological break-up of Diarrhoeal incidences reporting to Matlab rural Hospital in 1978 - 1979. (Courtesy of Glimpse, U:2, & ICDDR,B, Feb, 1982.)

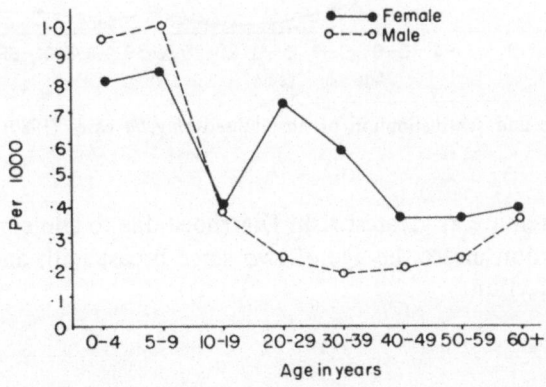

Fig. 7. Age & sex distribution of cholera cases Dacca city per 1000 per year, 1966 - 1975.

44

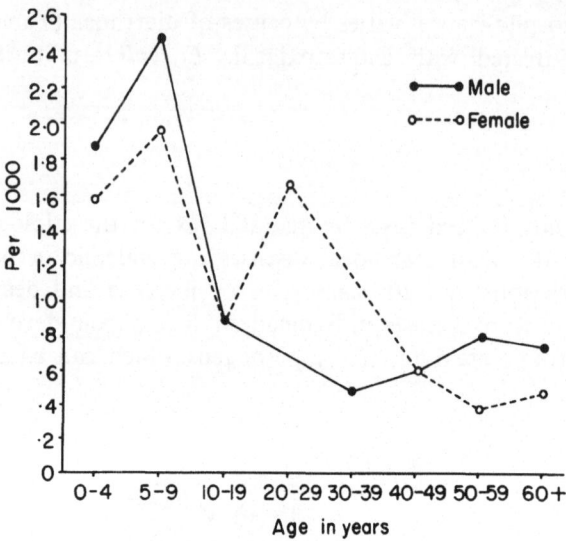

Fig. 8. Age & sex distribution of cholera cases/1000/year Matlab (Rural).

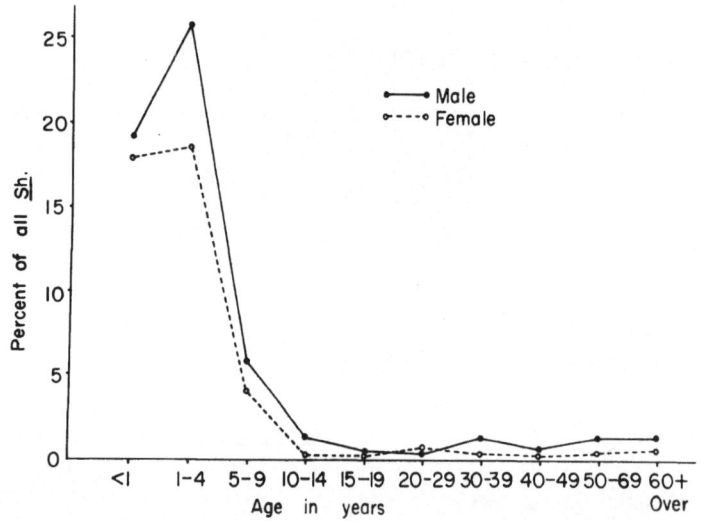

Fig. 9. Age and sex distibution of hospitalised *shigella* cases (1980), Dacca.

Bangladesh. Children are at greatest risk. Diarrhoea due to cholera may not reflect the extent of infection under the age of two since breast milk antibodies prevent illness but not infection.

Sex

The sex distribution by agent differs by age. The pattern of cholera, NAG,

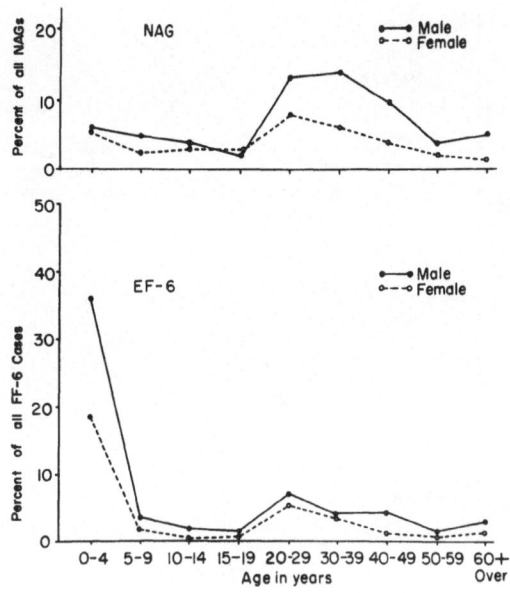

Fig. 10. Age and sex distribution of NAG and EF-6 infected diarrhoea patients. (From Ref. 21.)

Shigella and EF-6 are also shown in Figures 6-10. Male children upto 14 years of age have higher cholera attack rate than female children. But females aged 15-45 years have almost twice the attack rate of cholera as compared to males of the corresponding age group. NAG and EF-6 are twice as common in males aged 10 and over than females. But shigella is slightly higher in males than females.

Seasonality

Diarrhoea in Bangladesh due to specific bacteria or viruses has distinct seasonality. Cholera is a striking example of this (Fig. 4). There is a rise of cholera incidences during the spring months of March to May with the major epidemic peak after the monsoon (October through December). Before 1972 this peak was in December. Since the replacement of classical by El Tor biotype in 1973, the peak has shifted to October. The peak in Calcutta is during spring (March-May). Seasonality in Bangladesh has been observed for 2 decades with accurate information from the areas in which ICDDR,B and before it CRL works (Fig. 11). Diarrhoea due to other vibrios is high during spring and during early winter (Fig. 12, 13). Shigellosis occurs throughout the year with slight rise during spring and post monsoon seasons (Fig. 14). Rotavirus is most common during the winter months as in other countries. What was called "summer diarrhoea" in this country is caused principally by ETEC. The distribution of Toxin combinations for ETEC are shown in Table 2 and 4 (2, 8).

46

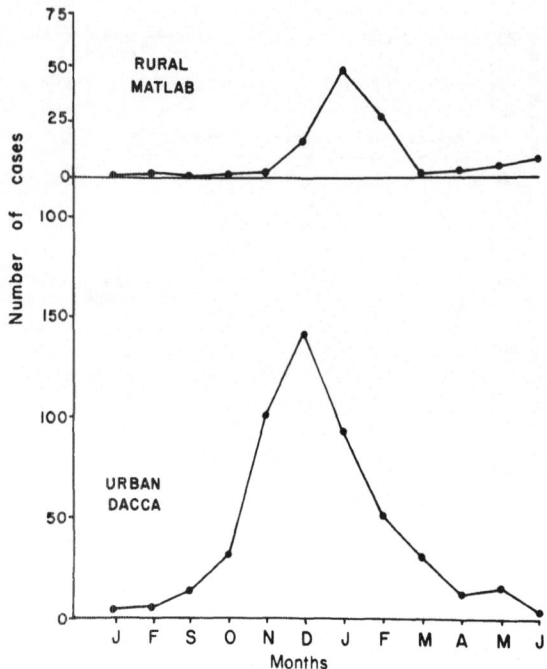

Fig. 11. Seasonality of cholera during 1964 & 1966 in a rural & an urban area.

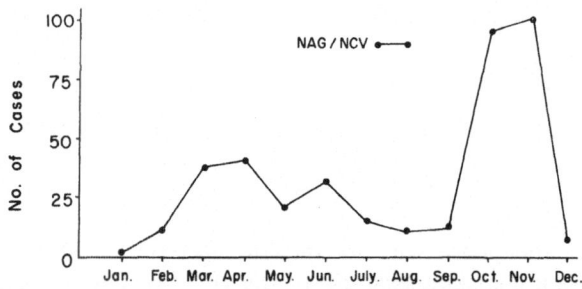

Fig. 12. Seasonality of NAGS (1970 - 1975), Dacca.

Spectrum of Diarrhoeal Illness

Many healthy people carry ETEC, Rotavirus and *Campylobacter*. One-third of the shigella infections are symptomatic. Of all shigella, *Shigella dyst.* Type 1 produces symptoms in a larger proportion of infected people. Half of the people infected with *Vibrio cholerae* produce symptoms and 5-12% need hospitalization for electrolyte replacement (Fig. 15). In other countries, 1-10% of the people infected with El Tor biotype become ill (Fig. 16). But recent studies in Bangladesh

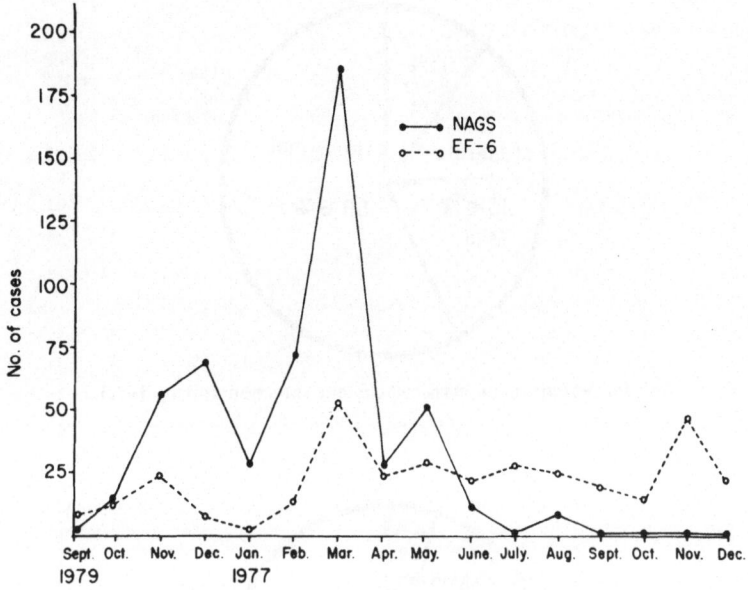

Fig. 13. Seasonal variation in incidence of NAGS and EF-6 1976 - 1977, Dacca.

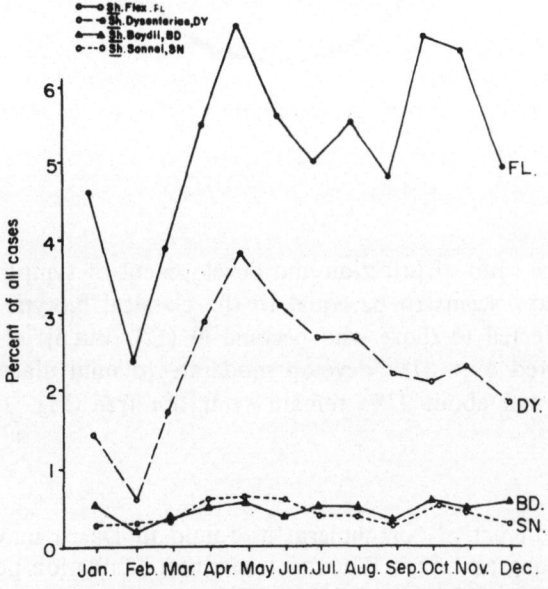

Fig. 14. Seasonality of shigellae in Dacca (11 years, Av) shown in proportion of all *shigella*.

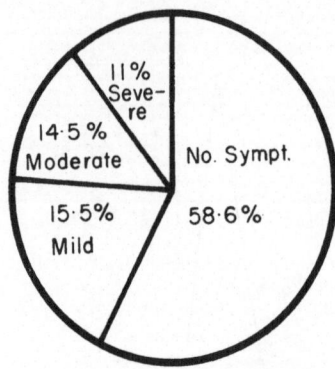

Fig. 15. Spectrum of classical cholera infection (up to 1972).

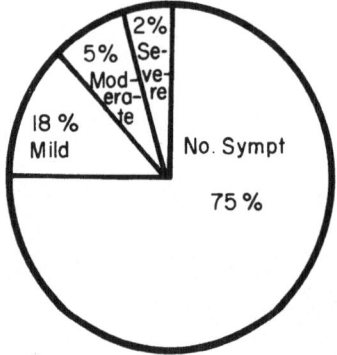

Fig. 16. Spectrum of Eltor cholera infection (up to 1972).

show a shift in the ratio of infection and development of symptoms. *V. cholerae* biotype El Tor now seems to be equal to the classical biotype (Fig. 17) in the ratio of those infected to those who become ill (12). But if all El Tor infected cases are considered over 57% develop moderate to mild diarrhoea, over 21% severe diarrhoea and about 21% remain symptom free (Fig. 18).

Incubation Period

The incubation period for cholera, as found in Dacca may be as short as 10 hours and as long as 4 days. The most common incubation period for cholera is 2-2.5 days, but ranged from 1-7 days. For non O1 group vibrios it may be 1-4 days, for rotavirus 1-7 days; for ETEC 0.5-3 days and for salmonella 6 hr. - 2 days. Although the incubation period of *E. histolytica* is 3-4 weeks it may be much shorter during epidemics. Shigella takes usually 2-3 days.

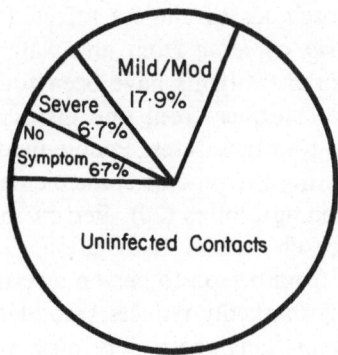

Fig. 17. Spectrum of El for cholera infection in family contacts (after 1972).

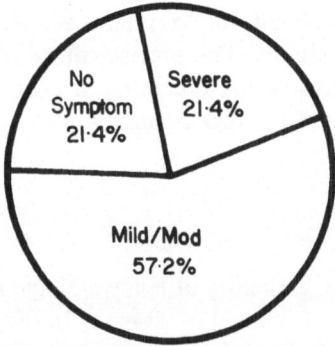

Fig. 18. Spectrum of all Eltor cholera infected persons (after 1972).

Immunity

Cholera in Bangladesh produce lasting immunity but there are instances of re-infection (13). When vaccinated parenterally, people develop immunity by 8 days (14) and are protected partially for only 4-6 months. Attack ratio decreases as vibriocidal titres rise with the increasing age (15). Since the local immune response is the principal mechanism for protection, circulating antibodies are only a partial guide to the state of host defenses. There is little information about other causes of diarrhoea although it appears that rotavirus infection may give long lasting immunity since few cases are seen after the age of three.

Transmission

Bangladesh is a fertile ground for all diseases which can be spread by the faecal-oral route. It being a deltaic country with the largest flux of fresh water in the world, water borne diarrhoeal diseases thrive. Normally surface or piped water do not yield *Vibrio cholerae*, it may be isolated from about one-third of all water sources from households of cholera infected families. Without cholera cases the presence of *Vibrio cholerae* from any water source is an exceptional event even with intense search. Patients have been found to carry cholera when travelling by boat, train or steamer from one district to another (16, 17, 18). Water use is closely related to attack rates. People living by the side of the canal have more cholera (19). During the time of epidemic people may contract cholera from food of charitable feeding centres (20). Person to person transmission have not been clearly shown for cholera in Bangladesh.

Shigella is transmitted from person to person directly by hand. A recent study confirms that hand washing markedly reduces secondary case and infection rates (21). Flies being abundant in Bangladesh may play a role in transmitting diarrhoeal diseases specially Shigella (22). It has been found that 8% and 6% of samples of flies carried Shigella and *V. cholerae* on their bodies during epidemics in Dacca (23). ETEC transmission is correlated with warmer temperature and food. Non O1 group vibrios are probably water related. Intensive work in collaboration with Dr. Rita Colwell of the University of Maryland is seeking to describe the natural ecology of vibiros in Bangladesh. The precise routes of transmission of rotavirus are not known. Salmonellosis is rare excepting *S. typhi*, perhaps because the main vehicle of transmission is the food processing industry, which is almost non-existent in Bangladesh.

Prevention

A principal goal for the gathering of epidemiologic knowledge is to intelligently focus cost-effective means of control of disease. In diarrhoea we know that while expensive technology such as the tubewells can fail, simple measures such as hand washing (Fig. 19) can drastically alter the spread of disease (24, 21).

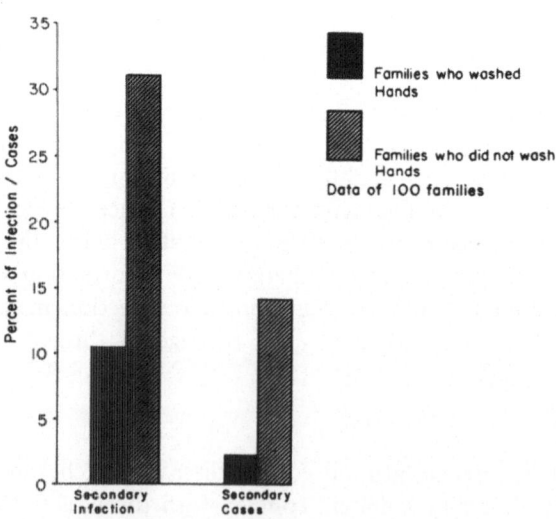

Fig. 19. Effect of washing hands with soap and water before meals and after defecation.

Table 6.   Proportions of children dead by
            women's education

Women's education level	Proportion of children dead
0	0.2767
1-5	0.2172
6-10	0.1653

From recent analysis of data relating to social and economic variables in Matlab it has been shown (Table 6) that the education of a mother is crucial to survival of children (25). The recently reported high degree of protection by a genetically engineering live vaccine against *salmonella typhi* indicates that biological as well as social interventions both hold promise and must progress side by side with equal emphasis to reduce the toll taken by diarrhoeal diseases (26).

REFERENCES

1.   Nytrop, R. F. 1975. Area Handbook for Bangladesh, U.S. Govt. Printing Office, Washington D. C., Editon 1975, pp. 65.

2.   Black, R. E., M. H. Merson, A. S. M. M. Rahman, M. Yunus, A. R. M. A. Alim, M. I. Huq, R. H. Yolken, and G. T. Curlin. 1980. A two years study of bacterial, viral and parasitic agents associated with diarrhoea in rural Bangladesh. J. Infect. Dis. **142**: 660–664.

3.   Khan, M. U., and M. Shanhidullah. 1980. Contrasting Epidemiology of Shigellae dysenteriae and Shigella flexneri, Dacca. Trans. Roy. Sco. Trop. Med. & Hyg. **74**: (4), 528–533.

4.   Black, R. E., M. H. Merson, M. I. Huq, A. R. M. A. Alim, and Yunus, M. 1981. Incidence and severity of rotavirus and Escherichia coli diarrhoea in Rural Bangladesh. Implication for vaccine development. Lancet, January 17, 1981.

5.   Oseason, R. O., A. S. Benenson, and M. Fahimuddin. 1965. Field trial of cholera vaccine in Rural East Pakistan. Lancet **1**: 450–453.

6.   Kennedy, E. 1978. Speech at WHO Conference on Primary Health Care. Alma Ata USSR, Sept. 6–12.

7.   Merson M. H., R. E. Black, M. U. Khan, and M. I. Huq. 1978. Epidemiology of cholera and enterotoxigenic *Escherichia coli* diarrhoea. Proceedings of 43rd. Nobel Symposium, Stockholm, pp. 34–35.

8.   Stoll, B. J., R. I. Glass, M. I. Huq, M. U. Khan, J. Holt, and H. Basu. Surveillance of patients attending on diarrhoeal disease hospital in Bangladesh, British Med. 5. **288**: 1185–88, October 23, 1982.

9.   Blaser, M. J., R. I. Glass, M. I. Huq, B. Stoll, and A. R. M. A. Alim. 1980. Isolation of Campylobacter fetus subsp jejuni from Bangladeshi children. J. Clin. Micro **12**: 744–747.

10. Khan, M. U., and M. Shahidullah. 1981. Epidemiological pattern of Diarrhoea caused by NAG vibrio and EF-6 organisms in Dacca. ICDDR,B working paper no. **21**:

11. Glass, R. I., S. Becker, M. I. Huq, M. U. Khan, M. H. Merson, and J. V. Lee. Endemic cholera in rural Bangladesh 1966–1980. Sent for Publication to Am. J. Epid.

12. Khan, M. U., and M. Shahidulla. 1980. Cholera due to El Tor biotype equals the classical biotype in severity and attack rates. J. Trop. Med. & Hyg. **83**:

13. Woodward, W. E. 1971. Cholera erinfection in man. J. Infect. Dis. **123**: 61–66.

14. Sommer, A., M. U. Khan, and W. H. Mosley. 1973. Efficacy of vaccination of family contacts of cholera cases. Lancet, I: 1230–1232.

15. Mosley, W. H., A. S. Benenson, and P. K. Barui. 1968. Serological Survey for cholera an-

tibodies in rural East Pakistan. 1. The distribution of antibody in control of a cholera vaccine field trial area and the relation of antibody titre to the pattern of endemic cholera. Bull. WHO, **38**: 327–334.

16. Khan, M. U., and W. H. Mosley. 1967. Role of boatman in the transmission of cholera. East Pak. Med. J. pp. 61–66.

17. Bart, K. J., Z. Huq, M. U. Khan, and W. H. Mosley. 1970. Sero-epidemiologic studies during a simultaneous epidemic of infection with El Tor Ogawa and classical Inaba *Vibrio cholerae.* J. Infect. Dis. **121**: Suppl. May S19–S23.

18. Mosley, W. H. et al. Epidemiology of cholera. T. C. Report 1965, Section III (d,h).

19. Khan, M. U., W. H. Mosley, A. M. Sarder, J. Chakraborty, and M. R. Khan. 1981. The relationship of cholera to water source and use in rural Bangladesh. Int. J. Epid. 10(1): 23–25.

20. Khan, M. U., G. T. Curlin, and M. Shahidullah. 1977. Urban cholera study, Dacca 1974 and 1975. Scientific report no. 7.

21. Khan, M. U. 1981. Interruption of shigellosis by hand washing. Trans. Roy. Soc. Trop. Med. & Hyg. V. 76: no. 2, pp. 167, 1982.

22. Khan, M. U., M. M. Rahaman, K. M. S. Aziz, and S. Islam. Epidemiologic investigation of an outbreak of Shiga Bacillus dysentery in an Island Population. SEA journal of Trop. Med. & Public Health. **6**: 2, pp. 215–256.

23. Khan, A. R., and F. Huq. 1978. Disease agents carried by flies in Dacca city. Bull. BMTC 4(2): pp. 86–93.

24. Curlin G. T., K. M. A. Aziz, and A. R. Khan. 1979. The intake of during tube well water on diarrhoea rates in Matlab Thana, Bangladesh, Cholera Research Laboratory, Bangladesh Workshop paper no. 1.

25. Stan D'Souza, B. Abbas, and R. Mizanur. 1980. Socioeconomic differentials in mortality in a rural area of Bangladesh. International Centre for Diarrhoeal Disease Research, Bangladesh. Scientific Report No. 40.

26. Wadhan Mit, Serie C, Cerisiery, Sallam S, and Germair R. A controlled field trial at live Salmonella typhi strain Ty 21A oral vaccine ageinst typhoid: Three years results. J. Infect. Dis. V. **145**: 3, March, 1982.

Bacterial Diarrheal Diseases, eds., Y. Takeda, T. Miwatani, 53–63.

EPIDEMIOLOGY OF BACTERIAL ENTERIC PATHOGENS IN RURAL THAILAND: APPLICATION OF A DNA HYBRIDIZATION ASSAY TO DETECT ENTEROTOXIGENIC *ESCHERICHIA COLI*

P. Echeverria[1], C. Tirapat[2], C. Charoenkul[2], S. Yangratoke[2] and W. Chaicumpa[3]

US Component, Armed Forces Research Institute of Medical Sciences, Rajvithi Road, Bangkok 4, Thailand[1]
Soongnern Training and Research Center, Faculty of Public Health, Mahidol University, Bangkok, Thailand[2]
Department of Microbiology, Faculty of Tropical Medicine, Mahidol University, Bangkok, Thailand[3]

Diarrhea continues to be a major public health problem in developing countries (1, 2). Although previous studies have implicated more than ten bacterial enteric pathogens in causing diarrhea, most of these studies have been performed over a short period of time and do not permit an accurate assessment of the relative importance of different enteric pathogens (3, 4). There have been few attempts to identify environmental sources of these pathogens so that meaningful sanitary intervention can be planned. We therefore prospectively studied individuals with diarrhea at a local hospital and in a village in northeastern Thailand to identify the relative importance and seasonality of bacterial enteric pathogens. Environmental sources of bacterial enteric pathogens were also sought. Molecular genetic technology proved to be a promising tool in identifying sources of organisms which carry structural genes for enterotoxin production. Although observations made in rural Thailand will not be universally applicable, this experience hopefully will expand our knowledge of the epidemiology of bacterial diarrheal disease in a rural setting in a tropical developing country.

Incidence of diarrhea in Soongnern

This study was conducted in Amphur Soongnern located 240 kilometers northeast of Bangkok. The Amphur has a population of approximately 57,000 persons. Between November 1,1980 and October 31,1981, 490 patients with diarrhea were investigated at Soongnern Hospital. An episode of diarrhea was defined as the passage of two or more liquid stools in a 24 hour period for less than 72 hours.

No patients were studied more than once in a three month period so each patient was considered as a single episode of diarrhea. Thirty-three percent of the patients with diarrhea were less than two years of age. Children under the age of two years had the highest incidence of hospital-treated diarrhea (Fig. 1). Diarrheal disease occurred throughout the year with increased numbers in March and April during the hot dry season and again in November and December during the coldest months of the year.

Since a variety of factors influence who comes to the hospital for treatment of diarrhea (severity of the disease, age, sex, occupation, distance from the hospital, financial resources, etc.), the incidence of diarrhea in a village in the district served by the hospital was also studied in 1981. Ban Pong, a rural farming community consisting of 625 inhabitants living in 125 homes, was visited six days each week. Stool specimens were collected from anyone with diarrhea, and the family member without diarrhea closest in age to the member with diarrhea (Control A). A person without diarrhea of the same age and sex as the individual with diarrhea was also selected from a home nearby as a control (Control B). In addition every two weeks age and sex matched controls for each case identified in the preceding two weeks were selected and cultured (Control C). This group was added because an appropriate control for the individual with diarrhea was often not present in an adjacent home. Thirteen percent (80/625) of people living in the village developed 132 episodes of diarrhea during the year. Stools from these 132 episodes of diarrhea, from 120 household contacts in control group A, from 45 without diarrhea in control group B, and from 130 without diarrhea in control group C were cultured. The age specific incidence of diarrhea for the village is shown in fig. 2. Children under two years of age had the highest incidence of diarrhea and 15 percent of

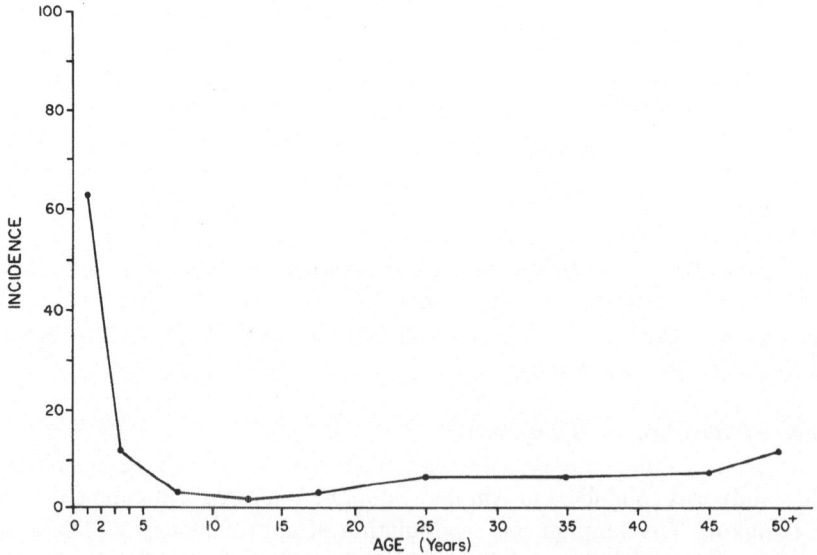

Fig. 1. Annual age specific incidence of hospital-treated diarrhea per 1,000 persons accessed by hospital surveillance (November 1980-October 1981).

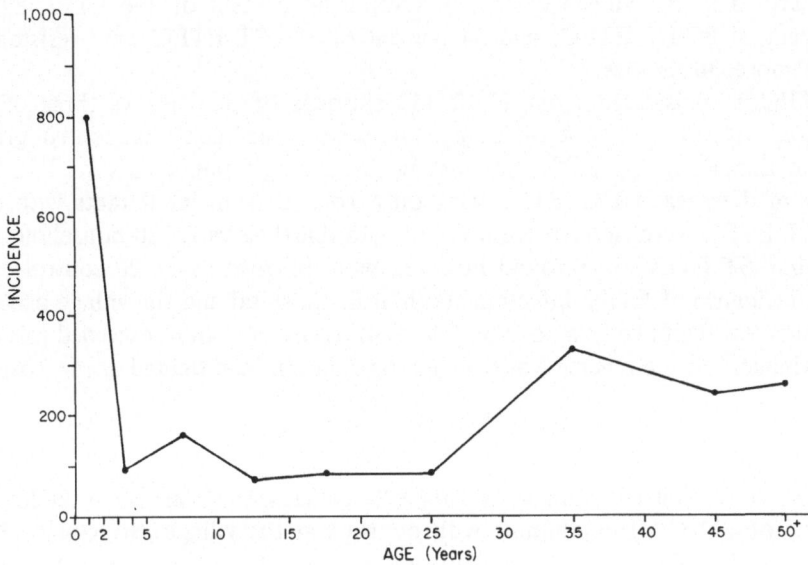

Fig. 2. Annual age specific incidence of diarrhea per 1,000 persons accessed by surveillacne of Ban Pong (January-December 1981).

children under two years of age experienced more than one episode. Diarrhea increased in March and April however there was no increase in diarrhea in November and December as had been found at the hospital the preceding year, in part reflecting the lower incidence of rotavirus in children in the village vs the hospital. In November and December rotavirus accounted for 60 percent of pediatric diarrhea cases at the hospital, but only ten percent of those in the village. Since only 132 episodes of diarrhea occurred in the village during one year, conclusions based on results from the Ban Pong study must be interpreted with caution.

Bacterial enteric pathogens Enterotoxigenic Escherichia coli

Enterotoxigenic *Escherichia coli* (ETEC) were isolated from 51 (10%) of 490 persons with diarrhea at the hospital and 15 (11%) of 132 episodes of diarrhea in inhabitants of the village. The proportion of LTST, LT, and ST ETEC infections was similar at the hospital and in the village. Twenty-nine percent of these ETEC produced heat-labile (LT) and heat-stable (ST) toxin, 33 percent produced LT alone, and 38 percent produced ST alone. Clinically there were no differences between individuals infected with ETEC which produced LT and ST, LT alone, or ST alone. ETEC infections were more common in April, May, and June (the hot dry season) at both the hospital and the village. Sixty-seven percent (34/51) of persons with diarrhea at the hospital vs 33 percent (5/15) of inhabitants with diarrhea at the village were infected with ETEC which were resistant to two or more antibiotics suggesting that individuals with diarrhea treated at the hospital had been exposed to more antibiotics prior to being investigated than inhabitants with diarrhea in the village (p<0.01). Overall 84 percent of 136 LTST ETEC, 50 percent of 86 LT ETEC, and 54 percent of 134 ST ETEC were resistant to two or more antibiotics.

ETEC were isolated from 15 of 132 episodes of diarrhea vs three of 120 household controls and none of 175 age and sex matched controls (control groups B&C) in Ban Pong (p<0.005) supporting the etiologic importance of ETEC as a cause of diarrhea. LTST ETEC were only isolated from inhabitants with diarrhea, LT ETEC were isolated from 6/132 with diarrhea vs 2/120 household controls while ST ETEC were found in 6/132 with diarrhea vs 1/120 controls. The highest incidence of ETEC infections both at the hospital and the village occurred in children less than two years of age (Fig. 3, 4). ETEC infections exceeded rotavirus in the village, but the reverse was true among children investigated at the hospital.

Shigella

Shigella was isolated from 94 of 490 (19%) patients with diarrhea at the hospital and nine of 132 (7%) inhabitants with diarrhea at the village. Sixty-nine (74%) of the *Shigella* isolated at the hospital were *S. flexneri*, 12 (13%) were *S. sonnei*, nine (10%) were *S. boydii*, and three (3%) were *S. dysenteriae*. Five (55%) of the *Shigella* isolated from persons with diarrhea in Ban Pong were *S. boydii*, three (33%) were *S. flexneri*, and one (11%) was *S. dysenteriae*. *Shigella* was the most common bacterial pathogen in patients over ten years of age at both the hospital and the village. *Shigella* exceeded ETEC infections at the hospital, but the reverse was true in the village. All *Shigella* were resistant to at least four antibiotics. There were no seasonal differences in the isolation rates of *Shigella* in patients

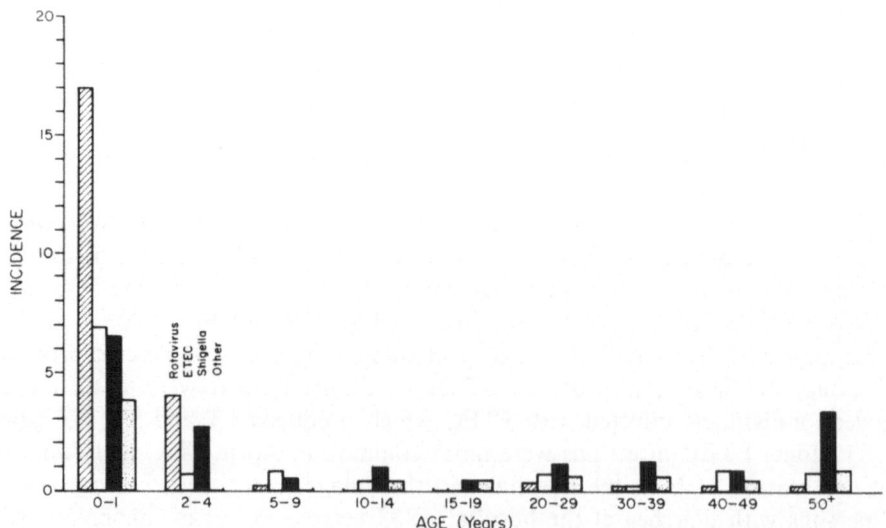

Fig. 3. Annual age specific incidence of diarrhea associated with different enteric pathogens per 1,000 persons accessed by hospital visits (November 1980-October 1981).

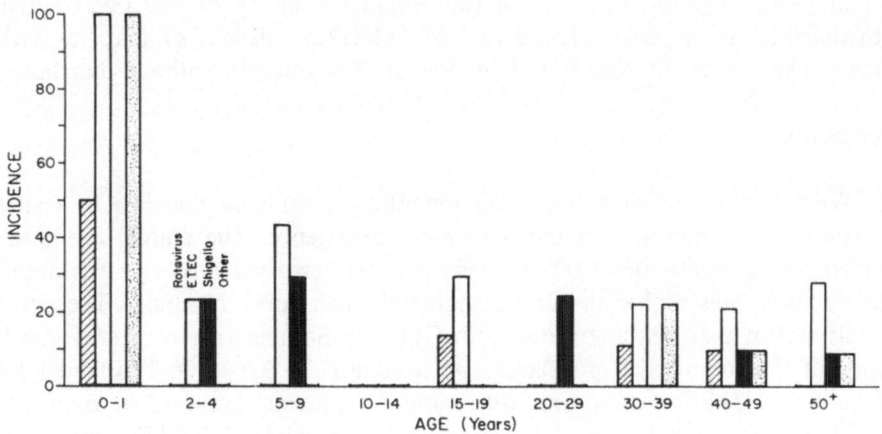

Fig. 4. Annual age specific incidence of diarrhea associated with different enteric pathogens per 1,000 persons accessed by daily visits to Ban Pong (January-December 1981).

with diarrhea at the hospital or in the village. In Ban Pong *Shigella* were isolated from three of 120 healthy household contacts closest in age to the individual with diarrhea (Control A) and two of 175 age and sex matched controls without diarrhea in the village (Control B, C).

Campylobacter jejuni

C. jejuni were isolated from six of 162 (4%) children with diarrhea less than two years of age at the hospital and two of 16 (12%) episodes of diarrhea which occurred in children of the same age with diarrhea at the village. This organism was isolated from one of 18 (5%) children without diarrhea less than two years of age at the village, but was not isolated during 116 episodes of diarrhea in older children and adults or from 295 inhabitants without diarrhea over two years of age (Control A, B, and C). *C. jejuni* was the third most common bacterial pathogen associated with episodes of diarrhea in young children at the hospital.

Other bacterial enteric pathogens

Non-typhoid *Salmonella* was isolated from seven of 490 (1%) patients with diarrhea at the hospital, but was not cultured from patients with diarrhea in the village. These bacteria were isolated from three of 295 inhabitants without diarrhea in the village (Control A, B, and C). *Salmonella* were equally distributed among all serogroups and only 44 percent were resistant to two or more antibiotics. *V. parahaemolyticus* was isolated from 16 of 490 (3%) patients with diarrhea at the hospital and during two of 132 episodes of diarrhea in Ban Pong. Ninety-four percent (17/18) of persons from whom this pathogen was isolated were over 20 years of age. This organism was isolated from one of 120 household contacts in Ban Pong. Non-O1 *V. cholerae* was isolated from 16 of 490 (3%) patients with diarrhea at the hospital and two of 132 (1%) episodes of diarrhea in the village. This organism was found in one of 295 villagers without diarrhea.

Conclusion

We are aware of only one other longitudinal study of diarrhea in a village in Asia (5) to compare with the Soongnern experience. The annual age specific incidence of diarrhea per 1,000 persons less than two years of age was approximately five times higher in rural Bangladesh than rural Thailand. The percent of episodes of diarrhea associated with ETEC in Soongnern (10 - 11%) was less than half that reported from Dacca and Matlab (23 - 32%). In Thailand LTST, LT, and ST ETEC were found with similar frequency however in Bangladesh ST ETEC accounted for the majority of ETEC isolates. LT ETEC are unusual in Bangladesh (2 - 4%), but accounted for 33 percent of ETEC in Soongnern. Antibiotic resistance among ETEC was also more common in Thailand than has been reported from the Indian subcontinent (6), but similar to what has been found elsewhere in the Far East (7). There was one similarity between Matlab and Soongnern. ETEC infection increased in the hot dry season prior to the onset of the rainy season in both Thailand and Bangladesh (8). While *V. cholerae* was isolated from 12 - 14 percent of episodes of diarrhea in Matlab (9), this enteric pathogen was not isolated in Soongnern in 1980 and 1981. Non-O1 *V. cholerae* was associated with 1-2 percent of episodes of diarrhea in Soongnern compared to seven percent reported from Bangladesh. *V. parahaemolyticus* (3%) and *Shigella* (19%) were more often isolated from a treatment facility in Soongnern than in Matlab (<1% and 6%). These differences between Soongnern and Matlab may reflect yearly variations in the incidence of enteric pathogens however the differences in the incidence and characteristics of ETEC suggest that there may also be regional differences in these bacteria.

Environmental sources of enteric pathogens

Environmental cultures of 332 leftover foods, 328 water samples, and 821 animals were collected from 125 homes of inhabitants with diarrhea, and 39 homes of an inhabitant of the same age without diarrhea. Pools of approximately 75 flies caught every two weeks in animal pens, yards, bathrooms, and kitchens in the village were also cultured. Lastly 180 chickens, 150 ducks, 150 pigs, 150 cattle, 100 dogs, and 20 cats were cultured selectively for *C. jejuni*.

In only two of 132 homes in which a person had diarrhea were we able to identify the same bacterial enteric pathogen from an inhabitant with diarrhea and either an environmental source or a family member without diarrhea within the home. In April LTST ETEC were isolated form an 85 year old man with diarrhea and ST ETEC were isolated from leftover fish in his home. In June LTST *E. coli* were isolated from a 17 year old girl with diarrhea while LT ETEC were isolated from her 19 year old asymptomatic sister. As shown in table 1, cultures of certain locations within the home were found to be potential sources of bacterial

Table 1. Enteric pathogens isolated from environmental sources in
a rural village in Thailand

	Water	Pigs	Cattle	Food	Flies
	(328) $^\Delta$	(431)	(390)	(332)	(144)
E. coli	150(46%)	431(100%)	390(100%)	33(10%)	126(87%)
Enteric pathogens					
ETEC	0	10/276°(4%)	7/184°(4%)	1(<1%)	2(1%)
Shigella	0	3(<1%)	7(2%)	1(<1%)	1(<1%)
Salmonella	5(1%)	0	2(<1%)	0	0
Non-O1 V. cholerae	25(8%)	38(9%)	1 (<1%)	3(2)$^+$(1%)	16(11%)

A number of specimens examined; ° number of specimens tested for ETEC
(+ two isolates of V. alginolyticus)

enteric pathogens. Although *C. jejuni* was not isolated from water samples, or
leftover foods collected in homes in Ban Pong, this enteric pathogen was isolated
form 22 of 47 puppies (39%), 68 of 180 chickens (38%), 51 of 150 ducks (34%),
ten of 47 adult dogs (23%), and four of 20 cats (20%) in the village.

Although we have been unable to show that bacterial enteric pathogens were
transmitted directly from animals to man (or whether those isolated from animals
are enteropathogenic to man), animals were a reservoir of enteric pathogens in
Soongnern. ETEC have previously been isolated from livestock living in close pro-
ximity to man in Bangladesh (10) and the Philippines (11) and livestock are often
infected with *Salmonella* worldwide (12). Non-O1 *V. cholerae*, Group F vibrio,
and *Shigella* were also found in pigs and cows in Soongnern. Although *C. jejuni*
were not found in pigs or cattle they were frequently isolated from birds, dogs,
and cats presumably because these animals' higher body temperatures are selective
for this enteric pathogen (13).

Quantitating *E. coli* in water by the millipore technique proved impossible
because of the presence of soil and large numbers of non-coliform bacteria, algae,
etc. in most water samples. Although *E. coli* were found in 46 percent of 328
water samples in Ban Pong, none of these isolates were enterotoxigenic. However
we have been able to isolate ETEC from two of 144 water samples (1%) by standard techniques and 13 of 144 (9%) by more modern techniques elsewhere in
Soongnern. *Salmonella* were isolated from five (1%) and non-O1 *V. cholerae* from
25 (8%) of 328 water samples collected in Ban Pong. Water is obviously important
in the dissemination of enteric pathogens in rural Thailand, however newer techniques (discussed below) will have to be used to obtain an accurate appraisal.

Contamination of food and flies with enteric pathogens also occurs, but is
probably of lesser importance. Further studies are in progress to determine how
often and by what routes ETEC, the most common bacterial enteric pathogen
in Thai villages, are spread from these sources in the community to man.

Application of the DNA hybridization assay

An assay in which clinical specimens were examined with a DNA hybridization technique for genes encoding for enterotoxins (14) was established in Thailand in April 1981. Initially stools from 110 children with diarrhea in Bangkok were examined by testing ten lactose positive colonies from each specimen with the Y-1 adrenal cell (15) and suckling mouse (16) assays and by spotting the stool directly on nitrocellulose paper in triplicate and examining the papers with the LT, ST-H, and ST-P probes. The same eight children were found to be infected with ETEC by both methods. Two children were infected with LTST, five with LT, and one with ST *E. coli*. The number of ETEC detected by the Y-1 adrenal and suckling mouse assays varied from one to ten. In three stools the LT probe detected DNA coding for LT when only one of ten isolates tested from the stool culture was positive in the Y-1 adrenal cell assay. The ST-H probe which detected all of the stools containing ST producing colonies was also able to detect a stool in which only one of ten colonies tested produced ST. None of the stools were positive with the ST-P probe.

Different proportions of non-ETEC, or *A. hydrophila* were mixed with LTST ETEC to determine if the DNA from other bacteria interfered in detecting genes coding for LT and ST. The DNA hybridization assay was positive when 10^9 *A. hydrophila* or non-ETEC were mixed with 10^5 LTST ETEC B2C (LT and ST-H probe positive) or a clinical isolated of LTST ETEC 12C-2 (LT, ST-H, and ST-P probe positive), spotted on nitrocellulose paper, and examined with the hybridization assay. To determine the sensitivity of the DNA hybridization assay in detecting ETEC in water containing other species of bacteria, soil, algae, etc. tenfold dilutions of LTST ETEC B2C were made in klong (canal) water. One ml of klong water contained 2.1×10^5 *Proteus*, 1.5×10^5 *Enterobacter*, 1.3×10^5 *Aeromonas*, 6.0×10^4 non-ETEC, 6.0×10^4 *Klebsiella*, and 3.2×10^4 *Pseudomonas*. The DNA hybridization assay was positive with both the LT and ST-H probes when ETEC B2C was diluted to contain ten ETEC/ml. To compare the sensitivity of the DNA hybridization assay with our standard method of detecting ETEC in water, similar dilutions passed through 0.45 mμ millipore and nitrocellulose filters were examined with the DNA hybridization assay and by picking ten *E. coli* from filters incubated on MFc media incubated anaerobically at 37°C. While picking ten random *E. coli* for toxin testing was able to detect ETEC at a dilution of 10^5 ETEC/ml of klong water the hybridization assay was able to detect as few as ten ETEC/ml.

To date 414 ETEC have been examined simultaneously with the DNA hybridization, Y-1 adrenal, and suckling mouse assays. One hundred and twenty nine LTST, 118 ST, and 167 ST *E. coli* were homologous with either the LT, ST-H and/or the ST-P probes (Table 2). Sixteen isolates which were originally thought to produce LT only were not homologous with the LT probe and were subsequently found to produce an exoprotein which is heat-labile and causes rounding of Y-1 adrenal cells which is not inhibited by *V. cholerae* antisera. Genes homologous with either the ST-P or ST-H probes were distributed among isolates of LTST *E. coli* from patients in different locations in Thailand. ST *E. coli* homologous

Table 2. Examination of 414 ETEC with the DNA
          hybridization assay

		Results of the probe assay		
ETEC	LT	ST-H	ST-P	ST-H + ST-P
LT+ST+ (129)*	129	74	24	31
LT+ST- (118)	118	0	0	0
LT-ST+ (167)	0	112	52	3

* number of specimens examined

with ST-H, but not ST-P were only isolated from individuals in rural Thailand.
The differences between the proportions of *E. coli* homologous with the ST-H
probe from rural vs urban Thailand (9/9 vs 4/12) was significant (p = 0.03 (Fischer's
exact test)).

Beginning in July 1981 we began to examine patients and potential environmental sources for ETEC in Soongnern with the DNA hybridization assay as well
as the Y-1 adrenal and suckling mouse assays. ETEC were identified in 29 of
199 human stools (15%), 13 of 144 water samples (9%), and in 11 of 130 animal
stools (8%) examined by both methods. Although four specimens which contained
ETEC as identified in the standard assay were negative in the probe assay, only
21 percent (11/53) of probe positive specimens could be verified by testing ten
individual *E. coli* in the standard assays from the same source, table 3. These
results were surprising since we were previously able, using the standard assays,
to identify ETEC from 100 percent of probe positive stools collected from children
with diarrhea. We are not sure why these discrepancies exist however the following
observations have been made.

Table 3. Detection of ETEC in specimens from
          Soongnern with standard assays and
          the DNA hybridization assay

	DNA hybridization assay	
Assay*	+	-
Water (144)**		
+	2	0
-	11	131
Animal stool (130)		
+	0	0
-	11	119
Human stool (199)		
+	9	4
-	20	166

* testing ten E. coli in the Y-1 adrenal and suckling
   mouse assays
** number of specimens tested

62

1. In *in vitro* experiments with klong water the probe assay is 10^4 times more sensitive than testing ten individual organisms in detecting ETEC. This observation probably also holds for stool and other environmental samples examined.

2. The ability to produce toxin is plasmid mediated and therefore theoretically labile. Since we tested *E. coli* in our standard assays several months after they had been isolated, plasmids coding for enterotoxin may have been lost.

3. The probe may have identified false positives. In a nick translation reaction as the probe becomes smaller specificity is lost. Adjusting the DNA and the DNase concentrations in the nick translation reaction are therefore critical for specificity of each newly made probe. By making multiple copies of the spotted nitrocellulose papers we are currently retesting and thus confirming probe positive specimens.

The DNA hybridization assay to detect ETEC is a novel application of molecular genetics and recombinant DNA technology. Not only does this technique increase the detection of ETEC, but also provides another marker which may be useful in epidemiologic studies of diarrhea caused by this enteric pathogen.

REFERENCES

1. Puffer, R. R., and C. V. Serrano. 1973. Patterns of mortality in childhood, Washington DC. Pan American Health Organization (PAHO Scientific Publication 262).

2. Oberle, M. W., M. H. Merson, M. S. Islam, A. S. M. Mizanur Rahman, D. H. Huber, and G. Curlin. 1980. Diarrheal disease in Bangladesh: epidemiology, mortality averted and costs at a rural treatment centre. 1980. Intern. J. Epidemiol. **9**: 341–348.

3. Ryder, R. W., D. A. Sack, A. Z. Kapikian, J. C. McLaughlin, J. Charkraborty, A. S. M. M. Rahman, M. H. Merson, and J. G. Wells. 1976. Enterotoxigenic *Escherichia coli* and reovirus-like agent in rural Bangladesh. Lancet. **i**: 659–663.

4. Leksomboon, U., P. Echeverria, C. Suvongse, and C. Duangmani. 1981. Viruses and bacteria in pediatric diarrhea in Thailand: A study of multiple antibiotic resistant enteric pathogens. Amer. J. Trop. Med. 30(6): 1281–1290.

5. Black, R. E., M. H. Merson, I. Huq, A. R. M. A. Alim, and M. D. Yunus. 1981. Incidence and severity of rotavirus and *Escherichia coli* diarrhoea in rural Bangladesh. Lancet. **i**: 141–143.

6. Sack, D. A., J. C. McLaughlin, R. B. Sack, F. Orskov, and I. Orskov. 1977. Enterotoxigenic *Escherichia coli* isolated from patients at a hospital in Dacca. J. Infect. Dis. **135**: 275–280.

7. Echeverria, P., L. Verhaert, C. V. Uylangco, M. T. Ho, S. Komalarini, F. Orskov, and I. Orskov. 1978. Plasmid-mediated antimicrobial resistance and enterotoxin production among isolates of *Escherichia coli* in the Far East. Lancet. **ii**: 589–591.

8. Merson, M. H., R. E. Black, M. Kahn, and I. Huq. 1978. Epidemiology of cholera and enterotoxigenic *Escherichia coli* diarrhea in cholera and related diarrhea. 43rd Nobel Symp. Stockholm pp. 34–45.

9. Black, R. E., M. H. Merson, A. S. M. M. Rahman, M. Yunus, A. R. M. A. Alim, I. Huq, R. H. Yolken, and G. T. Curlin. 1980. A two year study of bacterial, viral, and parasitic agents associated with diarrhea in rural Bangladesh. J. Infect. Dis. **142**: 660–664.

10. Black, R. E., M. H. Merson, B. Rowe, P. R. Taylor, A. R. M. Abdul Alim, R. J. Gross, and D. A. Sack. 1981. Enterotoxigenic *Escherichia coli* diarrhoea: Acquired immunity and transmission in an endemic area. Bull WHO 59(2): 263–268.

11. Echeverria, P., L. Verhaert, V. Basaca-Sevilla, T. Banson, and J. H. Cross. 1978. Prevalence of heat-labile enterotoxigenic *Escherichia coli* in humans, liverstock, food, and water in a community in the Philippines. J. Infect. Dis. **138**: 87–89.

12. Cohan, M. L., and E. J. Gangarosa. 1978. Non-typhoidal Salmonellosis. Southern Med. J. **71**: 1540–1545.

13. Blaser, M. J., and L. B. Reller. 1981. Campylobacter enteritis. N. Engl. J. Med. **305**: 1444–1452.
14. Moseley, S. L., I. Huq, A. R. M. A. Alim, M. So, M. Samadpour-Motalebi, and S. Falkow. 1980. Detection of enterotoxigenic *Escherichia coli* by DNA colony hybridization. J. Infect. Dis. **142**: 892–898.
15. Sack, D. A., and R. B. Sack. 1975. Test for enterotoxigenic *Escherichia coli* using Y-1 adrenal cells in miniculture. Infect. Immun. **11**: 334–336.
16. Dean, A. G., Y. C. Ching, R. G. Williams, and L. B. Harden. 1972. Test for *Escherichia coli* enterotoxin using infant mice: Application in a study of diarrhea in children in Honolulu. J. Infect. Dis. **125**: 407–411.

Bacterial Diarrheal Diseases, eds., Y. Takeda, T. Miwatani, 65–73.

EPIDEMIOLOGY OF BACTERIAL DIARRHOEAL DISEASES IN INDIA WITH SPECIAL REFERENCE TO *VIBRIO PARAHAEMOLYTICUS* INFECTIONS

S. C. Pal, B. K. Sircar, G. B. Nair and B. C. Deb

National Institute of Cholera and Enteric Diseases, P-33, C.I.T. Scheme XM, Beliaghata, Calcutta-700016, India

Acute diarrhoeal diseases constitute one of the major health problems in India. This will be evident from the fact that 40 - 50 percent beds in the Infectious Diseases Hospitals as well as in the children hospitals in the country are occupied by diarrhoea patients. Number of patients admitted in the Infectious Diseases Hospital, Calcutta during 1975 - 1979 are shown in Table 1.

Acute diarrhoeal disease has also been recognized as the major killer of infants and children under 5 years of age. According to 1971 Census, as many as 1.5 million children die of diarrhoeal diseases in India every year, apart from cholera.

The cases are primarily sporadic in nature and the children under 5 years suffer from at least 1 - 2 attacks of diarrhoea per year. 383 children under 5 years of age in a Calcutta community were kept under daily surveillance during 1977 - 1978 (1). The children under 2 years were found to suffer from 198 episodes of diarrhoea per 100 children per year. However, 99.5 percent of the diarrhoea cases were mild, with average number of 7 loose stools per episode for a mean duration of 35 hours. None of the patients was hospitalized and there was no death. Data collected from other parts of the country confirm the above findings. It is estimated that about one in every 200 - 300 community diarrhoea cases may require hospitalization. Overall case fatality rates of the hospitalized diarrhoea patients vary from 1 - 5 percent in different hospitals in the country.

Role of different microbial agents in the causation of sporadic acute diarrhoeal diseases were investigated by several workers. Intestinal pathogens were detected from 40 - 80 percent of these diarrhoea cases. These include *V. cholerae* biotype *ElTor*, rotavirus, toxigenic and enteropathogenic *E. coli*, *V. parahaemolyticus*, *Campylobacter jejuni*, Shigella, *E. histolytica* etc. Spectrum of microbial agents detected from 356 acute diarrhoea cases admitted in Infectious Diseases Hospital, Calcutta is shown in Table 2 (2). It will be seen that *V. cholerae* biotype *ElTor* is the commonest pathogen responsible for acute diarrhoeal diseases in Calcutta. In about 10 percent of the cases more than one pathogen was isolated. As for example on 5 out of 6 occasions *Campylobacter jejuni* was isolated along

Table 2. Spectrum of microbial isolates from 356
          hospitalised acute diarrhoea cases in Calcutta
          during 1981

Pathogens Detected	No. of cases Found positive	Percent
V. cholerae	132	37.1
Rotavirus	39	11.0
V. parahaemolyticus	27	7.6
EPEC	29	8.1
ETEC	20	5.6
A. hydrophila	14	3.9
Shigellae	8	2.2
Pl. shigelloides	7	2.0
Campylobacter fetus ssp. jejuni	6	1.7
Providencia stuartii	4	1.1
Group 'F' vibrios	2	0.6
E. tarda	1	0.3
Citrobacter freundii	1	0.3
Total	290	81.5

Table 1. Total admisiions in Infectious Diseases Hospital,
          Calcutta 1975 - 1979

Cases	1975	1976	1977	1978	1979
Gastroenteritis including cholera	10250 (52.5%)	8091 (47.8%)	8927 (50.1%)	7916 (46.6%)	6209 (40.5%)
Diphtheria	4788	4012	3800	4348	5392
Tetanus	3178	3388	3420	3275	2335
Rabies	110	115	137	142	155
Meningitis	710	865	988	817	1001
Smallpox	4	-	-	-	-
Chickenpox	134	60	92	127	50
Encephalitis	364	389	460	363	177
Total	19538	16920	17824	16988	15319

with *V. cholerae* biotype *ElTor*. The relative importance of these multiple pathogens in causation of diarrhoea could not be determined.

Recurrent outbreaks of infantile winter diarrhoeas have been reported from two distinct geographical areas in the country namely Manipur (3) in the East and Calicut (4) in the South. Children aged between 6 months to 18 months were the main victims of these outbreaks and rotavirus was isolated from 70 - 90 percent of the patients. Neither the cause of recurrence nor the mode of transmission of the disease could be determined.

Vibrio parahaemolyticus infection

Incidence

Vibrio parahaemolyticus infection constitutes one of the major health hazards for the Calcutta populations. Isolation of *V. parahaemolyticus* from a small number of acute diarrhoea cases in Calcutta was first reported by Chatterjee and co-workers (5) in 1970. However, Sakazaki and co-workers (6), while working at the Cholera Research Centre during July, 1969 to June, 1970 isolated 378 strains of *V. parahaemolyticus* from 3433 stool specimens of acute diarrhoea cases in Calcutta. *V. cholerae* was isolated from 38.2 percent and *V. parahaemolyticus* from 11.0 percent of the cases. Studies conducted during the subsequent years by the National Institute of Cholera and Enteric Diseases (7) showed that the problem of *V. parahaemolyticus* infection in Calcutta in only second to that of cholera. *V. parahaemolyticus* was detected from 3.5 to 23.9 percent of acute diarrhoea cases admitted to hospital during different months. Results of the studies also showed that *V. parahaemolyticus* infection are present all the year round and no distinct seasonal pattern could be observed.

Clinical features

Diarrhoea (100%) and vomiting (95%) are the two main presenting symptoms by which they closely simulate cholera. However, certain clinical features such as fever (54%), pain in abdomen (78%) and blood with mucus (25%) in stool distinguish *V. parahaemolyticus* infection as a separate clinical entity (8).

There is no significant difference in serum electrolytes level between cholera and *V. parahaemolyticus* cases. However, the general milder nature of the disease, presence of leucocytosis and higher concentration of protein in stool differentiate *V. parahaemolyticus* infection from cholera (Table 3) (7).

Incubation period of 163 cases studied, varied from 1 - 23 hours but in 77.3% of the cases it was within 12 hours (9).

Antibiotic sensitivity

Antibiotic sensitivity of the *V. parahaemolyticus* strains isolated from clinical

Table 3. Important biochemical features of 53 hospitalised acute diarrhoea cases in Calcutta

Groups	Means of concentrations on admission				
	In blood/plasma (MEQ/L) of				Of stool protein (MGM/ML)
	Na$^+$	K$^+$	HCO$_3^-$	Cl$^-$	
V. parahaemolyticus (25)	109.0	5.2	20.4	90.2	12.7
V. cholerae (15)	110.0	5.2	11.7	98.6	2.7
ETEC[1] (13)	109.0	6.1	14.9	96.8	7.6

[1] Enterotoxigenic E. coli
N.B. Figures in ( ) indicate number of cases studied in the group

cases suggests that the pathogen in highly susceptible to gentamycin (99.2%) and chloramphenicol (92.0%), moderately susceptible to tetracycline (42.2%) and doxycycline (17.8%), whereas insensitive to ampicillin and streptomycin (10).

Epidemiology

Unlike in Japan, USA and other developed countries *V. parahaemolyticus* infection in Calcutta communities are primarily sporadic in nature. However, a few small localized outbreaks involving 4 - 5 persons in each episode have also been reported (11). The sporadic cases are generally scattered all over the community. Over 89.4% of infected houses had a single case, 5.7% houses had 2 cases and 5.0% houses and three cases (9) (Table 4). The disease is prevalent among the people of low socio-economic status. The distribution of diarrhoea cases caused by *V. parahaemolyticus* favourably compares with that of cholera cases in the Calcutta communities.

Age and Sex

It is interesting to note that about 92% of the cases are among adults, though in Calcutta situation adults and children equally share the same meals. In one study 65% of the patients were found among females (8). However, other studies suggest that the cases are equally distributed among both sexes.

Carriers

Existence of carrier state or inapparent infection for *V. parahaemolyticus* in India was first reported by Deb (9) in 1975. 15.3% of the family contacts of *V. parahaemolyticus* diarrhoea cases were found to be excreting the organism for upto 5 days. Incidence of contact carriers in different age groups is shown in Table 5. It will be seen that there was no significant difference in the distribution of carriers among different age and sex groups. Most of the carriers (58.3%) were

Table 4. Percent distribution of houses with number of simultaneously occurring diarrhoea cases in the same house in Calcutta (Modified from Deb. 1975)

No. of cases in the same house	No. of houses having hospitalised diarrhoea cases due to	
	V. parahaemolyticus	V. cholerae
1	89.4 (126)	97.7 (258)
2	5.7 (8)	2.3 (6)
3	5.0 (7)	–
Total	100.0 (141)	100.0 (264)

N.B. Figures in ( ) indicate number of houses

Table 5. Incidence of contact carriers excreting
V. parahaemolyticus who did not suffer
from diarrhoea (Modified from Deb. 1975)

Age group (years)	No. of contacts sampled	No. found positive	Percent
≤4	28	4	14.3
5 - 9	21	2	9.5
10 - 14	21	4	19.0
≥15	87	14	16.1
Total	157	24	15.3

N.B. Difference between incidences of carriers in
two sexes was not statistically significant

found to be excreting only once. However, 16.7% of the carriers excreted *V. parahaemolyticus* 4 - 5 times during the period of 10 days.

The existence of carrier state was further confirmed by Sircar *et al.* (8) in 1976. 15 out of 100 contacts of 17 bacteriologically confirmed *V. parahaemolyticus* cases were found excreting the vibrios on more than one occasion. All the strains isolated from carriers and all except one isolate from the index cases were Kanagawa phenomenon positive. 21.7% of the isolates from cases and 46.7% from carriers belonged to the serotype O1:K56.

On further detailed studies on *V. parahaemolyticus* carriers it was observed that as many as four contact carriers could be detected in the same family (12). It was also noted that a carrier may excrete the vibrio for several days. Serotypic patterns of the strains isolated from index cases and carriers are shown in Table 6. It will be seen that in most of the families there was no correlation among the serotypes of the strains isolated from the index cases and their contact. It is also interesting to note that the same carrier was excreting different serotypes on different days both Kanagawa positive and negative strains. The strains isolated from the environmental samples collected from in and around these families did not show any similarity either in serotypes or Kanagawa phenomenon.

Environmental studies

Studies have been conducted in inland and coastal areas of India to locate the environmental reservoirs of *V. parahaemolyticus*. An in-depth study carried out in Calcutta (13) revealed the prevalence of this pathogen in a variety of environmental samples such as water, fish and crustaceans (Table 7). Uniquely different from elsewhere in the world, *V. parahaemolyticus* was isolated from fresh water fishes (13.0%), crabs (57.0%) and 5% of water samples with practically no salinity. Shrimps and pomfrets (sea fish) also showed a high percentage of isolation of *V. parahaemolyticus*. Results of the Calcutta study stimulated further studies under a multicentric project (ICMR) at four centres in India, namely, Bombay, Calicut, Bangalore and Port Blair. Of these, two centres were situated in

Table 6. Serotypes of different strains isolated from different
categories of samples in V. parahaemolyticus positive index
case houses (modified from Sircar et al., 1979)

Serotypes of strains isolated from index cases	Serotypes of strains isolated from carriers with dates of isolation			
	1st carrier	2nd carrier	3rd carrier	4th carrier
O4:K49 (19/4)	O1:K56 (20/4) O4:K49# (21/4) O4:K49# (22/4) O4:K49 (23/4) O3:K45# (24/4) O4:K49# (25/4) U.T. (26/4)	O1:K56 (20/4) O1:K56 (21/4) O1:K56 (23/4) O1:K56 (24/4)	–	–
O1:K38 (26/4)	O1:K56 (29/4)	O3:K31 (2/5)	O1:K56 (30/4) O2:K28# (2/5) O4:K9# (3/5)	O3:K57 (5/5)
O7:K19 (18/5)	O7:K19 (19/5) U.T. (21/5) O7:K19 (22/5) O3:K57 (23/5) O7:K19 (24/5) O7:K19 (25/5) O5:K17 (28/5)	U.T. (22/5)	–	–
O7:K19 (21/5)	O3:K57 (23/5) O3:K57 (26/5) O3:K57 (28/5)	O1:K38 (24/5) O7:K19 (25/5) O5:K17 (28/5) O5:K17 (30/5)	O1:K56 (27/5)	–
UT (29/7)	U.T. (30/7) O5:K17 (31/7) O5:K17 (1/8) U.T. (2/8) O5:K17 (3/8) O5:K49 (4/8) O1:K56 (7/8) O1:K56 (8/8)	–	–	–

\# Indicates Kanagawa negative strains
U.T. Untypable strains

the Western coast, one in the Bay of Bengal and the other one was located in inland area. The results of three years investigation indicated that *V. parahaemolyticus* was found abundantly in the environment in all the centres, but the incidence of diarrhoea due to *V. parahaemolyticus* was less than 1% in these areas (Table 8). This suggests that the problem of *V. parahaemolyticus* gastroenteritis is of singular importance only in Calcutta. The cause and significance of high prevalence rate of *V. parahaemolyticus* diarrhoea in Calcutta is still not clearly understood.

Along the Coromandel and West coast of India, *V. parahaemolyticus* has been frequently isolated from estuarine and marine environs (14, 15). Seasonal distribution of this organism in estuarine environs has been worked out in detail at Porto Novo (14). The annual cycle of *V. parahaemolyticus* in brackish waters

Table 7. Isolation of V. parahaemolyticus from
environmental samples in Calcutta
(Modified from De et al., 1977)

Categories of sample	No. of samples examined	No. found positive	Percent
Water	404	20	5.0
Fishes:			
Fresh water	484	63	13.0
Sea water	71	25	35.2
Crustaceans:			
Crabs	79	45	57.0
Shrimps	120	39	32.5
Mollusca:			
Mussels	76	2	2.6
Total	1234	194	15.7

N.B. From the same samples isolations of V. cholerae
and NAG vibrios were 0.2% and 68.9%, respectively

Table 8. Incidence of V. parahaemolyticus in different parts of India

Place	Diarrhoea cases (Hospitalised)		Fish and crustacean samples		Water samples	
	Number examined	No. +VE	Number examined	No. +VE	Number examined	No. +VE
Bombay	2992	27 (0.9)	2627	91 (3.5)	410	16 (3.9)
Bangalore	2033	8 (0.4)	315	81 (25.7)	90	3 (3.3)
Calicut	855	6 (0.7)	263	69 (26.2)	86	NIL (-)
Port Blair	172	2 (1.2)	585	200 (34.2)	500	42 (8.4)
Porto Novo (Natarajan et al. 1980)	ND	-	944	381 (40.4)	252	91 (36.1)
Mangalore (Sagar & Mohan Kumar, 1980)	ND	-	65	8 (12.3)	28	5 (17.8)

N.B. Figures in ( ) indicate percentage
ND = not done
39.3% of plankton samples examined at Porto Novo were positive

was found to be chiefly influenced by salinity, zooplankton and phytoplankton blooms.

Quantitation of *V. parahaemolyticus* in diarrhoeal stools and in the intestinal contents of fishes and crustaceans revealed a rather high density ranging from $>10^4$ to 10^6 organisms/ml (7). Likewise, Nair *et al.* (16) also observed preponderance of *V. parahaemolyticus* in the gastrointestinal tract of estuarine and marine fishes.

Kanagawa phenomenon

In Japan, most investigators have observed that over 90% of the isolates of *V. parahaemolyticus* from patients were Kanagawa positive while less than 1% of the isolates from sea-foods and sea-water were Kanagawa positive (17). In Calcutta, almost similar results have been documented wherein 88.2% strains isolated from human sources (case and carriers) were Kanagawa positive (12). On the other hand, less than 1% of strains isolated from environmental samples were Kanagawa positive (13). Higher Kanagawa positivity of environmental strains of the vibrio was, however, noted in Mangalore (25%), Port Blair (11.5%) and Porto Novo (6.7%) (15, 18, 14).

Transmission

V. parahaemolyticus gastroenteritis is primarily transmitted by raw or contaminated cooked sea-food or their products in Japan. The situation, in Calcutta, however, differs in that sea-foods are rarely consumed as fresh-water fish is normally preferred by the local population. Furthermore, epidemiological investigations in Calcutta have indicated that 33.3% patients suffering from *V. parahaemolyticus* gastroenteritis, denied consumption of any fish or sea-food seven days prior to onset of the disease (8). The predominant occurrence of single case in the family also points out that the disease is not of a common source origin (9). The exact mode of transmission of *V. parahaemolyticus* in Calcutta is not yet clearly established.

Conclusion

The problem of *V. parahaemolyticus* infection in Calcutta is therefore, distinctly different from that in Japan. The major points of differences are shown in Table 9. It may be concluded that diarrhoea due to *V. parahaemolyticus* in Japan,

Table 9. Comparison of Epidemiological features of V. parahaemolyticus infection in India and Japan

Features	India (Calcutta)	Japan
Disease pattern	Sporadic (mostly 1 case per family), scattered all over	Food-poisoning type (50-70% affected)
Frequency of isolation (HOSP.)	11-15%	24%
Age	Mostly above 15 years	-
Seasonality	Occur throughout the year (little variation)	Occur during summer (May - October)
Incrimination of any special food	None (33.3% occurred in Veg. families)	Sea fish, shell fish and their products
Inapparent infection (Carriers)	15.3% of family contacts are carriers	0.3% amongst healthy Japanese
Mode of transmission	Use of contaminated water sources (ponds, open wells)	Use of contaminated sea foods
Environmental reservoirs	Fresh water fishes, crabs, shrimps and mussels	Marine animals

USA and other developed countries is primarily food poisoning in nature. In countries within South East Asia, including India, the chances of food poisoning are rare as the methods of preparation of food are likely to eliminate the vibrios from the contaminated ingredients. However, lack of proper environmental sanitation and poor personal hygiene may be responsible for sporadic cases of diarrhoea caused by *V. parahaemolyticus* in the countries, namely, India, Indonesia, Thailand and Vietnam. Much remains to be studied to get an insight on the epidemiology of *V. parahaemolyticus* infection particularly in the developing situations.

REFERENCES

1. National Institute of Cholera and Enteric Diseases. Annual Report. 1978.
2. National Institute of Cholera and Enteric Diseases. Annual Report. 1981.
3. Sengupta, P. G., D. Sen, M. R. Saha, S. Niyogi, B. C. Deb, and S. C. Pal. 1981. An epidemic of rotavirus diarrhoea in Manipur, India. Trans. Roy. Soc. Trop. Med. Hyg. **75**: 521–523.
4. Paniker, C. K. J., S. Mathew, R. Dharmarajan, M. M. Mathan, and V. I. Mathan. 1977. Epidemic gastroenteritis in children associated with rotavirus infection. Indian J. Med. Res. **66**: 525–529.
5. Chatterjee, B. D., K. N. Neogy, and S. L. Gorbach. 1970. Study of *Vibrio parahaemolyticus* from cases of diarrhoea in Calcutta. Indian J. Med. Res. **58**: 234–238.
6. Sakazaki, R., K. Tamura, L. M. Prescott, Z. Bencic, S. C. Sanyal, and R. Sinha. 1971. Bacteriological examination of diarrhoeal stools in Calcutta. Indian J. Med. Res. **59**: 1025–1034.
7. Cholera Research Centre. Annual Report. 1976.
8. Sircar, B. K., B. C. Deb, S. P. De, A. Ghosh, and S. C. Pal. 1976. Clinical and epidemiological studies on *V. parahaemolyticus* infection in Calcutta (1975). Indian J. Med. Res. **64**: 1576–1580.
9. Deb, B. C. 1975. Studies on *Vibrio parahaemolyticus* infection in Calcutta as compared to cholera infection, pp. 490–502. *In* E. Jucker (ed.), Progress in Drug Research - Vol. 19, Tropical Diseases II. Birkhauser Verlag Basel und Stuttgart, Switzerland.
10. Sen, D., S. P. De, S. N. Ghosh, D. K. Chanda, A. Ghosh, and S. C. Pal. 1977. Antibiotic sensitivity of *V. parahaemolyticus* from cases of gastroenteritis. Indian J. Med. Res. **65**: 628–631.
11. Chatterjee, B. D., T. Sen, and A. C. Mukherji. 1974. Food poisoning associated with *Vibrio parahaemolyticus* serotype O5: Cal/Ka in Calcutta. Bull. Cal. Sch. Trop. Med. **22**: 1–3.
12. Sircar, B. K., S. P. De, P. G. Sengupta, S. Mondal, D. Sen, B. C. Deb, and S. C. Pal. 1979. Studies on transmission of *V. parahaemolyticus* infection in Calcutta communities : A preliminary report. Indian J. Med. Res. **70**: 898–907;.
13. De, S. P., M. Banerjee, B. C. Deb, P. G. Sengupta, J. Sil, B. K. Sircar, D. Sen, A. Ghosh, and S. C. Pal. 1977. Distribution of vibrios in Calcutta environment with particular reference to *V. parahaemolyticus*. Indian J. Med. Res. **65**: 21–28.
14. Natarajan, R., M. Abraham, and G. B. Nair. 1980. Distribution of *Vibrio parahaemolyticus* in Porto Novo environment. Indian J. Med. Res. **71**: 679–687.
15. Karunasagar, I., and K. C. Mohankumar. 1980. Occurrence of Kanagawa positive *Vibrio parahaemolyticus* strains around Mangalore (South India). Indian J. Med. Res. **72**: 619–621.
16. Nair, G. B., M. Abraham, and R. Natarajan. 1980. Distribution of *Vibrio parahaemolyticus* in Finfish harvested from Porto Novo (S. India) environs: a seasonal study. Can. J. Microbiol. **26**: 1264–1269.
17. Sakazaki, R., K. Tamura, T. Kato, Y. Obara, S. Yamai, and K. Hobo. 1968. Studies on the enteropathogenic, facultatively halophilic bacteria, *Vibrio parahaemolyticus*. III. Enteropathogenicity. Jap. J. Med. Sci. Biol., **21**: 325–331.
18. Lall, R., D. Sen, M. R. Saha, A. K. Bose, S. P. De, N. C. Palchowdhury, and S. C. Pal. 1979. Prevalence of *Vibrio parahaemolyticus* in Port Blair. Indian J. Med. Res. **69**: 217–221.

Bacterial Diarrheal Diseases, eds., Y. Takeda, T. Miwatani, 75–81.

ETIOLOGICAL STUDY OF DIARRHEAL DISEASES IN SHANGHAI

H. Sima

Shanghai Hygiene and Antiepidemic Center, 280 Chan Su Road, Shanghai, China

Diarrheal diseases have attracted attention internationally, because of their high morbidity and the complexity of pathogenic factors involved, especialy in countries or areas with poor sanitary condition. These disease frequently cause death of infants in some developing countries. Realizing the importance of public health in control of these diseases and the significance of recent scientific finding, the World Health Organization has launched a programme for control of diarrheal diseases.

Shanghai is the largest city in China. Within the past 30 years, medical and preventive services have been established in rural areas and so medical care has become much more generalized; for instance, there is now one commune hospital for every commune with a population of about twenty thousand. A commune usually comprising 10 - 15 brigades, and each of them has a health clinic with one doctor from the commune hospital and 4 - 5 barefood doctors responsible for health propaganda, family planning, childhood immunization visiting medical care and other health work. (This is somewhat similar to the WHO program for primary health care). We believe that generalization of basic medical facilities is of primary importance for improvement of the people's health and for reduction of morbidity and mortality from diarrhoeal diseases.

For many years there has been a communicable-disease reporting system, (as regards diarrheal diseases only those diagnosed as, or suspected of being, dysentery have been reported). Among the cases of diarrheal diseases, 20 - 30% are of *Bacillus* dysentery 7 - 10% of *V. parahaemolyticus* 3% of *Salmonella*, and about 50 - 70% of unknown causes. This shows that a more thorough study of diarrhoeal diseases is required with special attention to cases of unknown cause.

WHO reported that until the last decades, 80% of the cases of acute diarrheal diseases were described as "acute undifferentiated diarrhea", as existing knowledge did not permit recognition of the etiological agents. Since then the situation has completely changed. Today with recognition of several newer agents, a well equipped laboratory can demonstrate entero-pathogens in more than 70 % of the patients visiting treatment centers, and of more than one pathogen in 10 - 15% the cases. This helps in proper treatment and control of the disease. The above facts show that accurate diagnosis is important in prevention and control of diar-

Table 1. Sero-grouping of <u>Shigella</u> isolated in 1964, 1978 and 1979 in Shanghai

Year	Shigella sonnei Number of strains (%)	Shigella flexneri Number of strains (%)	Shigella dysenteriae* Number of strains (%)	Shigella boydi Number of strains (%)	Total Number of strains (%)
1964	1875 (72.8)	615 (23.9)	85 (3.2)	2 (0.1)	2577 (100)
1978	1483 (32.5)	3018 (66.6)	24 (0.6)	12 (0.3)	4537 (100)
1979	2589 (40.1)	3778 (58.5)	21 (0.3)	55 (1.1)	6443 (100)

* Serotype 2

rheal diseases, and that research on the etiology of diarrheal diseases is very important. As reported, *Campy. jejuni, Y. enterocolitica*, and pathogenic *E. coli* (including ETEC, EPEC and EIEC) and viral agents are important pathogenic factors. In reviewing past research work, we selected an area for studying the rate of isolation of common enteric pathogens. We also used diarrheal infants to study the isolation rates of *Campy. jejuni* and *Y. enterocolitica*. Doctors in the Division of Virology in our center also screened for Rotavirus in cases of infantile diarrhoea.

I. In previous etiological studies, *Shigella*, has been studied more extensively than *V. parahaemolyticus* or *Salmonella*. The most common serogroups of *Shigella* in the whole municipality of Shanghai are *sonnei* and *flexneri, Schmitzi* and *Boydi* being less common and *Shigella Shiga* being very rare with only twelve cases reported from 1954 to 1958. (All enquiries on *Shigella* patients were made in the Shanghai area). In 1962 only 3 strains of *Shiga* were isolated and since 1963 no Shiga strains have been isolated. In 1964, of all *Shigella* isolated 23.9% were of flexneri strains and 72.8% of *Sonnei* strain. In 1978 the percentages were 66.6% and 32.5% respectively, and in 1979 they were 58.5% and 40.1% respectively. Thus, cases of *Shigella Sonnei* infection seem to have increased, particularly among atypical cases and children. Typing showed that *Shigella flexneri* F2a and F3 were the most commonly encountered. (Table 1 and 2).

V. parahaemolyticus was isolated for the first time from patient who died from eating baked goose in 1958 in Shanghai. Subsequently studied the bacteriology, epidemiology, environmental dispersion and resistance of this organism. We found

Table 2. Typing of <u>Shigella flexneri</u>: percentages in 1978 and 1979 in Shanghai

Year	Fla	Flb	F2a	F2b	F3	Fx	Fy	Total
1978	3.9	5.9	50.9	2.0	31.4	3.9	2.0	100
1979	5.4	17.9	33.9	10.7	19.6	7.1	5.4	100

Table 3. Isolation of pathogenic bacteria from 678 cases of diarrheal
in Pudu District in Shanghai

Number of samples examined	Number of positives cultures	Rate (%)	Shigella			V. parahaemolyticus			Salmonella		
			Number of strains	Rate (%)	% of cases	Number of strains	Rate (%)	% of cases	Number of strains	Rate (%)	% of cases
678	161	23.7	83	12.2	51.5	61	9.0	37.9	17	2.5	10.6

that a large percentage of the cases of food poisoning in Shanghai were due to this organism. Now we have nearly controlled this kind of food poisoning.

Salmonella was responsible for only 3% of the cases of diarrheal. In 1980, we have isolated 9 groups and 29 serotypes of *Salmonella* in Shanghai. Among these, *S. typhimurium* Group B, and *S. anatum* Group E were the most common.

II. To determine isolation rates of common enteric pathogens in 1980 we examined 678 patients with acute diarrhoea in Nichuan Street Hospital in the Pudu District, which is adjacent to a rural area. The results were as follows. (Table 3, 4, 5, 6, 7).

III. Studies on other agents of diarrheal diseases.
1. Stool examination of cases of infantile diarrhea for agents such as *Campy. jejuni* and *Y. enterocolitica*. Untreated patients of under 3 years old were examined. Fecal samples and swabs were taken, put into Cary- Blair transport medium and sent to the laboratory. Three swab samples were taken from each patient. The first swab was used for direct streaking on SS and two MacConkey media (one in a 25°C incubator), and then enriched with SF enriched medium, and plated on SS agar after incubation for 12 - 18 hours. The second swab was used for direct streaking on *V. parahaemolyticus* selective medium and the last swab was streaked on Campy- BAP medium or Skirrow's medium (prepared by ourselves). The cultures were incubated for 48 hours at 42°C in an atmosphere of 5% oxygen, 10% carbon dioxide and 85% nitrogen, or put into a Campylobacter bag, made by Shanghai First Medical College. Colonies were tested for oxidase and catalase production and smear preparations were made when positive results were obtained to determine whether cells were. Gram negative, vibrio-like, S-shaped or spindle-shaped and whether the cells were motily. Then growth at 42°C and 25°C, tolerance

Table 4. Serogrouping of 83 strains of Shigella

Group	Number of strains	%
flexneri	42	50.6
boydi	7	8.4
sonnei	34	41.0
Total	83	100.0

Table 5.   Typing of 42 strains of <u>Shigella</u>
           <u>flexneri</u>

Type	Number of strains	%
F1a	1	2.4
F1b	5	11.9
F2a	13	30.9
F2b	2	4.8
F3	15	35.7
F4	1	2.4
F6	1	2.4
Fx	1	2.4
Fy	2	4.7
Not typable	1	2.4
Total	42	100.0

Table 6.   Typing of 17 strains of <u>Salmonella</u>

Group	Type	Number of strains	%
B	S. typhimurium	9	52.9
B	S. derby	1	5.9
C	not typable	1	5.9
C2	S. manhattan	1	5.9
C2	S. newport	1	5.9
D	S. London	1	5.9
E1	S. anatum	2	11.7
E1	S. meleagridis	1	5.9
Total		17	100.0

to glycine, tolerance to 3.5% NaCl, and H_2S production were examined and the TTC test was carried out.

In 1981, we isolated *Campy. jejuni* from 18 of 31 chicken samples (58.1%) and all 29 ducks samples (100%) tested. We also isolated *Y. enterocolitica* from pig feces. On the basis of these results, in May 1981 we isolated the first strain of *Campy. jejuni* from a four-year-old child and in June 1981 began planning to examine stools of children of 0 - 3 years old with diarrhea. *Campy. jejuni* was first isolated from a 4-year-old boy who became ill on May 18th, had fever for 2 days, and had been treated with sulfa drugs with no effect. He came to the out patient clinic with the symptoms of cough, nasal catarrh and swollen erythematous tonsils. The next day he had diarrhoea 4 times, first with watery stools and then with mucous and blood. Microscopic examination showed the presence of RBC, WBC and phagocytes. Cultures of stools showed *Campy. jejuni*, but not other enterobacteria. After treatment with Gentamycin, his temperature dropped to normal. The first serum sample in the first week showed no agglutination titer for *Campy. jejuni* but a second serum sample taken one month later had a titer of 1 : 640.

Table 7. Isolation of pathogenic bacteria from 678 cases (of different age groups) of acute diarrhea in Pudu District in Shanghai

Age group (years)	Number of samples	Number of positive cultures	Rate (%)	Shigella		V. parahaemo-lyticus		Salmonella	
				Number of strains	Rate (%)	Number of strains	Rate (%)	Number of strains	Rate (%)
0-4	118	20	16.9	15	12.7	3	2.5	2	1.7
5-9	20	3	15.0	1	5.0	0	0	2	10.0
10-19	63	12	19.1	7	11.1	4	6.3	1	1.6
20-29	167	40	23.9	19	11.4	14	8.4	7	4.2
30-39	89	.26	29.2	14	15.7	12	13.5	0	0
40-49	61	19	31.2	8	13.1	10	16.4	1	1.6
50-59	96	23	23.9	11	12.5	10	10.4	2	2.1
60-69	64	18	28.1	8	12.2	8	12.5	2	3.1
Total	678	161	23.7	83	12.2	61	9.0	17	2.5

In 396 cases of infantile diarrhea, enteropathogen was found in 49.7%, and *Campy. jejuni* in 10.9%. This percentage was second to that of *Shigella*, which also has a peak at the same time of year. In cases of *Shigella*, the proportion of *sonnei* is higher than that of *flexneri*. No *Y. enterocolitica* or *V. parahaemolyticus* was isolated from these samples. See Tables 8 and 9.

For age relation, see Table 10. The rate of incidence in infants of 0 and 3 years of age with diarrhea was apparently less than that in those below of 2 years old.

The seasonal peak of *Campy. jejuni* in Shanghai is August and September, and their are fewer cases in June and October (see Table 11).

The above samples were obtained at the Children's Hospital of Shanghai First Medical College, but from July 8th to September 12th, 94 samples were obtained

Table 8. Results of fecal culture of 396 cases of acute infantile diarrhea

Date of sample collection	Number of samples	Number of positive cultures	Rate (%)	Shigella				Campy. jejuni	Salmonella	EPEC	Y. enterocol-itica	V. para haemolyticus
				sonnei	flexneri	dysenteriae*	Total					
2, June-31, July	43	7	16.3	2	0	0	2	3	1	1	0	0
August	145	78	53.8	42	4	1	47	18	7	6	0	0
September	132	85	64.4	54	8	0	62	17	5	1	0	0
October	76	27	35.5	15	4	1	20	5	2	0	0	0
Total	396	197	49.7	113	16	2	131	43	15	8	0	0

* Serotype 2

80

Table 9. Rates of isolation and percentages of different enteric bacteria in positive samples from 396 cases

Strain of enteric bacterium	Number of positive cultures	Rate (%)	% of positive specimens
Shigella	131	33.1	66.5
Campy. jejuni	43	10.9	21.8
Salmonella	15	3.8	7.6
EPEC	8	2.0	4.1
Total	197	49.7	100.0

Table 10. Analysis of 396 cases of acute infantile diarrhea due to Campy. jejuni according to age (months)

Age (months)	Number of cases of diarrhea	Number of cases of Campy. enteritis	Rate (%)
0-5	73	4	5.5
6-11	111	16	14.4
12-23	129	20	15.5
24-36	83	3	3.6
Total	396	43	10.9

Table 11. Months of incidence of 396 cases of acute infantile diarrhea due to Campy. jejuni

Month	Number of cases of diarrhea	Number of cases of Campy. enteritis	Rate (%)
22, June-31, July	43	3	7
August	145	18	12.4
September	132	17	12.9
October	76	5	6.6
Total	396	43	10.9

in the outpatient clinic of Shanghai Municipal Children's Hospital. Of these 14 cases contained *Campy. jejuni* (positive rate 14.9%).

We found that patients with *Campy. enteritis* often had other entero-bacteria also (Table 12).

The isolation rate of *Campy. jejuni* from stool samples taken in September from 101 normal infants of 0 - 3 years old in nurseries was 1% (1/101). Electron microscopy or scanning microscopy showed that *Campy. jejuni* isolated from chickens, ducks or humans is mainly amphitrichated.

Rotavirus and other viruses were also found in stool samples taken from October to November, 1980, at the Division of Virology of our Centre. In diarrheal

Table 12. Patients with <u>Campylobacter</u> enteritis and <u>Shigella</u>
and/or <u>Salmonella</u> in the children's hospitals

Hospital	Number of patients with Campy. enteritis	Complication				
		Shigella		Salmonella	Total	%
		sonnei	flexneri			
Children's Hospital of Shanghai First Medical College	43	7	2	1	10	23.3
Shanghai Municipal Children's Hospital	14	6	2	0	8	57.1

Table 13. Rota and other viruses found by electron microscopy
in 63 cases of infantile diarrheal

Number of samples and %	Rotavirus positive					Adenovirus positive	Negative
	Total	Toravirus only	Rotavirus + Adenovirus	Rotavirus + Small round virus	Rotavirus + Astrovirus		
63 100%	51 81%	46	3	1	1	2 3.1%	10 15.9%

infants of 2 - 20 months old, the positive rate of Rotavirus was as high as 81%.
(Table 13).

REFERENCES

1. Enteric Infections due to *Campylobacter*, *Yercinia*, *Salmonella* and *Shigella*. Report of a Subgroup of the Scientific Working Group on Epidemiology and Etiology. WHO/DDC/EPE/80.4.
2. International Centre for Diarrhoeal Disease Research, Bangladesh. Special Publication No. 7 June 1980.
3. Butzler, J. P., and M. B. Skirrow. 1979. *Campylobacter* Enteritis. Clinics in Gastroenterology. **8**: 737.
4. Bokkenheuser, V. D., N. J. Richardson, *et al*. 1979. Detection of enteric Campylobacteriosis in children. J. Clin. Micro. **9**: 227.

Bacterial Diarrheal Diseases, eds., Y. Takeda, T. Miwatani, 83–93.
Copyright © 1985 by KTK Scientific Publishers, Tokyo.

CURRENT STATUS OF BACTERIAL DIARRHEAL DISEASES IN JAPAN

Y. Kudoh and S. Sakai

Department of Microbiology, Tokyo Metropolitan Research Laboratory of Public Health, 24-1, 3-chome, Hyakunin-cho, Shinjuku-ku, Tokyo 160, Japan

In Japan, the incidence of gastrointestinal infections such as bacillary dysentery, and typhoid and paratyphoid fevers has decreased remarkably since the early 1960s. However, the incidence of bacterial food poisonings has not decreased greatly during the last twenty years (1, 2, 3). Moreover, the incidence of diarrheal diseases brought by overseas travellers to this country has recently tended to increase (4).

In this paper, the current status of diarrheal diseases in all Japan and in Tokyo is discussed from epidemiological and bacteriological view points.

Bacillary dysentery

Fig. 1 shows the morbidity(case) rates per 100,000 head of population of bacillary dysentery, typhoid and paratyphoid fevers and food poisoning in Japan during the last 20 years (3). Until the early 1960s, bacillary dysentery, or shigellosis, was one of the most common communicable diseases in this country, and the incidence of this disease remained fairly constant. Since then, however, like the incidences of typhoid and paratyphoid fevers, that of shigellosis has decreased gradually year by year, and its case rate has recently become about 1.0.

This tendency is reflected in the change in frequency of detection of shigellae bacilli in healthy subjects. Table 1 shows results on this in Tokyo from 1961 - 1980. The recovery from food handlers has decreased year by year, and only one carrier has been detected since 1975.

Change in the incidence of shigellosis was accompanied by change in the predominant *Shigella* species or serogroups isolated (1, 2, 3). As shown in Fig. 2, in the early 1960s the most common *Shigella* species was *S. flexneri* (subgroup B). Later *S. sonnei* (subgroup D) became predominant, but recently *S. flexneri* again became predominant. The isolations of *S. dysenteriae* and *S. boydii* have also increased recently. These increases in frequency isolation of *S. flexneri*, *S. dysenteriae* and *S. boydii* mainly reflect recent increase in the number of imported cases.

During the past 10 years, there has been no seasonal variation in the incidence of shigellosis, but children of under 10 years old show the highest incidence.

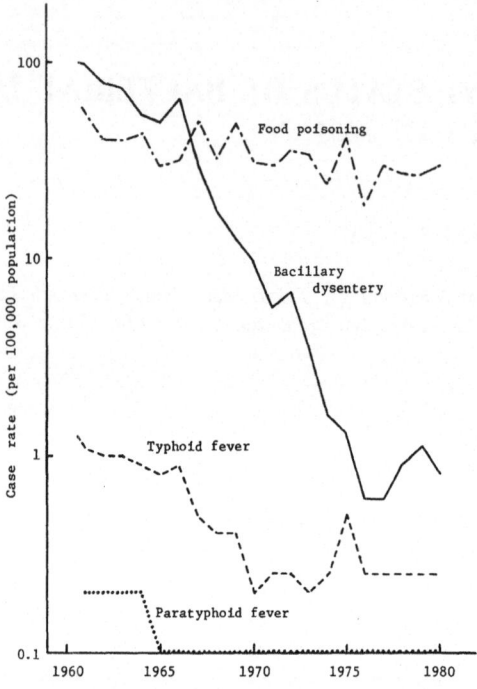

Case Rates of Bacillary Dysentery, Typhoid Fever, Paratyphoid
Fever and Food Poisonings in Japan (1961 – 1980)

Fig. 1

Table 1. Recovery of Shigella, S. typhi and Ss. paratyphi
A and B from Healthy Food Handlers in Tokyo
(1961 – 1980)

Year	No. of specimens examined	Number of positive with (%):	
		Shigella	S. typhi and Ss. paratyphi A and B
1961	213,906	589 (0.28)	–
1962	160,081	363 (0.14)	1 (0.0)
1963	310,307	555 (0.18)	–
1964	377,761	412 (0.11)	2 (0.0)
1965	304,776	243 (0.08)	5 (0.0)
1966	172,519	109 (0.06)	1 (0.0)
1967	170,534	50 (0.03)	3 (0.0)
1968	162,350	13 (0.01)	2 (0.0)
1969	155,372	9 (0.01)	7 (0.0)
1970	166,628	–	4 (0.0)
1971	141,391	1 (0.00)	3 (0.0)
1972	132,574	4 (0.00)	3 (0.0)
1973	131,200	1 (0.00)	1 (0.0)
1974	143,687	1 (0.00)	–
1975	99,406	–	–
1976	53,287	–	–
1977	36,495	–	–
1978	16,725	–	–
1979	12,630	–	–
1980	15,348	1 (0.00)	–

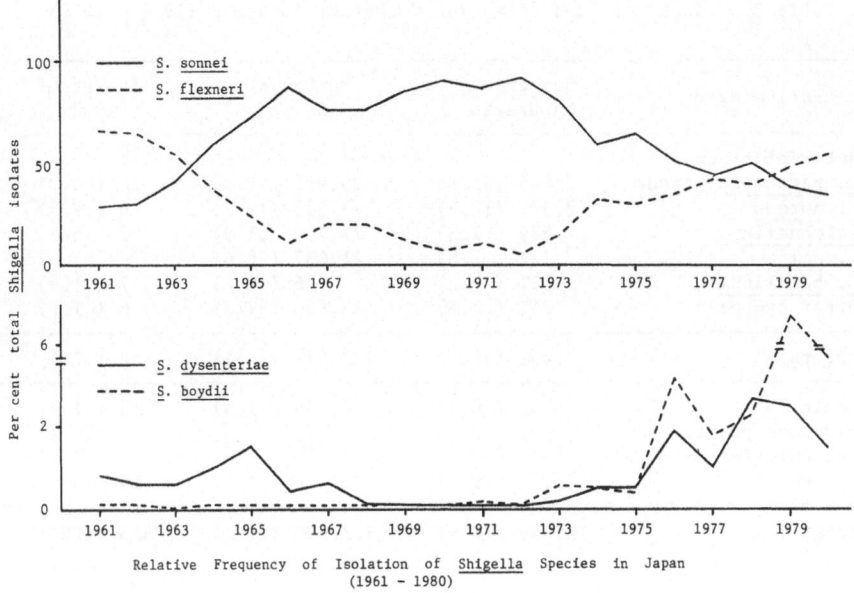

Relative Frequency of Isolation of Shigella Species in Japan
(1961 - 1980)

Fig. 2

Table 2.   Occurrence of Cholera During the Last Decade
in Japan

Year	Reported cases			Note
	Imported	Domestic	Total	
1971	–	–	–	· · · ·
1972	–	–	–	· · · ·
1973	–	–	–	· · · ·
1974	–	–	–	· · · ·
1975	3	–	3	· · · ·
1976	6	–	6	· · · ·
1977	11	99	110	Outbreak in Arida City
1978	17	53	70	Outbreak in Tokyo
1979	23	5	28	· · · ·
1980	33	7	40	Outbreak in Tokyo

Cholera

The occurrence of cholera in this country from 1971 - 1980 is shown in Table
2 (3). In Japan, cholera is not an endemic disease and except for 3 cases in 1964,
the source of infection of which is not known, there have been no reports of
indigenous cholera between 1974 and 1976. However, as indicated in the table,
in parallel with increasing import of food and international travel, not only imported cases but also suspected domestic cases have been observed every year since

Table 3.   Causes of Food Poisoning Outbreaks in Japan (1971 - 1980)

Causative agent	Number of outbreaks	Number of cases	Number of deaths
Bacterial			
V. parahaemolyticus	3,845 (31.3)	95,095 (29.4)	18 (5.0)
S. aureus	2,302 (18.8)	63,854 (19.7)	9 (2.5)
Salmonella	889 (7.3)	27,719 (11.9)	22 (6.1)
E. coli	222 (1.8)	21,687 (8.6)	–
C. botulinum	21 (0.2)	66 (0.0)	7 (1.9)
Other bacteria	212 (1.7)	23,650 (7.3)	6 (1.7)
Subtotal	7,491 (61.1)	232,071 (71.7)	62 (17.1)
Chemicals	82 (0.7)	4,539 (1.4)	5 (1.4)
Poisonous plants and animals	1,029 (8.4)	4,764 (1.5)	242 (66.7)
Unknown	3,654 (29.8)	82,234 (25.4)	54 (14.9)
Total	12,256 (100)	323,608 (100)	363 (100)

1977, and there have been outbreaks in Arida City, Wakayama Prefecture (1977), Ikenohata, Tokyo (1978) and Bunkyo, Tokyo (1980). The cause of these outbreaks could not be identified, but that in Ikenohata was suspected to be due to imported lobster from a cholera endemic area (5).

Other diarrheal diseases

Bacterial food poisoning outbreaks: In Japan, diarrheal diseases other than shigellosis or cholera are generally classified under the category of food poisoning, and outbreaks are regularly reported to the Ministry of Health and Welfare.

Table 3 shows the numbers of reported outbreaks of food poisoning in Japan during the last 10 years (1, 2, 3). During this period, the numbers of outbreaks, cases and deaths reported have remained relatively constant; there have been an average of about 1,200 outbreaks involving 32,000 cases and 36 fatal cases every year. The causes of 8,602, or 70.2%, of the outbreaks were determined. Bacterial pathogens accounted for 87% of the confirmed outbreaks and 96% of the cases. Among the bacterial pathogens, *Vibrio parahaemolyticus* was responsible for the most outbreaks (3,845), and the most cases (95,095). Other common pathogens were *Staphylococcus aureus* (2,302 outbreaks and 63,854 cases), *Salmonella* (889 outbreaks and 27,719 cases) and *Escherichia coli* (222 outbreaks and 21,687 cases). Information on the incidences of other pathogens however, is not available in annual reports (3).

Similar data on cases in Tokyo in 1979 - 1980 are shown in Table 4 (6, 7). In Tokyo, 296 outbreaks were reported and the cause of 219, or 74%, of them was determined. Bacterial infections accounted for 97% of the confirmed outbreaks and 95% of the cases. The main causative agents of bacterial food poisonings were also *V. parahaemolyticus*, *S. aureus*, *Salmonella* and *E. coli*. It is notewor-

Table 4. Causes of Food Poisoning Outbreaks in Tokyo
(1979 - 1980)

Causative agent	Number of outbreaks (%)	Number of cases (%)
Bacterial		
V. parahaemolyticus	86 (29.0)	2,115 (26.6)
S. aureus	75 (25.3)	1,505 (19.0)
Salmonella	30 (10.1)	336 (4.2)
C. jejuni	7 (2.4)	458 (5.8)
E. coli	6 (2.0)	897 (11.3)
B. cereus	4 (1.3)	13 (0.2)
C. perfringens	3 (1.3)	774 (9.7)
V. parahaemolyticus & Salmonella	1 (0.3)	64 (0.8)
Salmonella & S. aureus	1 (0.3)	2 (0.0)
Subtotal	213 (72.0)	6,164 (77.6)
Chemicals	6 (2.0)	289 (3.6)
Unknown	77 (26.0)	1,487 (18.7)
Total	296 (100)	7,940 (100)

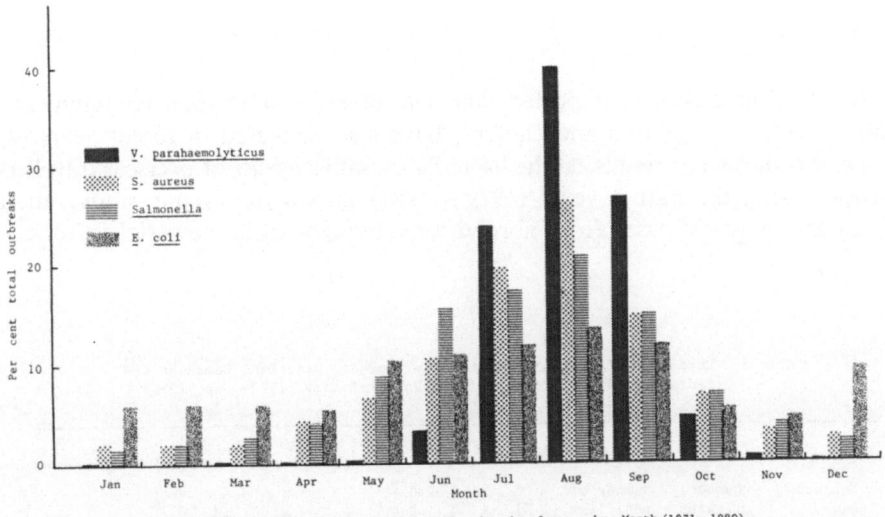

Major Bacterial Food Poisoning Outbreaks in Japan, by Month (1971 - 1980)

Fig. 3

thy that 7 outbreaks due to *Campylobacter jejuni* have occurred since surveillance of the disease started in 1979.

Fig. 3 shows the seasonal incidence of major outbreaks of bacterial food poisoning in Japan in the last 10 years. Bacterial food poisoning outbreaks have tended to be more frequent in summer months, and those associated with *V. parahaemolyticus* in particular have been concentrated in July and September.

In these outbreaks, fish and shellfish and their products were the most common vehicles of transmission of *V. parahaemolyticus*, grain, vegetables and their products were most often associated with *S. aureus* outbreaks, and meat, eggs, milk, and their products were the most common vehicles in *Salmonella* food poisoning. In *E. coli* outbreaks, no specific vehicles were recognized.

Outbreaks due to *V. parahaemolyticus, S. aureus* and *Salmonella* were mostly associated with foods eaten in homes or restaurants, but those associated with *E. coli* tended to occur in schools.

Sporadic diarrheal diseases: In contrast to the case with the bacterial food poisoning outbreaks described above, little information on the incidence of sporadic cases of diarrhea and their pathogens is available in Japan. However, several investigations so far reported have indicated that *V. parahaemolyticus, Salmonella* and *E. coli* were also the most common pathogens in sporadic cases (8), and recently, *C. jejuni/coli* has also emerged as an important cause of the disease in Japan.

Our recent studies conducted in collaboration with members of Tokyo Teishin General Hospital on the cause of sporadic diarrheal cases, especially in children, have shown that *C. jejuni/coli*, 3 types of diarrheagenic *E. coli* and *Salmonella* are the most common bacterial pathogens (Table 5). It is also noteworthy that rotavirus was found to be responsible for most cases in children of under 5 years old. Rotavirus-associated diarrhea was observed only in the winter months, but bacterial infections tended to occur more frequently in the summer months.

Imported diarrheal cases

As mentioned earlier, imported diarrheal diseases other than communicable diseases, such as shigellosis and cholera, have also increased in recent years (4).

Table 6 shows our results on the bacterial causative agents of overseas travellers' diarrhea during the past 3 years (1979 - 1981) in Tokyo. In our study, about 60% of the diarrheal cases from abroad were thought to be bacterial infections.

Table 5. Detection of Enteropathogens from Sporadic Diarrheal Cases at the Pediatric Clinic, Tokyo Teishin Hospital (Nov. 1980 - Feb. 1982)

Subjects (Age-groups)	Number of cases examined	Number of positives (%)	Number of cases with:							
			C. jejuni/coli	Salmonella	Enteropathogenic E. coli, serotype	Enteroinvasive E. coli	Enterotoxigenic E. coli	V. parahaemolyticus	Rota virus	Total
0 Year	96	30(31.3)	5	2	4	-	-	-	22	33
1-4 Year	159	61(38.4)	18	7	7	3	1	1	29	66
5-9 Year	92	26(28.3)	21	-	3	2	-	1	3	30
10 Year	29	10(34.5)	5	1	-	1	1	-	2	10
Unknown	9	2(22.2)	-	-	-	-	-	-	2	2
Total	385	129(33.5)	49 (34.8)	10 (7.1)	14 (9.9)	6 (4.3)	2 (1.4)	2 (1.4)	58 (41.1)	141 (100%)

Table 6. Detection of Enteropathogens from Travellers' Cases in Tokyo (1979 - 1981)

Month	No. of cases examined	No. of positives (%)	V. cholerae, 0-1	Shigella	Salmonella	Enterotoxigenic E. coli	Enteroinvasive E. coli	Enteropathogenic E. coli, serotype	V. parahaemolyticus	V. cholerae, non 0-1	V. fluvialis	C. jejuni/coli	Y. enterocolitica
January	73	35(47.9)	–	2	5	21	–	2	7	2	–	5	–
February	65	40(61.5)	1	5	7	24	1	–	9	–	–	4	–
March	89	45(50.6)	–	8	9	20	1	3	6	1	–	4	–
April	69	36(52.2)	–	7	4	23	1	2	3	–	–	–	1
May	89	56(62.9)	–	6	17	28	–	2	10	1	–	2	–
June	69	39(56.5)	–	6	11	22	1	1	5	1	–	2	–
July	77	51(66.2)	–	4	9	33	1	2	6	2	3	1	–
August	215	143(66.5)	3	10	29	82	1	2	32	6	2	6	–
September	120	75(62.5)	–	8	15	42	–	1	8	2	–	9	–
October	50	29(58.0)	–	4	2	16	1	2	8	2	–	–	–
November	53	29(54.7)	–	–	8	21	–	1	4	–	1	3	–
December	33	18(54.5)	–	2	3.	10	–	–	2	1	–	1	–
Total	1,002	596(59.5)	4	62	119	342	7	18	100	18	6	37	1

Table 7. Reported Isolation of Enteric Bacteria from Human Sources in Japan (1979 - 1980)

Organism	Number [a]	Percent
V. cholerae, 0 - 1	56 (31)	0.2
V. cholerae, non 0-1	172 (155)	0.6
V. parahaemolyticus	5,378 (763)	19.0
Shigella (Groups A-D)	1,056 (439)	3.7
S. typhi	727 (29)	2.6
S. paratyphi A	61 (12)	0.2
S. paratyphi B	123 (1)	0.4
Other Salmonella	11,297 (1,555)	40.0
E. coli	1,373 (435)	4.9
Y. enterocolitica	77 (14)	0.3
Y. pseudotuberculosis	3 (–)	0.0
C. jejuni/coli	1,193 (77)	4.2
P. shigelloides	20 (17)	0.1
A. hydrophila	4 (–)	0.0
S. aureus	5,097 (31)	18.0
C. perfringens	1,519 (1)	5.4
B. cereus	107 (–)	0.4
Total	28,263 (3,777)	100.0

[a] ( ) = Isolation from imported cases.

A total of 11 different pathogens were isolated, but no seasonality was observed in the frequency of bacterial isolations. Among the pathogens detected, the most common was enterotoxigenic *E. coli*, accounting for approximately 48% of the total bacterial isolations, followed by *Salmonella* (17%), *V. parahaemolyticus* (14%) and *Shigella* species (8.7%). *C. jejuni/coli*, which has been tested for since November 1979, also exhibited a fairly high frequency (5.2%). Similar results were reported recently from Osaka Airport Quarantine Station (9).

Enteropathogens responsible for diarrheal diseases

Since 1979, surveillance programs for isolation of causative agents responsible for major infectious diseases have been carried out by the National Institute of Health in collaboration with 67 prefectural/municipal public health laboratories, which cover all the country (10, 11).

Table 8. Reported Shigella Serotype from Human Sources
in Japan (1979 - 1980)

Species	Serotype	Number[a]	Percent
S. dysenteriae	2	13 (12)	1.2
	3	4 (4)	0.4
	7	1	
	9	1 (1)	
Subtotal		19 (17)	1.7
S. flexneri	1a	9 (3)	
	1b	132 (59)	12.1
	1	2 (2)	
	2a	216 (97)	19.9
	2b	34 (4)	3.1
	3a	52 (10)	4.8
	3b	5 (5)	
	3c	3 (2)	
	4a	35 (23)	3.2
	4b	2	
	5	2 (2)	
	6	18 (12)	
	X	11 (2)	
	Y	17	
Subtotal		538 (221)	49.4
S. boydii	1	5 (4)	
	2	11 (11)	1.0
	3	2 (2)	
	4	11 (7)	1.0
	5	1 (1)	
	7	1 (1)	
	8	1 (1)	
	10	3 (3)	
	12	1 (1)	
Subtotal		36 (31)	3.3
S. sonnei		495 (163)	45.5
Total		1,088 (432)	100

[a] ( ) = Numbers isolated from imported cases.

Table 7 shows the major enteropathogenic bacteria associated with human diarrheal diseases isolated between 1979 and 1980. In this period, a total of 28,263 isolations were reported, of which about 13% were from imported cases. Among the pathogens reported, *Salmonella* was the most common, accounting for approximately 40% of the total isolations. The next most common pathogens were *V. parahaemolyticus* (19.0%), *S. aureus* (18.0%), *C. perfringens* (5.4%), enteropathogenic *E. coli* (4.9%), and *C. jejuni/coli* (4,2%). These frequencies of isolation of enteric pathogens reflect the recent situation of bacterial diarrheal diseases in Japan.

Table 8 lists reported *Shigella* serotypes isolated from human sources in Japan in the same period. A total of 28 different serotypes were reported, of which *S. sonnei* accounted for approximately 46%, *S. flexneri* 2a for 19.9%, *S. flexneri* 1b for 12.1% and *S. flexneri* 3a for 4.8%, although there were noticeable differences between the serotype distributions of domestic and imported cases.

The most frequently reported *Salmonella* serotypes from human sources in Japan are shown in Table 9. A total of 155 different serotypes were identified and reported. The 10 most frequently reported serotypes accounted for 7,583 (63,2%) of the 11,996 isolates reported and the next 10 most frequently reported

Table 9. Most Frequently Reported <u>Salmonella</u> Serotypes from Human Sources in Japan (1979 – 1980)

Rank	Serotype	Number[a]	Percent
1	S. <u>typhimurium</u>	1,931 (75)	16.1
2	S. <u>enteritidis</u>	1,761 (11)	14.7
3	S. <u>typhi</u>	805 (64)	6.7
4	S. <u>litchfield</u>	760 (11)	6.3
5	S. <u>java</u>	464 (20)	3.9
6	S. <u>infantis</u>	463 (35)	3.9
7	S. <u>braenderup</u>	440 (17)	3.7
8	S. <u>agona</u>	420 (106)	3.5
9	S. <u>thompson</u>	298 (11)	2.5
10	S. <u>panama</u>	241 (16)	2.0
	Subtotal	7,583 (366)	63.2
11	S. <u>anatum</u>	229 (137)	1.9
12	S. <u>derby</u>	228 (149)	1.9
13	S. <u>newport</u>	187 (72)	1.6
14	S. <u>virchow</u>	172 (40)	1.4
15	S. <u>tennessee</u>	152 (11)	1.3
16	S. <u>paratyphi</u> B	151 (4)	1.3
17	S. <u>london</u>	131 (47)	1.1
18	S. <u>senftenberg</u>	125 (71)	1.0
19	S. <u>heiderberg</u>	113 (28)	0.9
20	S. <u>cerro</u>	107 (44)	0.9
	Subtotal	9,178 (955)	76.5
All Other serotypes (135 types)		2,818 (843)	23.5
Total		11,996 (1,798)	100

[a]( ) = Numbers isolated from imported cases.

Table 10. Serotype of Diarrheagenic E. coli from Human Sources
in Tokyo (1967 - 1981)

Type / O serotype		Number in type (%) :	
		Outbreaks	Imported cases
ETEC: ST only	O 27	11 ⎫	13 ⎫
	0148	2 ⎬ 21	42 ⎬ 225
	0159	7	7
	Others or not tested	1 ⎭	163 ⎭
LT only	O 25	- ⎫	15 ⎫
	0148	- ⎬ 0	6 ⎬ 102
	0159	-	3
	Others or not tested	- ⎭	78 ⎭
LT + ST	O 6	11 ⎫	38 ⎫
	O 25	-	4
	0148	1 ⎬ 12	3 ⎬ 139
	Others or not tested	- ⎭	94 ⎭
Subtotal		33 (56.9)	466 (84.1)
EIEC	O 28	2	3
	0124	4	5
	0136	2	4
	0164	-	4
	Others	-	3
Subtotal		8 (13.8)	19 (3.4)
EPEC	O 44	2	15
	O 55	1	10
	0111	2	6
	0125	5	2
	0127	3	5
	0128	1	8
	Others	3	23
Subtotal		17 (29.3)	69 (12.5)
Total		58 (100)	554 (100)

serotypes accounted for 1,595 isolates (13,3%). Likewise *Shigella*, serotypes have shown different distributions in domestic isolates and imported isolates; i.e., the 5 most common serotypes of domestic isolates were *S. typhimurium*, *S. enteritidis*, *S. lichfield*, *S. typhi* and *S. java*, while those of imported isolates were *S. derby*, *S. anatum*, *S. agona*, *S. typhimurium* and *S. newport*.

Table 10 summarizes results on causative strains of *E. coli* and their serotypes isolated from domestic outbreaks and imported sporadic cases in Tokyo between 1967 and 1981. Although no definitive information is available for the whole country, in our studies in Tokyo, all three types of *E. coli* (i.e., enterotoxigenic, enteropathogenic (serotype) and enteroinvasive strains) were identified in 58 outbreaks and 554 sporadic cases. Among them, enterotoxigenic strains, especially those producing ST only, were found to be the most common in both outbreaks and sporadic cases, followed by enteropathogenic *E. coli* (serotype) and enteroinvasive *E. coli*. The most frequent O serogroups of enterotoxigenic *E. coli* were

O27, O148 and O159 for ST strain, O25 for LT strain and O6 for LT/ST strain.

This paper briefly reviews the current status of bacterial diarrheal diseases in Japan. The data show that the incidences of communicable diseases such as bacillary dysentery have decreased remarkable in recent years, but that imported cases have tended to increase. The occurrence of bacterial food poisoning outbreaks has remained fairly stable over the last 20 years. The most common pathogens responsible for disease have been *V. parahaemolyticus*, *S. aureus*, *Salmonella* and *E. coli*, and in addition *C. jejuni* has also been found to be an important cause.

For more complete understanding of the incidence of bacterial diarrheal diseases, a system for surveillance of diarrheal diseases, including sporadic cases, must be developed.

REFERENCES

1. Kudoh, Y., and M. Ohashi. 1982. Current status of gastrointestinal infections in Japan, pp.15-24. *In* Proc. 8th SEAMIC Seminar, Singapore, 1980. South East Asian Medical Information Center (Publication No. 27), Tokyo.

2. Ministry of Health and Welfare. 1981. Communicable disease and food poisoning in Japan, Annual summary, 1979. Statistics and Information Department, Tokyo (Text in Japanese).

3. Ministry of Health and Welfare. 1982. Communicable disease and food poisoning in Japan, Annual summary, 1980. Statistics and Information Department, Tokyo (Text in Japanese).

4. Kudoh, Y., S. Matsushita, S. Yamada, M. Tsuno, K. Ohta, A. Kai, S. Sakai, and M. Ohashi. 1980. Travellers' diarrhea and enterotoxigenic *Escherichia coli* - A survey in 1977 - 1979 in Tokyo, pp.225-236. *In* Proc. 15th Jt. Conf. Cholera, U.S.-Japan Coop. Med. Sci. Program, Bethesda, 1979.

5. Ohashi, M. 1980. Laboratory aspects on the cause of the cholera outbreaks in Japan, originating from a public wedding hall in November 1978, pp.334-345. *In* Proc. 15th Jt. Conf. Cholera, U.S.-Japan Coop. Med. Sci. Program, Bethesda, 1979.

6. Bureau of Public Health, Tokyo Metropolitan Government. 1980. Food poisoning in Tokyo, Annual summary, 1979 (Text in Japanese).

7. Bureau of Public Health, Tokyo Metropolitan Government. 1981. Food Poisoning in Tokyo, Annual Summary, 1980 (Text in Japanese).

8. Kudoh, Y. 1981. Epidemiology of *Escherichia coli* diarrheal disease. Modern Media **27**: 299–309 (Text in Japanese).

9. Abe, H., T. Kanda, Y. Yanai, S. Hashimoto, R. Ogawa, Y. Miyata, M. Shinbo, K. Harada, T. Tsukamoto, Y. Kinoshita, M. Arita, Y. Takeda and T. Miwatani. J. J. A. Inf. D., **35**: 679–690 (Text in Japanese).

10. Scientific Working Group for Laboratory-depending information on causative agents of infectious diseases. 1980. Laboratory confirmed agents for infectious diseases in Japan, Annual summary, 1979 (Text in Japanese).

11. Scientific Working Group for Laboratory-depending information on causative agents of infectious diseases. 1981. Laboratory confirmed agents for infectious diseases in Japan, Annual summary, 1980 (Text in Japanese).

Bacterial Diarrheal Diseases, eds., Y. Takeda, T. Miwatani, 95-102.
Copyright © 1985 by KTK Scientific Publishers, Tokyo.

EPIDEMIOLOGICAL ASPECTS OF CAMPYLOBACTER ENTERITIS

M. B. Skirrow

*Department of Microbiology, Worcester Royal Infirmary, Worcester, WR1 3AS.
U.K.*

Campylobacter enteritis is now recognized as a common disease of worldwide distribution. Wherever it has been sought it has been found and in several countries it has emerged as the commonest form of acute bacterial diarrhoea. Since the regular reporting of *Campylobacter* isolations to the Communicable Disease Surveillance Centre* (CDSC) began in 1977, the annual totals (England and Wales) have steadily increased to culminate in a 1981 total of 12,496, which is substantially more than the salmonella total of 10,745 (Fig. 1).

Seasonal variation

The CDSC figures also show that there was a rise in the incidence of *Campylobacter* infection each summer. This rise roughly paralleled the rise in salmonella infections except that it was less pronounced - at least until 1981 when it was of equal size but earlier occurrence (Fig. 1). This latter rise was observed throughout the country; moreover, in the Worcester district the excess isolations were almost all of *Campylobacter jejuni* biotype 2, which is particularly associated with poultry (see below). A high summer incidence has also been reported from Europe, the USA, and Australia. The increase of salmonellosis in summer is generally held to be due to the heightened risk of bacterial multiplication in food occasioned by high ambient temperatures. But this can hardly be the reason in the case of campylobacters, since they would need a temperature of at least 32°C in order to multiply in food and, in general, survival tends to vary inversely with temperature (1).

Age distribution

The CDSC reports show a fairly even distribution of infection from infancy, including the newborn, to extreme old age. The true incidence by age cannot be calculated from these national figures because denominators are unknown. However, more complete data from local studies show that the incidence of infection is somewhat higher in older children and young adults than other age groups (2).

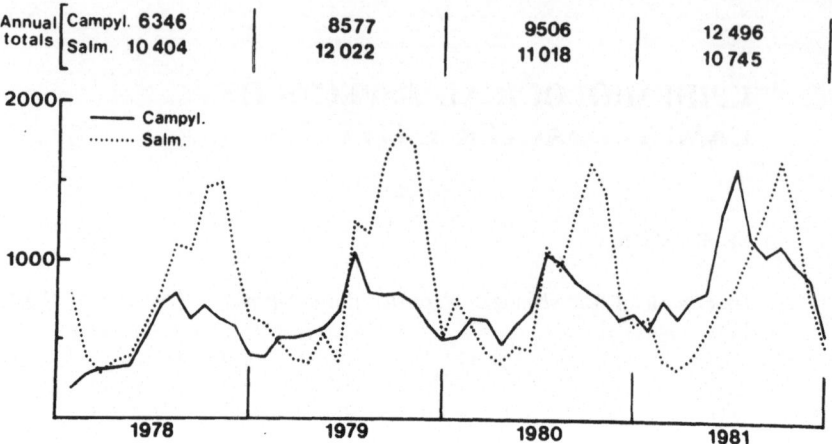

Annual totals	Campyl. 6346	8577	9506	12 496
	Salm. 10 404	12 022	11 018	10 745

Fig. 1. *Campylobacter* and *Salmonella* isolations reported to CDSC from laboratories in England and Wales (4-weekly totals).

This general pattern, which is seen in other technically advanced countries where standards of hygiene are good, contrasts with the state of affairs in developing countries where the burden of infection falls on infants and young children (3-6). Here the disease is far less frequent in older children and adults, presumably owing to immunity acquired through repeated exposure to infection at an early age. Whatever the reason there is little doubt that *Campylobacter* enteritis is a major cause of infantile diarrhoea in the Third World. High prevalence in such areas is also reflected in the frequency with which travellers from technically advanced countries suffer from *Campylobacter* enteritis when they visit these areas; and nowhere is the difference more striking than in Scandinavia where at least half of all cases of *Campylobacter* enteritis are acquired abroad - 75% in the case of Sweden (7).

Incidence in the sexes

Reports to CDSC show that up to the age of 14 there is a preponderance of infections in boys girls in the ratio of about 1.6:1. In adults there is a slight excess of infections in men (1.1:1), but over the age of 65 years the ratio is reversed (0.7:1) which probably merely reflects the excess of old women in the population.

SOURCES AND TRANSMISSION OF INFECTION

Like salmonellosis, *Campylobacter* enteritis is a zoonosis with a complex pattern of transmission. Complex because many animal species may harbour campylobacters and thereby form potential sources of human infection. Fundamental to the understanding of the epidemiology of infectious disease is the ability to identify strains of infecting organisms, and our inability to do so in the case of campylobacters - at least until recently - has been a severe handicap. Therefore this section begins with a description of the main groups of *Campylobacter* associated with enteritis.

Campylobacter groups and their distribution

The Approved Lists of Bacterial Names (8) recognizes two species of *Campylobacter* equivalent to King's original 'related vibrios' (the name *C. fetus* subsp. *jejuni* is no longer recognized). They can be differentiated by means of the hippurate hydrolysis test: *C. jejuni* hydrolyses hippurate, *C. coli* does not (9). Furthermore *C. jejuni* can be divided into two biotypes according to the ability to produce H_2S in a certain iron-containing medium (9). Since the techniques of performing these tests have been sightly modified since their original description, they are given in an appendix to this paper.

In addition, a group of 'thermophilic' campylobacters characterised by nalidixic acid resistance (NARTC) have been described occurring in wild seagulls of the genus *Larus* (10). They are occasionally found in other animals including man, but so far they have not been associated with disease.

Recent DNA hybridization experiments indicate that *C. jejuni*, *C. coli*, and probably the NARTC group are distinct spacies (11).* The principal differentiating features of these groups are shown in Table 1 which also includes *C. fetus*. The distribution of these groups in man and animals in Britain is shown in Fig. 2. It will be seen that *C. jejuni* biotype 1 is the predominant organism in all animals except pigs, *C. jejuni* 2 is found most often in chickens, and *C. coli* accounts for almost all of the strains found in pigs. This does not tell us much about the sources of human infection, except that pigs are not a major source in Britain.

Table 1. Principal tests for the identification of the common intestinal campylobacters

	C. fetus	NARTC[a]	C. jejuni biotype 1	C. jejuni biotype 2	C. coli
Control NCTC strains	5850	11352	11168	11392	11353
Growth at: 25.0°C	+	-	-	-	-
43.0°C	-	+	+	+	+
Nalidixic acid (30 µg disc)	R	R	S	S	S
Cephalothin (30 µg disc)	S	R	R	R	R
Hippurate hydrolysis[b]	-	-	+	+	-
H_2S in FBP medium[b]	-	+ or ±	-	+	-

R = resistant (0 mm); S = sensitive (> 6 mm from edge of disc)
a Nalidixic acid-resistant 'thermophilic' campylobacter (10)
b See appendix

*The NARTC group have since been named *C. laridis* (Benjamin, J., S. Leaper, R. J. Owen, and M. B. Skirrow. Curr. Microbiol. **8**: 231–238).

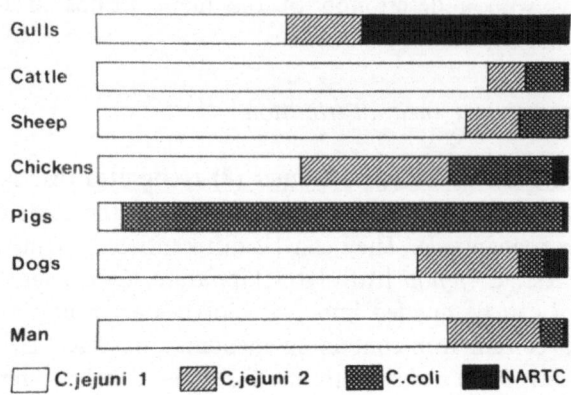

Fig. 2. Distribution of campylobacter groups in animals and man in Britain.

Sources of infection as revealed by outbreaks

Outbreaks of infection provide special opportunities for tracing sources and transmission of infection. Raw or inadequately treated cows' milk and unchlorinated water are both outstanding as causes of major outbreaks of *Campylobacter* enteritis. Food has been associated with smaller outbreaks.

Milk: Over 20 milkborne outbreaks have been reported in Britain during the last three years, and a general account of the more striking ones has been given by Robinson and Jones (12). In most cases the evidence implicating milk was only circumstantial but nevertheless strong. In all but one outbreak the cows' milk was knowingly distributed unpasteurized (it is still legal to do so in Britain) either from customer's choice, or because of power failures and transport problems caused by severe winter weather. In the one case the milk was distributed as pasteurized but there were faults at the dairy (13). Milkborne outbreaks have also been reported from the USA and Canada. People who habitually drink raw milk probably develop immunity to infection; a high proportion of students at a college of agriculture in England were found to have antibody to *C. jejuni* (14).

In these outbreaks milk is the vehicle rather than the source of infection. *C. jejuni* does not seem to be capable of multiplying in milk - at least at usual ambient temperatures - but strains can survive for three weeks in autoclaved cows' milk held at 4°C (15). The milking cows themselves are thought to be the source of the organism, but the ways in which they get into the milk are unknown. The possibilities are faecal contamination at the time of milking, or excretion of organisms from an infected udder. The sheer size of some of the outbreaks - an estimated 3500 people affected in one (13) - suggests the latter, but although *Campylobacter* mastitis with gross shedding of bacteria has been produced experimentally (16), naturally occurring infections have not been reported. It is worth noting that in several of the British outbreaks the methods used by the dairy farms were blameless. Pasteurization kills *C. jejuni* (1, 17) and this, or some other form of heat treatment, is the obvious solution to the problem.

Water: Two major waterborne outbreaks have been reported, one in the USA (18) and the other in Sweden (19). Inadequate chlorination in the first case, and an inflow of untreated surface water into the main supply when the pressure was unusually low in the second case were thought to have caused these outbreaks. The ingestion of natural untreated water while engaged in the pursuit of outdoor activities - e.g. camping and water sports - features in the histories of patients with *Campylobacter* enteritis too often to dismiss as coincidental. *C. jejuni, C. coli*, and NARTC strains have all been found in natural water, both fresh and marine. While it is easy to see how contamination from birds, other animals, and man occurs, it is surprising that organisms that die so readily when exposed to air in the laboratory are able to survive so well in water (15).

Food: Although there have been a few outbreaks associated with the consumption of particular meals, campylobacters are not food poisoning organisms in the strict sense. As already pointed out they do not multiply under 'kitchen' conditions, yet the infective dose is small and simple contamination is probably sufficient for the transmission of infection. Nine outbreaks have been reported from Tokyo, one of them associated with the consumption of clam salad (101 of 118 affected) and another with chicken meat (20). Another large outbreak has also been reported from Japan (21) but the item of food responsible was not detected. Undercooked chicken was thought to have been the most likely source in a small outbreak among people who attended a dinner dance in Britain (22). Chickens were responsible for an unusual outbreak among military cadets in the Netherlands, but in this case infection probably resulted from the handling and preparation of raw carcasses under field conditions as much as by the consumption of the meat (23). Also reported from the Netherlands was an outbreak attributed to eating chicken liver fondue (24), and another associated with consumption of raw hamburgers (25). An outbreak in the USA was traced to an apparently contaminated birthday cake (26).

Sources of sporadic infections

The sources and pathways of sporadic infections are much more difficult to trace than outbreak sources which, of course, may also give rise to sporadic infections under the right circumstances. But some are known.

Direct contact with animals: In Britain probably less than 10 percent of infections are caused by direct animal contact. They are conveniently considered under two headings: occupational, and domestic.

Occupational infection has been strikingly shown by the high prevalence of antibody in meat process workers (chicken and duck processing, up to 68%; cattle processing, 36%) and veterinary assistants (18%) (27). The equivalent figures for women attending antenatal clinics in a rural and urban community were 5% and 2% respectively.

In a domestic context, the animals involved are nearly always a sick puppy or occasionally a kitten. Typically the animal is newly acquired and it either has diarrhoea on arrival in the household or develops it soon afterwards (28). Human infection from a healthy dog or cat is rare.

Man as a source of infection: Person-to-person infectivity of *Campylobacter* enteritis is low. Secondary cases in outbreaks are few even among close family contacts, and when transmission does occur it is usually from a small child. Failure of transmission is probably due to poor survival of the organisms outside the body where they are exposed to atmospheric oxygen and desiccation. Since infectivity is low even when there is profuse diarrhoea, it can safely be assumed that it is far lower once the stools have become formed again, and the risks of infected but symptomless food handlers transmitting infection via food are negligible. When such people have been allowed to continue work no infection has resulted (7) and it would be difficult to justify a policy of exclusion.

Other sources of sporadic infections: We are still left with the majority of day-to-day sporadic infections to account for. They are probably acquired via the food chain from raw animal products but this conclusion is arrived at more by deduction than hard evidence. Most of the poultry bought at retail outlets is contaminated with campylobacters; this is true in Europe and the USA, indeed wherever poultry has been examined for these organisms. Raw red meats are contaminated less often. In a large multicentre survey in Britain, *C. jejuni* or *C. coli* were isolated from only one percent of raw red meat samples (mainly beef, lamb, and pork) bought from retail shops (29), although higher figures have been reported from Sweden (30) and in abattoir samples (31).

There are three ways in which infection could be acquired from campylobacters brought into a kitchen in this way: by eating raw or undercooked meat; by eating other foods that have become cross-contaminated from contact with raw meat or its juices; by accidental ingestion of organisms picked up on the hands of those handling raw meats in the kitchen. We have seen how the first of these has caused outbreaks of infection, the second is probably common though difficult to prove, and there is evidence that the third might also be a frequent mode of transmission; in a swedish survey a significant number of patients who had prepared chicken were the only members of their families to have become infected despite the fact that all of them ate the chicken (7).

PREVENTION

Certain preventive measures, such as the heat treatment of milk and proper purification of drinking water are clearly called for. Good hygienic practice in the handling of animals, and the separation of sick family pets from children and food preparation areas are obvious and simple measures that should be observed. Good hygienic practice in the kitchen, in particular adequate cooking of meats and the separation of raw meats from cooked foods and salads, would probably prevent many sporadic infections.

Attempts to reduce the prevalence of campylobacters in animals bred for food might pose greater problems. Any control measures would almost certainly increase production costs, so it would be essential that their effectiveness and feasibility be assured. Moreover, one would need to be sure that control in a particular type of animal would result in a reduction of human infection, and on existing knowledge we cannot be confident that this would be so. Hopefully, the application of typing techniques now under development will help to provide some answers to these pressing questions.

APPENDIX

Hippurate hydrolysis test

Suspend a 2 mm loopful of growth from an overnight blood agar culture (37°C) in 2 ml sterile phosphate buffer pH 7.0. Add 0.5 ml of a freshly prepared 5% aqueous solution of sodium hippurate to the suspension, mix and place in a water bath at 37°C for 2 hours. Then add 1 ml of freshly prepared ninhydrin solution (ninhydrin 3.5 g; acetone 50 ml; butanol 50 ml) and leave for a further 2 hours at 37°C before reading: deep purple colour - positive; colourless or pale mauve - negative.

H_2S production in iron metabisulphite medium

Inoculate a large lump of growth (about the size of a small pea) from an overnight blood agar culture (37°C) into FBP broth (Oxoid Nutrient Broth No. 2, 1 litre; New Zealand agar, 1.2 g; $FeSO_4.7H_2O$, 0.5 g; sodium metabisulphite, 0.5 g; sodium pyruvate, 0.5 g; buffer to pH 7-2); do not disperse. Leave at room temperature and examine for blackening around the lump of growth after 2 hours, and again after 24 hours before discarding unchanged tubes as negative. *N.B.* it is essential that the blood agar plates (Oxoid BA Base No. 2) are incubated in an atmosphere containing not more than 7% oxygen.

I with to thank Dr. N. S. Galbraith for permission to publish data collected by the Communicable Disease Surveillance Centre (Public Health Laboratory Service), London.

REFERENCES

1. Doyle, M. P., and D. J. Roman. 1981. Growth and survival of *Campylobacter fetus* subsp. *jejuni* as a function of temperature and pH. J. Food Protect. **44**: 596–601.

2. Butzler, J. P., and M. B. Skirrow. 1979. *Campylobacter* enteritis. Clin. Gastroenterol. **8**: 737–765.

3. Ricciardi, I. D., and M. C. S. Ferreira. 1980. The age distribution in children with *Campylobacter* enteritis (letter). Trans R. Soc. Trop. Med. Hyg. **74**: 687.

4. Ringertz, S., R. C. Rockhill, O. Ringertz, and A. Sutomo. 1980. *Campylobacter fetus* subsp. *jejuni* as a cause of gastroenteritis in Jakarta, Indonesia. J. Clin. Microbiol. **12**: 538–540.

5. Blaser, M. J., R. I. Glass, M. I. Huq, B. Stoll, G. M. Kibriya, and A. R. M. A. Alim. 1980. Isolation of *Campylobacter fetus* subsp. *jejuni* from Bangladeshi children. J. Clin. Microbiol. **12**: 744–747.

6. Billingham, J. D. 1981. *Campylobacter* enteritis in The Gambia. Trans. R. Soc. Trop. Med. Hyg. **75**: 641–644.

7. Norkrans, G., and Å. Svedhem. 1982. Epidemiological aspects of *Campylobacter jejuni* enteritis. J. Hyg., Camb. **89**: 163–170.

8. Approved Lists of Bacterial Names. 1980. V. B. D. Skerman, V. McGowan, and P. H. A. Sneath (ed.) Int. J. Syst. Bact. **30**: 270–271.

9. Skirrow, M. B., and J. Benjamin. 1980. Differentiation of enteropathogenic *Campylobacter*

102

(letter). J. Clin. Path. **33**: 1122.

10. Skirrow, M. B., and J. Benjamin. 1980. '1001' Campylobacters: cultural characteristics of intestinal campylobacters from man and animals. J. Hyg., Camb. **85**: 427-442.

11. Owen, R. J., and S. Leaper. 1981. Base composition, size and nucleotide sequence similarities of genome deoxyribonucleic acids from species of the genus *Campylobacter*. FEMS Microbiol. Letts. **12**: 395-400.

12. Robinson, D. A., and D. M. Jones. 1981. Milk-borne campylobacter infection. Br. Med. J. **282**: 1374-1376.

13. Jones, P. H., A. T. Willis, D. A. Robinson, M. B. Skirrow, and D. S. Josephs. 1981. *Campylobacter* enteritis associated with the consumption of free school milk. J. Hyg., Camb. **87**: 155-162.

14. Jones, D. M., D. A. Robinson, and J. Eldridge. 1981. Serological studies in two outbreaks of *Campylobacter jejuni* infection. J. Hyg., Camb. **87**: 163-170.

15. Blaser, M. J., H. L. Hardesty, B. Powers, and W. L. Wang. 1980. Survival of *Campylobacter fetus* subsp. *jejuni* in biological milieus. J. Clin. Microbiol. **11**: 309-313.

16. Lander, K. P., and K. P. W. Gill. 1980. Experimental infection of the bovine udder with *Campylobacter coli/jejuni*. J. Hyg., Camb. **84**: 421-428.

17. Gill, K. P. W., P. G. Bates, and K. P. Lander. 1981. The effect of pasteurization on the survival of *Campylobacter* species in milk. Brit. Vet. J. **137**: 578-584.

18. Vogt, R. L., H. E. Sours, T. Barrett, R. A. Feldman, R. J. Dickinson, and L. Witherell. 1982. *Campylobacter* enteritis associated with contaminated water. Ann. Int. Med. **96**: 292-296.

19. Mentzing, L. O. 1981. Waterborne outbreaks of *Campylobacter* enteritis in central Sweden. Lancet **ii**: 352-354.

20. Itoh, T., K. Saito, Y. Yanagawa, S. Sakai, and M. Ohashi. 1982. *Campylobacter* enteritis in Tokyo. pp. 5-12. *In* Campylobacter: Epidemiology, Pathogenesis and Biochemistry. Ed. Newell, D. G. MTP Press, Lancaster.

21. Yanagisawa, S. 1980. Large outbreak of *Campylobacter* enteritis among school children (letter). Lancet **ii**: 153.

22. Skirrow, M. B., R. G. Fidoe, and D. M. Jones. 1981. An outbreak of presumptive food-borne *Campylobacter* enteritis. J. Infect. **3**: 234-236.

23. Brouwer, R., M. J. A. Mertens, T. H. Siem, and J. Katchaki. 1979. An explosive outbreak of *Campylobacter* enteritis in soldiers. Ant. van Leeuw. **45**: 517-519.

24. Mouton, R. P., J. J. Veltkamp, S. Lauwers, and J. P. Butzler. 1982. Analysis of a small outbreak of campylobacter infections with high morbidity. pp. 129-134. *In* Campylobacter: Epidemiology, Pathogenesis and Biochemistry. Ed. Newell, D. G. MTP Press, Lancaster.

25. Oosterom, J., H. J. Beckers, L. M. van Noorle Jansen, and M. van Schothorst. 1980. Een explosie van *Campylobacter*-infectie in een kazerne, waarschijnlijk veroorzaakt door rauwe tartaar. Ned. Tijdschr. Geneesk. **124**: 1631-1634.

26. Blaser, M. J., P. Checko, C. Bopp, A. Bruce, and J. M. Hughes. 1981. *Campylobacter* enteritis associated with foodborne transmission. Am. J. Epidemiol. **116**: 886-894.

27. Jones, D. M., and D. A. Robinson. 1981. Occupational exposure to *Campylobacter jejuni* infection (letter). Lancet **i**: 440-441.

28. Skirrow, M. B. 1981. *Campylobacter* enteritis in dogs and cats: a 'new' zoonosis. Vet. Res. Comm. **5**: 13-19.

29. Turnbull, P. C. B., and P. Rose. 1982. *Campylobacter jejuni* and salmonella in raw red meats. A Public Health Laboratory Service Survey. J. Hyg., Camb. **88**: 29-37.

30. Svedhem, Å., B. Kaijser, and E. Sjögren. 1981. The occurrence of *Campylobacter jejuni* in fresh food and survival under different conditions. J. Hyg., Camb. **87**: 421-425.

31. Stern, N. J. 1981. Recovery rate of *Campylobacter fetus* subsp. *jejuni* on eviscerated pork, lamb, and beef carcasses. J. Food Sci. **46**: 1291-1293.

Bacterial Diarrheal Diseases, eds., Y. Takeda, T. Miwatani, 103–116.
Copyright © 1985 by KTK Scientific Publishers, Tokyo.

EPIDEMIOLOGY OF *SALMONELLA* AND *SHIGELLA* INFECTIONS IN THE UNITED STATES

Roger A. Feldman and Lee W. Riley

Division of Bacterial Diseases, Center for Infectious Disease, Centers for Disease Control, Public Health Service, Department of Health and Human Services, Atlanta, Georgia 30333, U. S. A.

The epidemiologic characteristics of *Salmonella* and *Shigella* infections in the United States have been studied by examination of data from 3 major sources: a national laboratory-based surveillance system, outbreak investigations, and carefully designed field studies. In this presentation we will separately discuss *Salmonella* and *Shigella* infections and for each give examples of contributions from these 3 sources that have allowed identification of specific problems and development of appropriate control measures.

Salmonella Infections

In 1963, a cooperative voluntary program was begun among the 50 states, Centers for Diseases Control (CDC), Food and Drug Administration, and U. S. Department of Agriculture which called for reporting *Salmonella* isolates from all sources, with CDC serving as the coordinating center. The national program developed after 2 widespread outbreaks of salmonellosis, the first involving *S. thompson* contamination of commercial cake mixes (1) and the second involving *S. derby* contamination of eggs and egg products (2). The purpose of the national program was to allow study of the changes in endemic patterns of *Salmonella* infections, and detection of interstate epidemics of *Salmonella* infections.

Information reported to the national *Salmonella* surveillance system includes the age, sex, and state of residence of the patient, the specimen from which the isolate was cultured, the year and month of report, and the serogroup or serotype of the isolate. Even though the system has been in existence for almost 20 years, there are still many reports that do not include all of the requested information, and many states or hospitals that do not perform serogrouping or serotyping. In addition to omission of requested data, some important additional information is not reported. For example, it is not possible to differentiate whether the isolate is obtained from an ill person, or an asymptomatic person cultured in a household in which someone else was ill. The data may also include surveillance bias: for example, the ages of persons from whom *Salmonella* isolates are obtained are perhaps not representative of all persons ill with salmonellosis, since an infant with a diarrheal illness is more likely than an adult to be brought to a doctor, and it is possible that the doctor is more likely to obtain a stool culture from a child than an adult. Age may also affect the type of specimens obtained since when fever accompanies the diarrhea, blood cultures may be obtained more frequently from infants and from persons over 60 than they are from other age groups.

Using the available data, with all their imperfections, we make a series of continuing analyses concerning magnitude of the national problem, age-specific attack rates, seasonality, most frequently identified serotypes, and interrelated epidemiologic variables.

The number of isolates reported each year has risen slowly from 24,216 in 1970 to 30,004 in 1980 (Table 1). The number of isolates per 100,000 population has risen from 12 per 100,000 in 1970 to 13.6 per 100,000 in 1980. The highest isolation rates are from children under 1 year of age, with the peak at age 2-3 months (Fig. 1). The median age is another way to characterize the ages of persons from whom salmonellae are isolated. When this is done separately for each common serotype, large variations in median ages are noted (Table 2). The summer and fall have had the largest number of isolates, although the characteristics of the seasonal peak may vary with the individual serotype. For example, there is a prominent fall peak in reported isolates of *S. newport* which is more than 3 times as high as the number in the winter (Fig. 2). There is a prominent summer and fall peak in the number of isolates of *S. javiana*, with almost no isolates in the winter (Fig. 3). *S. choleraesuis* has no obvious seasonality.

Although over 1,400 *Salmonella* serotypes have been recorded, there are rarely more than 400 reported to the national surveillance system in any year, and usually 10 serotypes make up 70% of the total isolates (Table 2). *S. typhimurium* has been consistently the commonest serotype, often accounting for more than 30% of the total isolates.

Using the data available through this system, admittedly flawed by a variety of surveillance artifacts, we have made analyses of the ratio of blood (3) and

Table 1. Annual number and rate of reported Salmonella isolates, United States, 1970 - 80.

Year	Number	Rate (per 100,000)
1970	24,216	12.0
1971	25,694	12.5
1972	26,110	12.5
1973	26,693	12.7
1974	23,838	11.3
1975	23,445	11.1
1976	23,285	10.8
1977	27,462	13.1
1978	28,748	13.6
1979	31,123	14.1
1980	30,004	13.6

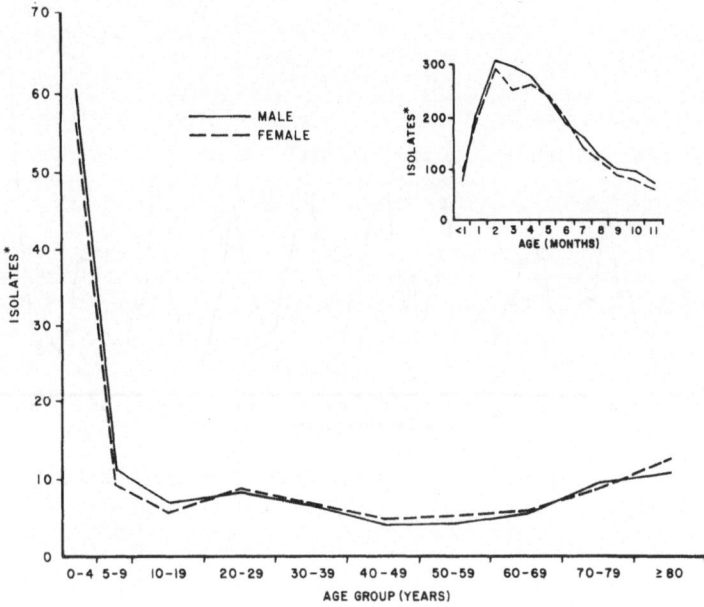

Fig. 1. Rate of reported isolates of *Salmonella*, by age, United States, 1980. *Per 100,000 population.

Table 2. The 10 <u>Salmonella</u> serotypes most frequently
isolated from humans, united States, 1980

Serotype	Number of isolates	Percent	Median age of patients (years)
<u>S</u>. <u>typhimurium</u>*	10,443	34.8	9
<u>S</u>. <u>heidelberg</u>	1,975	6.6	3
<u>S</u>. <u>enteritidis</u>	1,904	6.3	18
<u>S</u>. <u>newport</u>	1,651	5.5	14
<u>S</u>. <u>infantis</u>	1,428	4.8	4
<u>S</u>. <u>agona</u>	1,402	4.7	7
<u>S</u>. <u>saint-paul</u>	757	2.5	20
<u>S</u>. <u>montevideo</u>	665	2.2	17
<u>S</u>. <u>typhi</u>	605	2.0	24
<u>S</u>. <u>oranienburg</u>	503	1.7	14
Subtotal	21,333	71.1	12
Others	8,671	28.9	
Total	30,004	100.0	11

* Includes <u>S</u>. <u>typhimurium</u> var. <u>copenhagen</u>

cerebrospinal fluid isolates (4) to total isolates, and showed how this ratio varies
with the age of the patient and the *Salmonella* serotype. For example, the age-
specific ratio of blood to stool isolates shows little variation with age for *S. typhi*,
S. dublin, and *S. choleraesuis*, while with *S. agona*, *S. blockley*, *S. derby*, *S.
enteritidis*, *S. heidelberg*, *S. infantis*, *S. javiana*, *S. newport*, *S. saint-paul*, and

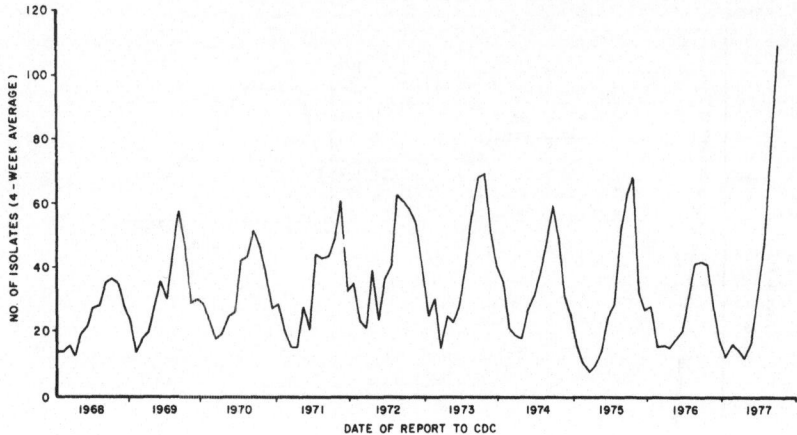

Fig. 2. Reported human *Salmonella newport* isolations, by 4-week average, United States, 1968-1977*.
*Through September

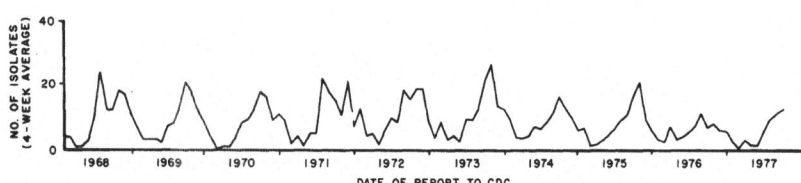

Fig. 3. Reported human *Salmonella javiana* isolations, by 4-week average, United States, 1968-1977*.
*Through September

S. typhimurium, the highest ratios were for children younger than 3 months of age and for adults, especially those over 60 years of age. Similar analyses have been done using ratios for CSF to stool isolations (Table 3) which suggest that the serotypes themselves vary in the frequency of their effects on man.

Another value of storing data over many years in a surveillance system derives from the ability to recognize quickly a rapid increase in the occurrence of a serotype with a known frequency of isolation. Knowledge of the background number of isolates helped in the study of outbreaks, for example, *S. newbrunswick* associated with powdered milk (5), and *S. eastbourne* associated with chocolate candy (6), and then case-control studies identified the vehicles. The investigation and reporting of outbreaks provides a second major source of epidemiologic information. Data concerning outbreaks of salmonellosis, particularly common-source foodborne outbreaks, have been maintained by a foodborne disease surveillance activity in combination with the laboratory based data on *Salmonella* isolates. These data show that in most outbreaks, food is the mode of spread, although person-to-person transmission may occur. The commonest vehicles associated with salmonellosis in the United States (Table 4) are meats (beef and pork), poultry,

Table 3. Ratio of isolates of <u>Salmonella</u> from cerebrospinal
fluid (CSF) and stool, by age of patient and
serotype, United States, 1968-1979

Age of patient	Serotype of Salmonella				
	typhi-murium	heidel-berg	enteri-tidis	typhi	panama
0-2 mo	3.7(11)	20.1(22)	16.0(11)	125.0 (1)	34.5 (5)
3-5 mo	1.5 (5)	6.8(10)	2.6 (2)	111.1 (1)	26.5 (4)
6-11 mo	0.8 (3)	4.9 (6)	1.2 (1)	0	5.5 (1)
1-9 yr	0.5(12)	1.5 (6)	0	12.0 (7)	1.7 (1)
10-59 yr	1.0(23)	1.3 (5)	0.8 (5)	6.0(10)	1.3 (1)
$\geq$ 60 yr	3.1(10)	1.0 (1)	2.6 (3)	0.8 (1)	0
Total	1.1(64)	3.9(50)	1.6(22)	5.8(20)	6.2(12)

Data are number of CSF isolates per 1,000 stool isolates
(no. of CSF isolates) in indicated age group. From Wilson
& Feldman, J. Infect. Dis., 1981.

Table 4. Vehicles involved in 475 human
Salmonella outbreaks in the United
States, 1970 - 1979

Vehicle	Number of outbreaks	Percent of total
Meat	78	16
Poultry	61	13
Human Contact	43	9
Dairy Products	33	7
Eggs	12	3
Pets	7	1
Other Known	112	24
Unknown	129	27
Total	475	100

and other miscellaneous foods, while pets and eggs and egg products, historically
important vehicles, are now uncommon. Unusual vehicles have also been identified. In a recent study of a widespread common-source outbreak, marijuana
was shown to be the vehicle (7).

An outbreak in which the known vehicle has been studied quantitatively in
the laboratory can allow estimation of the number of salmonellae that would be
needed to initiate an infection in man; otherwise this could only be determined
by volunteer experiments. The early volunteer data (8) suggested that all serotypes
required large numbers of *Salmonella* to initiate an infection (Table 5). Outbreak
data indicate that there is a wide range in the infective dose (Table 6). From
studies of outbreaks, it appears that secondary spread of *Salmonella* is less common than that of *Shigella*. The frequency of secondary spread appears to be related
to the age of the index case. Even when the index case is an infant, it appears

Table 5. Range of doses of <u>Salmonella</u> fed to volunteers

			Lowest dose causing	
Serotype	Vehicle	No.	clinical	positive
S. bareilly	eggnog	6	1.3×10^5	1.3×10^5
S. newport	eggnog	6	1.5×10^5	1.5×10^5
S. anatum	eggnog	6	5.9×10^5	1.2×10^4
S. meleagridis	eggnog	6	1.0×10^7	1.0×10^6
S. typhimurium	water	2	2.0×10^9	only 1 dose

Adapted from Blaser and Newman, Rev. Infect. Dis., in press.

Table 6. Range of calculated doses of <u>Salmonella</u> in outbreaks in which a quantitative culture of the vehicle was obtained

serotype	Vehicle	Number of patients	Calculated no. of organisms
S. typhimurium	water	16,000	1.7×10^1
S. typhi	"killed" bacteria	10	9.0×10^1
S. eastbourne	chocolate balls	114	2.5×10^2
S. heidelberg	cheese	339	1.0×10^3
S. cubana	carmine capsules	28	1.5×10^4
S. infantis	ham	8	1.2×10^6

Adapted from Blaser £ Newman, Rev. Infect. Dis., in press.

that an adult with a previously unstudied diarrheal illness may be the source of the infection in the infant (9) (Table 7). Additionally, when an infant infected in a hospital nursery returns to the family (Table 8), others in the family may become infected (10).

A third source of data is a carefully designed field study. Such studies have often concerned pathogenesis, regional and secular trends, specific risk factors, and antimicrobial resistance patterns. One recent national study of *Salmonella* antimicrobial resistance, in which the isolates were obtained throughout 1 year from a randomly selected group of countries, showed 12% overall resistance to 1 or more antimicrobials (Table 9). In previous studies it was found that antimicrobial resistance was 9-10% in 1960 (1), 28-29% in 1962 (12), 22% in 1967 (13), and 31% in 1975 (14). The isolates in the most recent study were not selected in the same manner as those used in the earlier studies, so that direct comparisons of earlier and recent results were not possible. Data from a laboratory analysis of these recent isolates suggest that the *Salmonella* antimicrobial resistance developed in the animal reservoir (Table 10).

109

Table 7. Frequency of prior diarrheal illness (PDI) in families of
          infant and 5 to 9-year-olds with salmonellosis, by number
          of other children in the family

No. of other children in the family	Families of patients with salmonellosis					
	Infant index case		5-9 yr old index			
	No. of families	No. (%) with PDI	No. of families	No. (%) with PDI	Odds Ratio	P Value*
0	74	24 (32)	23	0 (0)		.0007
1+	113	49 (43)	135	20 (15)	4.4	<.0001
Total	187	73 (39)	158	20 (13)	4.4	<.0001

* Fisher's exact test, two-tailed. From Wilson, et al., Pediatrics, 1982.

Table 8. Secondary Salmonella panama infections
          when index infection was in an infant

Family size*	No. of families	No. of other family members	Percent infected
3	13	26	50
4	15	45	51
5	12	48	35
6+	10	64	30
3-11	50	183	39

* Including the infant index case. From Leeder, Ann. N. Y. Acad. Sci., 1956.

Table 9. Antimicrobial resistance pattern of
          Salmonella for randomly selected
          counties, United States, 1979-1980

Serotype	Number studied	% resistant to 2 or more antimicrobials
S. heidelberg	47	45
S. typhimurium V. copenhagen	23	33
S. newport	56	20
S. typhimurium	299	14
S. saint-paul	14	14
S. infantis	25	7
S. agona	44	2
S. enteritidis	48	0
Others	252	4
Total	808	12

Table 10. Similarity of <u>Salmonella</u> plasmid profiles with the same antimicrobial sensitivity pattern, isolated from widely separated states in the United States

Serotype State	Antimicrobial resistance*						Plasmid molecular wts (in megadaltons)					
	A	C	K	S	Su	T	>100	70-99	40-69	10-39	5-9	<4.9
S. typhimurium												
PA	+	0	+	+	+	+	140			3.9		
FL	+	0	+	+	+	+	140			3.9		
CO	+	0	+	+	+	+	140			4		
RI	+	0	+	+	+	+	140			3		
TX	+	0	+	+	+	+	140			3		
VA	+	0	0	+	0	+		65	11	–	3.7	2.8
NC	+	0	0	+	0	+		65		–	3.7	2.8
PA	+	0	0	+	0	+		65		4.7	3.6	–
S. heidelberg												
TX	0	0	0	+	0	+		32,29		2.5	2.1	1.9 1.8
NY	0	0	0	+	0	+		32,29	5	2.5	–	1.9 1.8

* A=Ampicillin, C=Cephalothin, K=Kanamycin, S=Streptomycin, Su=Sulfadiazine, T=Tetracycline (disc sensitivity test) +=Resistant, 0=sensitive; CO=Colorado, FL=Florida, NC=North Carolina, NY=New York, PA=Pennsylvania, RI=Rhode Island, TX=Texas, VA=Virginia.

All 3 sources of data on *Salmonella* infections have been useful in studying salmonellosis. One example has been the program to control turtle-associated salmonellosis in the United States. Case studies indicated that contact with pet turtles and turtle water often preceded cases of salmonellosis, especially in small children. Carefully designed field studies showed that in several states turtle associated salmonellosis was a significant part of the *Salmonella* problem in the state, especially in children (15). Finally, national surveillance data showed that several uncommon serotypes were almost always identified with turtle-associated cases of salmonellosis. Using data from the 3 sources, we showed that the effect of eliminating of sale all pet turtles (Fig. 4) resulted in a significant reduction in the problem of salmonellosis in children (16). These sources have also enabled us to estimate the number of cases that occur annually in the United States by comparing the number of isolates recorded in the surveillance system from large carefully investigated outbreaks with the actual number of persons ill in the outbreaks. This analysis suggested that there are approximately 100 persons ill with salmonellosis for each isolate reported to the system. This allows an estimate of over 2 million cases of salmonellosis each year in the United States. Using data developed during an epidemic-related field study, which concerned the average age-related direct and indirect cost per case during an outbreak of salmonellosis (17), we estimated that the annual cost of salmonellosis in the United States was over 600 million dollars.

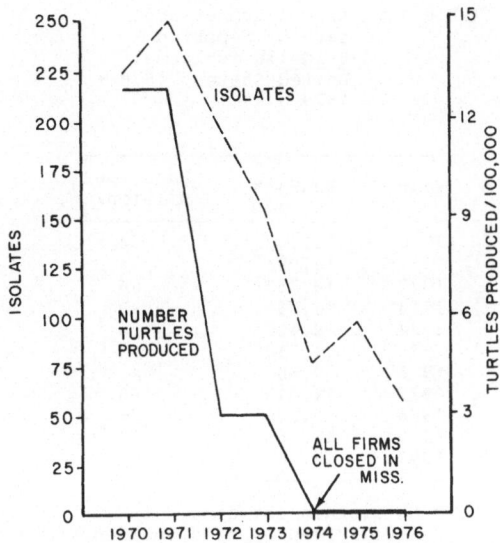

Fig. 4. Isolates of *Salmonella* serotypes*, associated with turtles, from children aged 1-9 and turtle production in Mississippi, 1970-1976. **S. urbana, S. litchfield, S. java.*

Shigella infections

The system for collecting data on *Shigella* infections developed in a manner similar to that for *Salmonella*, with national collection of reports from the states. These reports contain data on age, sex, source of specimen, state, month, year, and serogroup or species. An additional question concerns whether the residence is private, a medical facility, or an Indian reservation.

Using these data, we found that over the last 10 years the number of isolates apparently increased, with 10,903 isolates reported in 1970 and 14,168 in 1980 (Table 11). The reported isolation rate has gone from 54 per million in 1970 to 64 per million in 1980. There has been little change since 1975.

The age-specific isolation rates show a peak in the age group 1-3 years, with the highest isolations in the 2-year age-group (Fig. 5). The largest number of isolates are reported in the fall months for all species of *Shigella*, and for all regions of the country. There has been some shift in the percentage distribution of *Shigella* isolates by species in the last 2 decades. In 1964, 38% of the isolates were *Shigella sonnei*. In 1980, the species most commonly isolated was *S. sonnei*, with almost 70% of the isolates, followed by *S. flexneri*, with 27%, and *S. dysenteriae*, and *S. boydii* with less than 2% each.

Like *Salmonella*, a second major source of epidemiologic data concerning *Shigella* are from outbreak investigations. The majority of reported outbreaks are in homes for retarded children, mental institutions, and on Indian reservations; person-to-person transmission has been the commonest mode of spread identified. Secondary spread appears related to the age of the index case, as has been shown

Table 11. Annual number and
rate of reported
Shigella isolates,
United States, 1970 –
1979

Year	Number*	Rate (per million)
1970	10,903	54
1971	12,988	64
1972	13,752	66
1973	16,868	90
1974	19,420	76
1975	14,757	69
1976	7,907	41
1977	14,019	65
1978	15,336	71
1979	15,265	70
1980	14,468	64

* California isolates not
totally represented between
1970 – 1973.

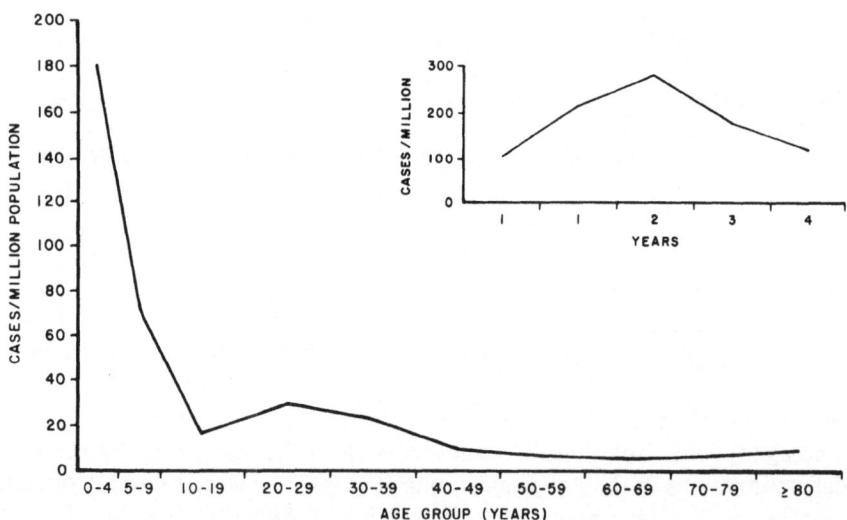

Fig. 5. Rate of reported isolates of _Shigella_, by age, United States*, 1980. *Excludes California.

in a recent study using routinely collected surveillance data (18) (Table 12). Common-source food- or water borne outbreaks, just as sporadic cases, are most frequently due to _S. sonnei_ (Table 13).

The infective dose of some strains of _S. flexneri_ and _S. dysenteriae_ have been studied in volunteers and shown to be relatively low (Table 14). However, there

Table 12. Relationship of age of the index patient with shigellosis to
age of persons with secondary cases reported to the Wisconsin
Department of Health and Social Services, 1975 - 1979

Age of index patient (years)	No. of index patients	No. of household members (% ill) in indicated age group (years)				
		<1	1-4	5-9	10-14	>15
<1	9	1 (0)	9 (44)	4 (25)	0	20 (10)
1-4	167	14 (21)	86 (55)	107 (32)	43 (26)	335 (21)
5-9	65	4 (0)	36 (42)	51 (27)	30 (0)	139 (18)
10-14	22	0	4 (25)	17 (6)	17 (12)	56 (4)
>15	175	13 (54)	43 (14)	48 (10)	42 (7)	287 (9)
Total	438	32 (31)	178 (41)	127 (24)	132 (12)	837 (15)

From Wilson et al., J. Infect. Dis., 1981.

Table 13. Foodborne and waterborne
common-source outbreaks due
to Shigella by species
United States* 1963 - 1979

Shigella species	Number of outbrekas	
	foodborne	waterborne
S. sonnei	33	10
S. flexneri	19	3
S. boydii	1	0

* From CDC Surevillance Data.

Table 14. Responses of man* to various doses of S.
dysenteriae 1 and S. flexneri 2a

Strain	Oral doses**	No. persons tested	Percent ill
Antimicrobially-sensitive endemic strain A1 of S. dysenteriae 1	200	4	25
	100,000	6	33
Antimicrobially-resistant pandemic strain M131 of S. dysenteriae 1	10	10	10
	200	4	50
	10,000	6	83
Virulent strain 2457T of S. flexneri 2a	180	36	22
	5,000	49	57
	10,000	88	59
	100,000	24	58

* From DuPont et al; J. Infect. Dis., 1972 and Levine et
al; J. Infect. Dis., 1973.
**In milk, after bicarbonate.

114

are no data that compare the infective dose of *S. sonnei* and *S. flexneri*, the 2 commonest species in the United States, and no data that compare the infective doses of the various serogroups of *S. flexneri*. It may be that the most infectious *Shigella* species is *S. sonnei*, and that this explains the persistence of this species in the United States, when *S. flexneri* is disappearing.

Field studies are a third major source of data. The pattern of antimicrobial resistance found among *Shigella* species identified in several different geographic regions of the country was studied in 1978 (Table 15). Isolates of *S. sonnei* from the eastern portions of the country (New York, New Jersey, Michigan, Illinois,

Table 15. Number and percent of S. sonnei with a common colicin type that have the common antimicrobial resistance pattern 10 State Shigella Study, 1978

State*	Common colicin type	Common antimicrobial resistance pattern	Percent with colicin type and common antimicrobial resistance pattern
WA	9	Strep-Su, Strep-Su-Tet	31,46
AZ	9	Strep-Su, Strep-Su-Tet	29,35
NM	9	Strep-Su, Strep-Su-Tet	55,35
TX	9	Strep-Su, Strep-Su-Tet	22,50
LA	UT	Amp	83
MO	UT	Amp, Ceph-Amp	24,59
IL	UT	Amp-Strep-Tet	43
MI	UT	Amp-Strep-Tet	35
NJ	UT	Amp-Strep-Tet	68
NY	UT	Amp-Strep-Tet	77

*AZ=Arizona, IL=Illinois, LA=Louisiana, MI=Michigan, MO=Missouri, NJ=New Jersey, NM=New Mexico, MY=New York, TX=Texas, WA=Washington.

and Louisiana) were predominantly colicin type untypable (UT) and had a series of common patterns of multiple or single antimicrobial resistance, (Amp-Strep-Tet, Ceph-Amp, Amp). *S. sonnei* isolates from the western portion of the country (Texas, New Mexico, Arizona, and Washington) were predominantly colicin type 9 and had a different combination of multiple antimicrobial resistance (Strep-Su, Strep-Su-Tet). The combinations of colicin type and antimicrobial resistance patterns emphasize the possible clonal nature of the organism that causes this highly transmissible infections. Different patterns of antimicrobial resistance were found in the *S. flexneri* identified in these regions of the country.

National laboratory-based surveillance has shown that problems with *Shigella* are predominantly limited to a few high-risk population groups; outbreak investigations have shown that person-to-person spread is more common than transmission by food and water, and field studies have shown that antimicrobial resistance patterns show marked regional variations. In contrast to control efforts for *Salmonella*, which are based on knowledge that the reservoir is in animals, and the major mode of spread is by food, control of *Shigella* is based on the knowledge that the major mode of spread is person to person, and that the major reservoir is man. As a result, control of *Shigella* infection is predominantly on the local rather than the national level, and based on personal hygeine, particularly hand-washing, rather than control of foods.

REFERENCES

1. Butler, R. W., and J. E. Josephson. 1962. Egg-containing cake mixes as a source of *Salmonella*. Can. J. Public Health **3**: 478.
2. Proceedings: National Conference on *Salmonella*, interstate outbreak of *Salmonella derby* gastroenteritis, March 1964.
3. Blaser M. R., and R. A. Feldman. 1981. *Salmonella* bacteremia: Reports to the Centers for Disease Control, 1968-1979. J. Infect. Dis. **143**: 743–746.
4. Wilson, R., and R. A. Feldman. 1981. Reported isolates of *Salmonella* from cerebrospinal fluid in the United States, 1968-1979. J. Infect. Dis. **143**: 504–506.
5. Collins, R. N., M. D. Treger, J. B. Goldsby, J. R. Boring, D. B. Coohon, and R. N. Ban. 1968. Interstate outbreak of *Salmonella new-brunswick* infection tracted to powdered milk. JAMA **203**: 838–844.
6. Craven, P. C., D. D. C. Mackel, W. B. Baine, W. H. Barker, and E. J. Gangarosa. 1975. International outbreak of *Salmonella eastbourne* infection traced to contaminated chocolate. Lancet **1**: 788–793.
7. Taylor, D. N., I. K. Wachsmtuh, Y. Shangkuan, E. V. Schmidt, T. J. Barrett, J. S. Schrader, C. S. Scherach, H. B. McGee, R. A. Feldman, D. J. Brenner. Salmonellosis Associated with Marijuana. A Multistate Outbreak Traced by Plasmid Fingerprinting. N. Engl. J. Med. **306**: 1249–1253.
8. Blaser, M. J., and L. S. Newman. Reviews of human salmonellosis: infective dose. Rev. Infect. Dis., in press.
9. Wilson, R., R. A. Feldman, J. Davis, and M. LaVenture. 1982. Salmonellosis in infants: the importance of intrafamilial transmission. Pediatrics, **69**: 436–438.
10. Leeder, F. S. 1956. An epidemic of *Salmonella panama* infections in infants. Ann. NY Acad. Aci. **56**: 54–60.
11. Ramsey, C. H., P. R. Edwards. 1961. Resistance of salmonellae isolated in 1959 and 1960 to tetracycline and chloramphenicol. Appl. Microbiol., **9**: 389–391.
12. McWhorter, A., M. G. Murrell, and P. R. Edwards. 1963. Resistance of salmonellae isolated in 1962 to chlortetracycline. Appl. Microbiol. **11**: 368–370.
13. Schroeder, S. A., P. H. Terry, and J. V. Bennett. 1968. Antibiotic resistance and transfer factor in *Salmonella*, United States 1967. JAMA **205**: 903–906.
14. Ryder, R. W., P. A. Blake, A. C. Murlin, G. P. Carter, R. A. Pollard, M. H. Merson, S. D. Allen, and D. J. Brenner. 1980. Increase in antibiotic resistance among isolates of *Salmonella* in the United States, 1967-1975. J. Infect. Dis., **142**: 485–491.
15. Lamm, S. H., A. Taylor, and E. J. Gangarosa. 1972. Turtle-associated salmonellosis: I. An estimation of the magnitude of the problem in the United States, 1970-1971. Am. J. Epid. **95**: 511–517.
16. Cohen, M. L., M. Potter, M. Pollard, and R. A. Feldman. 1980. Turtle-associated salmonellosis in the United States: effect of public health action, 1970 to 1976. JAMA **243**: 1247–1249.
17. Cohen, M. L., R. E. Fontaine, R. A. Pollard, S. D. VonAllman, T. W. Vernon, and E. J. Gangarosa. 1978. An assessment of patient-related economic costs in an outbreak of salmonellosis. N. Engl. J. Med. **299**: 459–460.
18. Wilson, R., R. A. Feldman, J. Davis, and M. LaVenture. 1981. Family illness associated with *Shigella* infection: the interrelationship of age of the index patient and the age of household members in acquisition of illness. J. Infect. Dis. **143**: 130–132.

Bacterial Diarrheal Diseases, eds., Y. Takeda, T. Miwatani, 117-123.
Copyright © 1985 by KTK Scientific Publishers, Tokyo.

THE CHOLERA/COLI FAMILY OF ENTEROTOXINS

B. A. Marchlewicz and R. A. Finkelstein

Department of Microbiology, University of Missouri School of Medicine, Columbia, Missouri 65212, U.S.A.

Numerous studies have reported immunological, structural, and functional similarities between the heat-labile enterotoxin(s) (LTs) of *Escherichia coli* and the enterotoxin (choleragen) of *Vibrio cholerae*[1-6]. These enterotoxins activate adenylate cyclase, leading to an increase in intracellular levels of cyclic 3',5'-adenosine monophosphate (cAMP)[7,8], and they each are believed to bind, through their B-regions, with host cell membrane receptors containing ganglioside G_{M1}[9,10]. There are, however, structural and immunological differences among choleragen (CT), LT produced by a human strain of enterotoxigenic *E. coli* (H-LT), and LT produced by porcine strains of enterotoxigenic *E. coli* (P-LT)[11,12].

The neutralization of a porcine *E. coli* LT by antisera to cholera enterotoxin was first reported by Gyles and Barnum[1]. Since then, there have been several reports of the neutralization of LT activity by anti-cholera serum; in rabbit ileal loops[13], in permeability factor assays[14], and on adrenal cells[15]. In those studies, crude preparations of LT were used and the degree of neutralization was not quantitated. In a previous report[16], Hardegree summarized the antitoxin titers and other properties of five anti-choleragen sera with the aim of defining a common reference standard. That study, though meticulously performed, did not compare the effectiveness of those sera against *E. coli* enterotoxins. In the present report, we attempt to evaluate the relative effectiveness of homologous and heterologous sera, as well as immuno-purified sera, in the neutralization of biological activity of CT, H-LT, and P-LT.

The sera used in this study include: the U.S. Standard Lot 1 goat anti-cholera toxin (obtained from Hardegree[16]); the Swiss Serum and Vaccine Institute (SSVI) equine anti-cholera immunoglobulins; equine anti-choleragenoid[17]; goat anti-choleragenoid[18]; goat anti-choleragen (Chemo-Sero-Therapeutic Research Institute (CSTRI) Lot G5156-11, Kumamoto, Japan); CSTRI equine anti-choleragen Lot E1006-10-A21, both obtained from N. Ohtomo; specific rabbit antisera directed

---

[1]Experimental data are reported in detail in Marchlewicz, B. A., and R. A. Finkelstein. 1983. Immunological differences among the cholera/coli family of enterotoxins. Diagn. Microbiol. Infect. Dis. 1: 129-138.
[2]Present address: Abbott Laboratories, Chicago, IL., U.S.A.

against isolated choleragen A and B subunits[19], respectively, (prepared by M. Boesman-Finkelstein in this laboratory); goat anti-H-LT[12] directed against LT isolated from strain H74-114; and goat anti-P-LT[3] directed against LT isolated from strain 711/FILT. CT, H-LT, and P-LT were purified to homogeneity as described previously[20, 12, and 2 respectively]. In the Ouchterlony assays, the purified toxins were used at 20 ug per 50 μl well.

In Ouchterlony double immuno-diffusion assays, the antisera were shown to recognize CT, H-LT, and P-LT with the expected spurs, demonstrating unique determinants of homologous over heterologous antigens (a representative sample is shown in Fig. 1). The most pronounced spurs were seen between P-LT and either of the other two toxins. This indicates, as previously described[3,12], that CT and H-LT appear more closely related to each other immunologically than either toxin is to P-LT.

The relative abilities of the sera to neutralize the homologous as well as the heterologous pure toxins were tested using the Y-1 adrenal cell assay[21,22]. Briefly, serial dilutions of the sera were made in Ham F-10 medium[22]; a 100 μl sample containing 10 ED_{50} doses (for CT, 1 ED_{50} = 6pg; for both LTs, 1 ED_{50} = 12pg after trypsin activation as described in[2]) of toxin in Ham F-10 medium was added to the diluted sera; and the toxin-sera mixtures were incubated at room temperature for 15 min. The culture medium on the Y-1 cells was removed by aspiration and toxin-sera mixtures added to each well (final volume 220 ul). The Y-1 cell plates

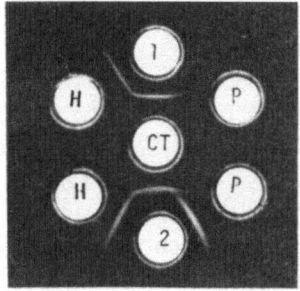

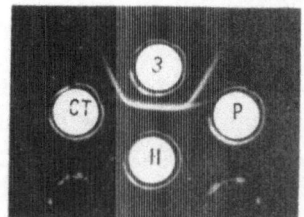
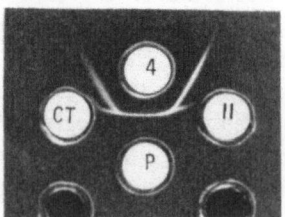

Fig. 1. CT, H, P, denote choleragen, Human and porcine LT respectively.
1 U.S. standard cholera antitoxin (lot 1).
2 Goat anti-choleragenoid
3 Goat anti-H-LT (H74-114)
4 Goat anti-P-LT (711(F1LT)).

were incubated at 37°C for 6 hr in a 5% CO_2 atmosphere. After incubation, each plate was scored for cell rounding using an inverted phase contrast microscope. The end point of the titration was the highest dilution of serum which allowed a 50% rounding of the Y-1 cells. The neutralization data were summarized as the relative potencies of the heterologous reactions as compared with the homologous system and can thus be reported as per cent cross-reactivity.

The data showed that sera directed against choleragen or choleragenoid neutralized H-LT considerably more effectively than they neutralized P-LT. For example, the U.S. Standard Cholera Antitoxin and the goat anti-choleragenoid or anti-choleragen sera (G5156-11) neutralized H-LT 70–90% as effectively as they neutralized CT. The same sera neutralized P-LT only 5–28% as effectively as they neutralized CT. Some sera (e.g., horse anti-choleragen (H1006-10-A-21) and rabbit anti-choleragen B subunit) appeared to neutralize H-LT better than the homologous toxin. These differences, which were at most two-fold, may be attributable to experimental variability, or they could reflect fundamental differences in the availability or number of common antigenic sites recognized by the particular antisera.

With the exceptions of the horse anti-choleragen and the rabbit anti-cholera A subunit, each of the sera against cholera toxin antigens neutralized the porcine LT much less effectively than they neutralized CT or H-LT, with the relative potencies vs P-LT ranging from 3 to 19 per cent. The rabbit anti-cholera A subunit serum neutralized both H-LT and P-LT to a similar degree suggesting that the A subunits of these three toxins may be more closely related than the B subunits. The higher relative potency of the horse anti-choleragen for P-LT may thus reflect its anti-A activity.

The goat anti-H-LT was relatively equally potent against both CT and P-LT (43% and 34%, respectively). Its content of anti-subunit A activity is not yet known.

Again reflecting the antigenic divergence of the porcine-LT, its antiserum was relatively ineffective against both CT and H-LT (12% and 21%, respectively), even though it had previously been shown to contain precipitating antibody against P-LT subunit A[3].

When the same sera have been tested, our results, on neutralization of cholera toxin by anti-cholera sera, are quite compatible with those summarized by Hardegree[16].

Honda and co-workers[23] have reported the preparation of antisera against the common and unique determinants of CT and LT. Using immunoaffinity column chromatography, we prepared sera which were specific for the unique and shared determinants of CT, P-LT, and H-LT. Each of three goat antisera, anti-choleragenoid, goat anti-H-LT, and anti-P-LT, was applied to an immunoaffinity column on which the homologous toxin was coupled to cyanogen bromide-activated Sepharose 4B (Pharmacia Fine Chemicals, Inc.) to yield specific homologous antibody preparations. Subsequently, a sample of goat anti-choleragenoid was applied to immunoaffinity columns on which either purified H-LT or P-LT were bound. The flow through (adsorbed sera) contained immunoglobulins directed against unique antigenic determinants not found on the bound toxin. The eluted immunoglobulin recognized common determinants on all the toxins. In a similar manner, each of the other sera was passed through columns containing heterologous toxins.

The immunological specificities of the various serum preparations were examined in Ouchterlony double diffusion tests. The unchromatographed sera recognized all three toxins with typical spur formation indicating the presence of unique antigenic determinants in the homologous systems. Similar spurring was also seen when immuno-affinity-purified sera were reacted with heterologous toxins. In each case, the immuno-adsorbed serum did not recognize the toxin bound to the column. Anti-H-LT serum, eluted from a choleragen column, gave a line of identity with all three toxins. However, the serum which had been adsorbed with CT recognized H-LT and, to a lesser degree, P-LT. Thus, H-LT and P-LT have antigenic determinants which are not present on CT. The CT-adsorbed anti-P-LT serum recognized P-LT more strongly than it recognized H-LT. Thus even though the LTs have shared determinants not present on CT, they each also have unique specificities. The choleragen-eluted anti-P-LT precipitated CT and H-LT but gave a barely visible line of precipitation with P-LT. Anti-CT adsorbed with H-LT recognized CT but only reacted with P-LT weakly while the eluted antibody recognized all the antigens similarly. Anti-P-LT adsorbed with H-LT recognized CT very weakly. The eluted serum was only weakly reactive. These observations further indicate that CT and H-LT are more closely related antigenically than are CT and P-LT. Further, anti-choleragenoid, adsorbed with P-LT, still recognized the other toxins strongly. Thus much of the antibody is directed against components which are not available on P-LT although on elution the adsorbed antibodies were strongly reactive with all three toxins.

Adsorption of anti-H-LT with P-LT left activity against both CT and H-LT, and the eluted antibody was again reactive with all three toxins.

Neutralization studies with these immuno-specific sera gave results similar to those demonstrated in the Ouchterlony assays. Adsorption of goat anti-choleragenoid serum with either H-LT or P-LT removed most of the homologous related antibody activity, as expected, but left nearly original titers of neutralizing activity against the other toxins. The eluted antibody was effective in neutralization of all three toxins.

Similarly, with anti-H-LT, a single adsorption with the heterologous toxins removed most of the neutralizing activity for the individual adsorbing toxin but left residual homologous and heterologous activity. In the case of adsorption with P-LT, 10% of the activity against H-LT remained but the titer against CT was only slightly affected.

Similar trends were observed with the anti-P-LT although, because of the relatively low cross-neutralization activity, the results were less striking.

DISCUSSION

The present data confirm and extend previous reports on both the immunologic relatedness as well as the immunologic differences among members of the cholera/coli family of ADP-ribosylating, adenylate cyclase-activating, heat-labile enterotoxins.

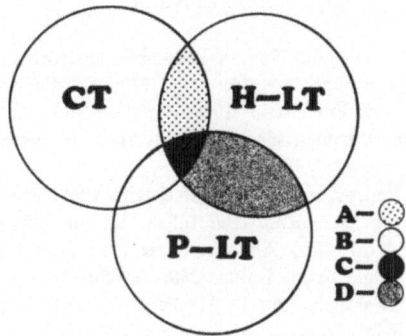

Fig. 2. Artistic representation (not drawn to scale) of the distribution of unique and common antigenic determinants of CT, H-LT, and P-LT.
A = Antigen(s) shared by CT and H-LT, exclusively.
B = Antigen(s) shared by CT and P-LT, exclusively.
C = Antigen(s) common to all three toxins.
D = Antigen(s) shared by P-LT and H-LT exclusively.

Ouchterlony-type precipitin analyses and neutralization tests with specifically immuno-affinity purified and adsorbed antisera, indicate that the three pure enterotoxins examined all share common antigens and, at the same time, each has its own unique antigenic determinants.

The current results are compatible with the operational model depicted in Fig. 2. Each of the samples of the three enterotoxins studied is depicted as having common determinants which are shared with the other two. Each has unique determinants. Each may also share determinants with one, but not the other toxin. And, (although it is not so clear from this drawing) choleragen and H-LT appear to be more closely related to each other than P-LT is to each of the others. The observed immunologic differences probably reflect differences in the amino acid composition of the three toxins[12], as well as differences in the conformation of the toxin molecules and availability of antigenic sites.

Deficiencies of the present study, which we hope to rectify in the future, are that we have, thus far, worked only with a limited number of polyclonal sera and these three holotoxin molecules.

It will be of interest to apply the absolute specificity of hybridoma-derived monoclonal antibodies to the identification of the common and the unique antigenic determinants of each of the subunits of the three toxin species. It will also be important to determine the full extent of the antigenic and structural drift in the cholera/coli family of heat-labile enterotoxins. The results may lead to the development of synthetic antigens which will be capable of affording equal protection against all the members of the family. These are our goals for the future.

This work was supported in part by U.S. Public Health Service grants AI-16776 and AI-17312 (to R.A.F.) under the U.S.-Japan Cooperative Medical Science Program from the National Institute of Allergy and Infectious Diseases.

REFERENCES

1. Gyles, C. L., and D. A. Barnum. 1969. A heat-labile enterotoxin from strains of *Escherichia coli* enteropathogenic for pigs. J. Infect. Dis. **120**: 419–426.
2. Clements, J. D., and R. A. Finkelstein. 1979. Isolation and characterization of homogeneous heat-labile enterotoxin with high specific activity from *Escherichia coli* cultures. Infect. Immun. **24**: 760–769.
3. Clements, J. D., R. J. Yancey, and R. A. Finkelstein. 1980. Properties of homogeneous heat-labile enterotoxins from *Escherichia coli*. Infect. Immun. **29**: 91–97.
4. Dallas, W. S., and S. Falkow. 1980. Amino acid sequence homology between cholera toxin and *Escherichia coli* heat-labile toxin. Nature **288**: 499–501.
5. Holmes, R. K., M. C. Bramucci, and E. M. Twiddy. 1980. Genetic and biochemical studies of heat-labile enterotoxin of *Escherichia coli*, pp. 187–201. *In* Proceedings of the 15th Joint Conference on Cholera, U.S.-Japan Cooperative Medical Science Program Symposium NIH Publication No. 80-2003.
6. Kunkel, S. L., and D. C. Robertson. 1979. Purification and chemical characterization of the heat-labile enterotoxin produced by enterotoxigenic *Escherichia coli*. Infect. Immun. **25**: 586–596.
7. Evans, D. J., L.C. Chen, G. T. Curlin, and D. G. Evans. 1972. Stimulation of adenylate cyclase by *Escherichia coli* enterotoxin. Nature (London) New Biology **236**: 137–138.
8. Moss, J., and M. Vaughan. 1979. Activation of adenylate cyclase by choleragen. An. Rev. Biochem. **48**: 581–600.
9. Holmgren, J. 1973. Comparison of the tissue receptors for *Vibrio cholerae* and *Escherichia coli* enterotoxins by means of gangliosides and natural cholera toxoid. Infect. Immun. **8**: 851–859.
10. Moss, J. J., P. H. Garrison, and S. H. Richardson. 1979. Gangliosides sensitize fibroblasts to *Escherichia coli* heat-labile enterotoxin. J. Clin. Invest. **64**: 381–384.
11. Gill, D. M., J. D. Clements, D. C. Robertson, and R. A. Finkelstein. 1981. Subunit number and arrangement in *Escherichia coli* heat-labile enterotoxin. Infect. Immun. **33**: 677–682.
12. Geary, S. J., B. A. Marchlewicz, and R. A. Finkelstein. 1982. Comparisons of heat-labile enterotoxins from porcine and human strains of *Escherichia coli*. Infect. Immun. **36**: 215–220.
13. Smith, N. W., and R. B. Sack. 1973. Immunologic cross-reactions of enterotoxins from *Escherichia coli* and *Vibrio cholerae*. J. Infect. Dis. **127**: 164–170.
14. Evans, D. G., D. J. Evans, Jr., and S. J. Gorbach. 1973. Identification of enterotoxigenic *Escherichia coli* and serum enterotoxin activity by the vascular permeability factor assay. Infect. Immun. **8**: 731–735.
15. Donta, S. 1974. Neutralization of cholera enterotoxin-induced steroidogenesis by specific antibody. J. Infect. Dis. **129**: 284–288.
16. Hardegree, M. C. 1979. Joint report of working groups for standardization of antitoxins, pp. 165–168. *In* Proceedings of the 14th Joint Conference of the U.S.-Japan Cooperative Medical Science Program Symposium on Cholera, (eds., K. Takeya and Y. Zinnaka). Fuji Printing Co., Tokyo.
17. Finkelstein, R. A. 1970. Monospecific equine antiserum against cholera exo-enterotoxin. Infect. Immun. **2**: 691–697.
18. Clements, J. D., and R. A. Finkelstein. 1978. Immunological cross-reactivity between a heat-labile enterotoxin(s) of *Escherichia coli* and subunits of *Vibrio cholerae* enterotoxin. Infect. Immun. **21**: 1036–1039.
19. Finkelstein, R. A., M. Boesman, S. H. Neoh, M. K. LaRue, and R. Delaney. 1974. Dissociation and recombination of the subunits of the cholera enterotoxin (choleragen). J. Immunol. **113**: 145–150.
20. Finkelstein, R. A., K. Fujita and J. J. LoSpalluto. 1971. Procholeragenoid: an aggregated intermediate in the formation of choleragenoid. J. Immunol. **107**: 1043–1051.
21. Donta, S. T., H. W. Moon, and S. C. Whipp. 1974. Detection of heat-labile *Escherichia coli* enterotoxin with the use of adrenal cells in tissue culture. Science **183**: 334–336.
22. Sack, D. A., and R. B. Sack. 1975. Test for enterotoxigenic *Escherichia coli* in miniculture.

Infect. Immun. **11**: 334–336.

23. Honda, T., Y. Takeda, and T. Miwatani. 1981. Isolation of specific antibodies which react only with homologous enterotoxins from *Vibrio cholerae* and *Escherichia coli*. Infect. Immun. **34**: 333–336.

Bacterial Diarrheal Diseases, eds., Y. Takeda, T. Miwatani, 125–135.
Copyright © 1985 by KTK Scientific Publishers, Tokyo.

RECENT ADVANCES IN THE STUDY OF HEAT-LABILE ENTEROTOXINS OF *ESCHERICHIA COLI**

R. K. Holmes, E. M. Twiddy, and R. J. Neill

Department of Microbiology, Uniformed Services University of the Health Sciences, 4301 Jones Bridge Road Bethesda, Maryland 20814, U.S.A.

The seventh pandemic of cholera began in the early 1960s and provided a stimulus for increased research on the pathogenesis of secretory diarrheal diseases caused by infectious microorganisms. Cholera enterotoxin, the protein toxin of *Vibrio cholerae* that acts on the intestinal mucosa to produce the diarrhea of cholera, was purified to homogeneity in 1969[1]. The availability of purified cholera enterotoxin made it possible for many investigators to perform detailed studies of its structure and biologic activities, and cholera toxin is now one of the best studied bacterial protein toxins[2].

During the late 1960s veterinary microbiologists identified enterotoxin-producing strains of *Escherichia coli* as the causative agents of several economically important diarrheal diseases in animals[3]. It soon became apparent that some strains of *E. coli* associated with diarrhea in man or animals can produce heat-labile enterotoxins related to cholera toxin[4]. Neutralization by antibodies against cholera toxin became accepted as an important criterion for identifying these heat-labile enterotoxins of *E. coli*[5]. The role of Ent plasmids in determining enterotoxigenicity in *E. coli* was also recognized during the late 1960s[6]. Throughout the 1970s the tools of molecular biology were applied successfully for isolating and characterizing the enterotoxin genes from several Ent plasmids[7,8].

Efforts to purify heat-labile enterotoxin from *E. coli* remained unsuccessful until 1979, when several investigators described purified *E. coli* enterotoxins with biologic, structural and immunochemical similarities to cholera toxin[9-11]. Studies of the heat-labile enterotoxins of *E. coli* in our laboratory have been directed primarily toward analysis of genetic regulation of toxin production[11-15] and characterization of enterotoxins produced by *E. coli* strains isolated from humans and animals[11,16]. The main purpose of this report is to summarize the results of our recent studies on the structure and immunochemistry of the heat-labile enterotoxins of *E. coli*.

---

*The opinions expressed are those of the authors and do not necessarily reflect those of the Uniformed Services University of the Health Sciences or the Department of Defense.

Genetic considerations

The bacterial strains and plasmids used in our studies are summarized in Table 1. The structural genes for the heat-labile enterotoxins that we have studied are located on Ent plasmids. All of the Ent plasmids considered here are conjugative. Plasmid pCG86, originally isolated from a porcine enteropathogenic strain of *E. coli*, also has determinants for resistance to several antibiotics. Plasmids pTD2Tc and pTP235Km are derived from Ent plasmids from *E. coli* strains of human origin. The ancestral Ent plasmids pTD2 and pTP235 were modified by insertion of the transposons Tn*10* and Tn*5*, respectively. Tn*10* has determinants for resistance to tetracycline, and Tn5 has determinants for resistance to kanamycin. The antibiotic resistance determinants in these Ent plasmids provide a convenient means of selecting for plasmid transfer in conjugative mating experiments. We have previously demonstrated that chromosomal mutations in *E. coli* can affect the regulation of production of heat-labile enterotoxin[14]. Strain HE12 is derived from *E. coli* KL320(pCG86) and has a chromosomal *htx* mutation that increases the yield of the heat-labile enterotoxin coded by the resident Ent plasmid. Strain HE22 is a cured variant of HE12 that still has the chromosomal *htx* mutation. We transferred plasmids pTD2Tc and pTP235Km into HE22; and we used strains HE12, HE22(pTD2Tc), and HE22(pTP235Km) to produce heat-labile enterotoxins for

Table 1. Plasmids and bacterial strains

Designation	Characteristics	Reference
Plasmids		
pCG86	LT$^+$, ST$^+$, multiply drug resistant plasmid from porcine *E. coli*	22
pTD2	Ent plasmid from human *E. coli* Throop D	this study
pTD2Tc	plasmid pTD2 with insertion of transposon Tn*10*	this study
pTP235	LT$^+$ plasmid from human *E. coli*	23
pTP235Km	plasmid pTP235 with insertion of transposon Tn5	23
E. coli strains		
KL320	*trp, his, met, pro, lac, rps*L; derived from *E. coli* K12	14
KL320 (pCG86)	KL320 harboring plasmid pCG86	14
HE12	hypertoxinogenic (*htx*) mutant of KL320 (pCG86)	14
HE22	derived from HE12 by curing of pCG86	14
Throop D	enterotoxigenic strain of human origin	24
HE22(pTD2Tc) HE22(pTP235Km)	HE22 harboring plasmid pTD2Tc	this study
SA53	HE22 harboring plasmid pTP235Km isolated from water buffalo; produces LT-like toxin	this study from P. Echeverria

purification and characterization. These procedures enabled us to compare the properties of the plasmid-coded, heat-labile enterotoxins produced by isogenic and hypertoxinogenic *E. coli* strains.

Purification and properties of heat-labile enterotoxins

Heat-labile enterotoxins were extracted from bacterial cells grown to stationary phase in glucose-syncase medium. Washed bacteria were disrupted by sonication, and particulate debris was removed by centrifugation. Enterotoxins in the extracts were purified by affinity chromatography on agarose[9], followed by dialysis and ion exchange chromatography on phosphocellulose[11]. For convenience the heat-labile enterotoxin coded by plasmid pCG86 was designated pLT, and the enterotoxins coded by plasmids pTD2Tc and pTP235Km were designated hLT1 and hLT2, respectively. Purified cholera enterotoxin used for comparative studies was prepared from supernatants of cultures of *V. cholerae* 569B Inaba according to published methods[17]. Cholera enterotoxin was designated CT.

Some of the properties of our purified *E. coli* heat-labile enterotoxins and cholera toxin are summarized in Table 2. The doses of CT, pLT, hLT1, and hLT2 needed to induce rounding of cultured Y1 adrenal tumor cells were comparable and were about 25 picograms per assay (125 picograms/ml). Antiserum prepared against purified CT, pLT, or hLT1 neutralized the cytotoxicity of the homologous and heterologous enterotoxins tested. Each of these enterotoxins was composed of two kinds of polypeptide chains designated A and B. CT was purified in the nicked form with some of the A subunit cleaved to fragments A1 and A2. In

Table 2. Properties of purified heat-labile enterotoxins of *V. cholerae* and *E. coli*

Property	Enterotoxin			
	CT	pLT	hLT1	hLT2
Cytotoxicity for Y1 cells				
Cytotoxic Dose	25 pg	25 pg	25 pg	25 pg
Potentiated by Trypsin	no	no	no	no
Neutralization				
Anti-CT	yes	yes	yes	n.t.[a]
Anti-pLT	yes	yes	yes	n.t.
Anti-hLT1	yes	yes	yes	n.t.
Form of toxin purified	nicked	intact	intact	intact
Molecular weight				
Subunit A	30,000	30,000	30,000	30,000
Fragment A1	21,000	21,000	22,000	22,000
Subunit B	11,600	11,600	12,100	12,100
Isoelectric point[b]				
Holotoxin	7.0	8.0	7.4	n.t.
Subunit A	n.t.	5.9	5.7	n.t.
Subunit B	n.t.	8.7	8.2	n.t.

a) n.t. = not tested b) average value of 2–8 determinations

contrast pLT, hLT1, and hLT2 were purified in the unnicked form with their A polypeptides intact. Treatment of these toxins with trypsin under appropriate conditions converted them quantitatively to the nicked form. The toxicity of the nicked forms of the *E. coli* heat-labile enterotoxins for Y1 adrenal cells in the assay system used[18] did not differ from the toxicity of the intact forms of these enterotoxins. In contrast, the NAD-dependent ADPR-transferase activity of these toxins, measured *in vitro* with (^{125}I)-guanyltyramine as the acceptor molecule[19], was activated by treatment of the toxins with trypsin and reducing agents and was associated with the Al fragment. Analysis of the electrophoretic mobilities of the polypeptide subunits and fragments of these toxins in polyacrylamide gels in the presence of sodium dodecylsulfate demonstrated that the Al fragments and the B subunits of hLT1 and hTL2 had slightly slower mobilities than the corresponding polypeptides of CT and pLT (Fig. 1). We performed intramolecular crosslinking experiments and demonstrated that the stoichiometry of the subunits in pLT is AB_5. Isoelectric focussing of the (^{125}I)-labeled toxins or their (^{125}I)-labeled subunits also revealed differences between CT, pLT, and hLT1. The pIs of pLT and hLT1 were 8.0 and 7.4, respectively, and were significantly higher than the pI of 7.0 determined for CT. The A subunits of pLT and hLT1 had pIs of 5.9 and 5.7. The pIs of the B subunits of pLT and hLT1 were 8.7 and 8.2. Thus pLT and hLT1 differ significantly from each other and also differ from CT in their isoelectric points.

Immunochemistry of E. coli heat-labile ecterotoxins

Antisera prepared against purified CT, pLT, and hLT1 neutralized the biologic

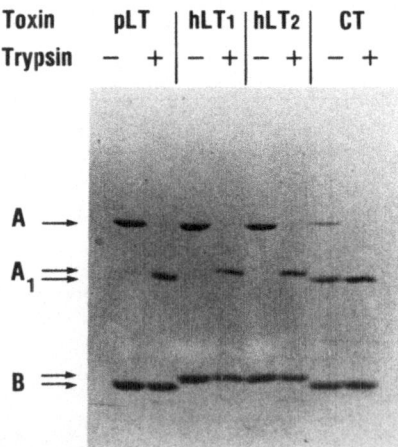

Fig. 1. Analysis of purified heat-labile enterotoxins by SDS-polyacrylamide gel electrophoresis. Samples containing 5 μg of purified pLT, hLT1, hLT2, or CT with or without pretreatment with trypsin were boiled in sample treatment mix in the presence of 2-mercaptoethanol and subjected to electrophoresis in polyacrylamide gels in the presence of sodium dodecylsulfate (SDS). The A, Al, and B polypeptides of pLT comigrated with the corresponding polypeptides of CT, whereas the Al and B polypeptides of hLT1 and hLT2 migrated slightly more slowly than the corresponding polypeptides of CT and pLT.

activity of CT, pLT, and hLT1 in Y1 adrenal cell assays. Neutralization tests with hLT2 and anti-hLT2 have not yet been completed. In each case the neutralizing titer of the antiserum was greatest for the homologous enterotoxin antigen. For each serum, neutralization titers with pLT and hLT1 did not differ by more than 2-fold, whereas neutralization titers with CT and either pLT or hLT1 as antigens differed by 8-fold to 16-fold[16]. Thus the antigenic determinants of CT, pLT, and hLT1 that are important for neutralization reactions are cross-reacting but not identical.

Purified CT, pLT, hLT1 and hLT2 were compared as antigens in immunodiffusion tests (Fig. 2). The antisera used for these studies were prepared by hyperimmunization of rabbits with purified CT, pLT, hLT1, or hLT2. With each of these antisera hLT1 and hLT2 produced reactions of identity, although both hLTs gave cross-reactions with pLT and with CT. The directions of the spurs in the cross-reactions indicated that anti-CT detected determinants on hLT1 and hLT2 that were absent on pLT and that anti-pLT detected determinants on hLT1 and hLT2 that were absent on CT. Additional experiments showed that the anti-hLT sera detected determinants on pLT that were not present on CT. These studies demonstrate that CT, pLT, and the hLTs represent three antigenically different subgroups of heat-labile enterotoxin that have both shared and unique antigenic determinants.

A solid phase radioimmunoassay for heat-labile enterotoxins[14] was modified and used for more quantitative comparisons of the cross-reactions between CT, pLT, hLT1 and hLT2 (Fig. 3). Each antiserum reacted most strongly with the homologous enterotoxin antigen. For each antiserum the reactions with hLT1 and

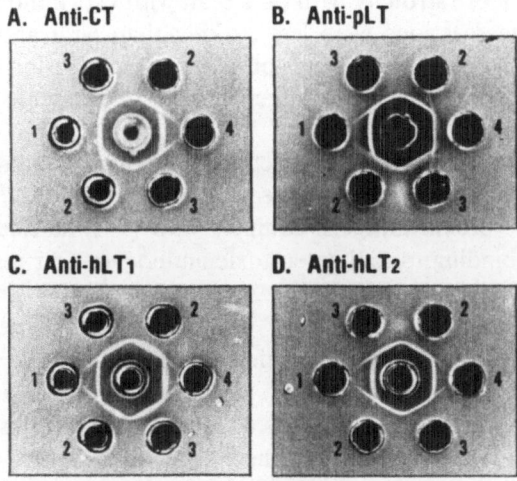

Fig. 2. Comparison of purified heat-labile enterotoxins of *V. cholerae* and *E. coli* by immunodiffusion tests. The antitoxins were from rabbits immunized with purified enterotoxins and were placed in the center wells as follows: A) Anti-CT serum A23 (1:2), B) Anti-pLT serum A45, C) Anti-hLT1 serum B59, and D) anti-hLT2 serum G48. The purified enterotoxin antigens were used at concentrations of 200 μg/ml and were arranged as follows: 1) CT, 2) hLT1, 3) hLT2, and 4) pLT.

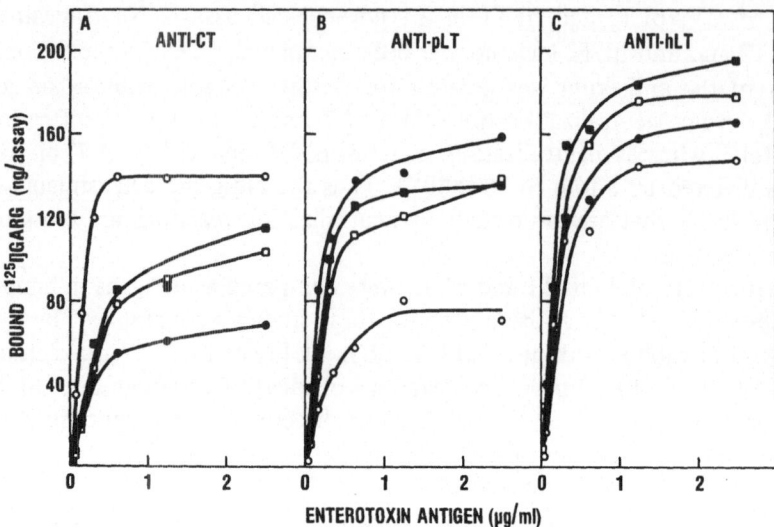

Fig. 3. Comparison of purified heat-labile enterotoxins of *V. cholerae* and *E. coli* by solid phase radioimmunoassays. The assay was modified from a published method[14] by sensitizing the plates with ganglioside G_{MI} instead of purified equine anti-choleragenoid and by using rabbit anti-enterotoxin and goat anti-rabbit IgG (GARG) at saturating concentrations (1:200 for anti-CT serum A23, or 1:100 for anti-pLT serum A45, or 1:100 for anti-hLT1 serum B59, and 25 μg/ml for [^{125}I]-labeled GARG). The purified enterotoxin antigens were as follows: CT:(o—o), pLT (•—•), hLT1 (□—□), and hLT2 (■—■). Under these conditions the maximum amount of (^{125}I)GARG bound with each antigen reflects the number of binding sites on that antigen for antibodies in the antiserum tested.

hLT2 were very similar. Anti-CT reacted more strongly with hLT1 and hLT2 than with pLT. Anti-pLT reacted more strongly with hLT1 and hLT2 than with CT. Anti-hLT1 reacted more strongly with pLT than with CT, although the differences in the extent of the reactions were less striking than with anti-CT or anti-pLT. These results confirmed the conclusions of the immunodiffusion tests and indicated that pLT and the two hLTs share a larger number of antigenic determinants with each other than with CT.

We have previously described competitive-binding radioimmunoassays specific for the A and B subunits of *E. coli* heat-labile enterotoxins[16]. In these assays nonradioactive enterotoxin antigens compete with (^{125}I)-labeled A or B subunits of enterotoxin for binding to anti-enterotoxic antibodies. Our results demonstrated that the antigenic determinants of the A subunits of pLT and hLT1 were indistinguishable, whereas the B subunits of pLT and hLT1 were partially cross-reacting[16]. Only subsets of the antigenic determinants of the A and B subunits of pLT and hLT1 were present on CT. These studies have now been extended by comparing purified hLT1 and hLT2 as competing antigens in similar competitive-binding radioimmunoassays (Fig. 4). These data demonstrate that hLT2 has all of the antigenic determinants associated with both the A subunit (Fig. 4A) and the B subunit (Fig. 4B) of hLT1. Figure 4B also confirms the observation that there is only partial cross-reactivity between the B subunits of pLT and hLT1.

In summary, our immunochemical data demonstrate that there are two antigenically distinct subclasses of *E. coli* heat-labile enterotoxin, one represented

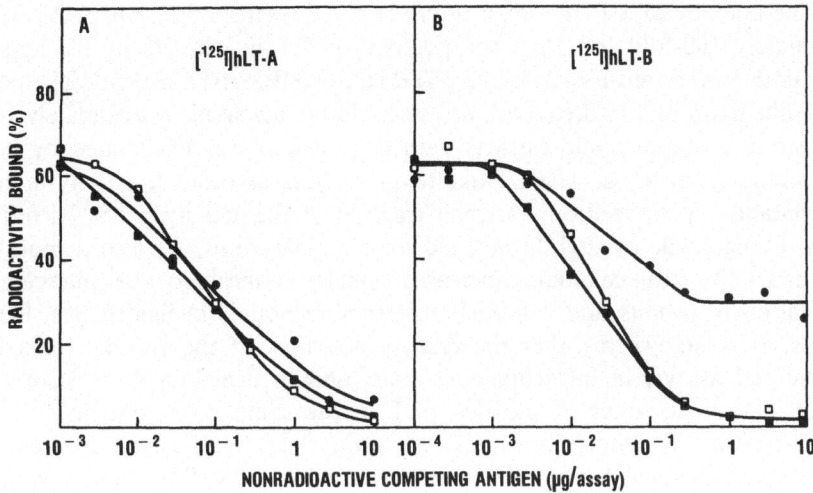

Fig. 4. Comparison of purified heat-labile enterotoxins of *E. coli* by competitive-binding radioim-munoassays. The assay system was based on published methods[16, 21]. Reaction mixtures contained trace amounts of the (^{125}I)-labeled A or B subunit of purified hLT1, a sufficient amount of anti-hLT1 to bind about 60% of the labeled ligand in the absence of competing antigen, and varying amounts of the purified antigen to be tested. Immune complexes containing IgG were adsorbed to protein A-bearing *S. aureus*, and the percent of total radioactivity bound in the immune complexes was deter-mined. The nonradioactive competing antigens were as follows: pLT (•—•), hLT1 (□—□), and hLT2 (■—■).

tigenically distinct subclasses of *E. coli* heat-labile enterotoxin, one represented by purified pLT and the other represented by purified hLT1 and hLT2. A similar conclusion has been reached independently by Honda and his collaborators[20]. Our data also indicate that the antigenic differences between pLT and the hLTs are probably restricted to determinants located on their B subunits.

A new heat-labile toxin of E. coli

To extend our studies on the range of antigenic variation among heat-labile enterotoxin of *E. coli*, we obtained strains that had been collected by several in-vestigators from various geographic locations, both from humans and from a number of different animals. All of these *E. coli* strains had been classified as enterotoxigenic based on bioassays. When these bacteria were tested in our laboratory, we discovered that several of the strains collected in Thailand by Dr. Peter Echeverria from rectal cultures of water buffalo had an unusual phenotype. Although sonic extracts of these bacteria induced morphologic changes in Y1 adrenal cells that were similar to the effects of classical *E. coli* heat-labile enterotoxins, the extracts did not contain enterotoxin antigen that could be detected in our solid phase radioimmunoassay. Furthermore, the activities in the extracts that caused Y1 adrenal cells to become rounded could not be neutralized by any of the hyperim-mune antisera against CT, pLT, or hLT1 that were available in our laboratory. We selected *E. coli* strain SA53 for further studies. For convenience we have designated the toxic activity of strain SA53 as LT-like toxin.

The potency of LT-like toxin in crude sonic lysates of *E. coli* SA53 was approximately 100-fold less than the potency of LT in extracts of the hypertoxinogenic *E. coli* strain HE12, HE22(pTD2Tc), or HE22(pTP235Km). The potency of LT-like toxin in Y1 adrenal cell assays could be increased approximately 10-fold by treatment of the crude extracts with trypsin and was inactivated by heating for 10 minutes at 60°C. The LT-like toxin was cell-associated; activity in culture supernatants represented only a small fraction of the activity in the bacterial extracts. Using crude or slightly purified toxin preparations, we also demonstrated that the LT-like toxin can induce increased vascular permeability after intracutaneous inoculation in rabbits and can elicit secretory responses in ligated ileal loops in rabbits. It is noteworthy that the relative activities of the LT-like toxin in Y1 adrenal cell assays, in intracutaneous tests, and in ileal loop tests were similar to the relative activities of purified pLT in the same assay systems.

The chemical properties of LT-like toxin were significantly different from those of the classical heat-labile enterotoxins of *E. coli*. We tested a variety of methods for purifying the LT-like toxin, including ammonium sulfate fractionation, ion exchange chromatography, gel filtration chromatography, isoelectric focussing, and other electrophoretic techniques. The LT-like toxin did not bind to agarose under conditions where pLT, hLT1, or hLT2 bound to agarose; and the isoelectric point for biologically active LT-like toxin was about 6.5.

We have purified the LT-like toxin approximately 940-fold with 3% yield. The ability of the toxin to be potentiated about 10-fold after treatment with trypsin was retained throughout the purification. The dose of the purified LT-like toxin required to produce a morphologic response in Y1 adrenal cell assays was approximately 17 nanograms (without trypsin treatment). The morphologic changes in Y1 adrenal cells induced by the LT-like toxin were accompanied by increases in the intracellular pool of cyclic-3',5'-adenosine monophosphate, and the time courses of the morphologic and biochemical changes were similar for the LT-like toxin and for pLT (Fig. 5). Although the LT-like toxin appears to be a protein, we have not yet determined its structure. The purified material remained heterogeneous, and only small amounts of the purified material were available for study. We radioiodinated a sample of the purified LT-like toxin and analyzed the distribution of biologic activity and radioactivity after analytical isoelectric focussing (Fig. 6). The active LT-like toxin did not correspond to any of the major (^{125}I)-labeled components. If the specific toxicity of the LT-like toxin were comparable to purified pLT, hLT1 or hLT2, then LT-like toxin would represent about 0.1% of the protein in the purified preparation.

CONCLUSION

We have purified and characterized several heat-labile enterotoxins coded by plasmids isolated from porcine and human enterotoxigenic strains of *E. coli*. These heat-labile enterotoxins are closely related to cholera enterotoxin in structure and mode of action, share antigenic determinants with CT, and are cross-neutralized by anti-CT antibodies. Immunochemical studies demonstrated that CT and LTs from human and porcine enterotoxigenic *E. coli* strains represent three different

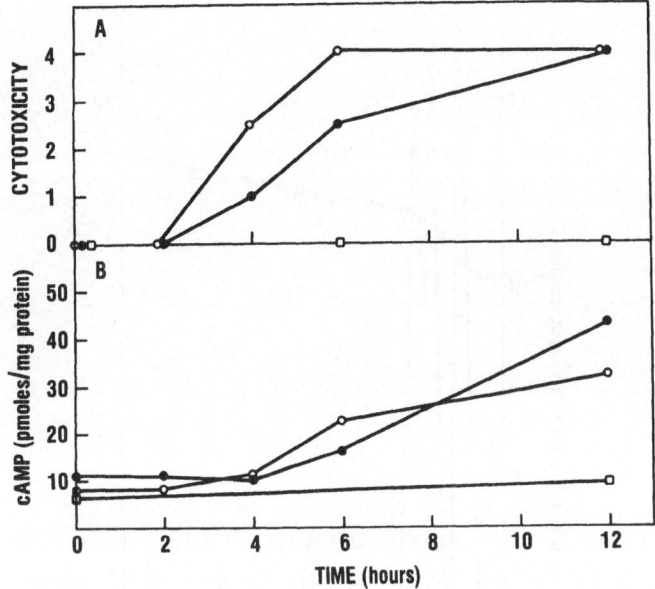

Fig. 5. Time course of changes in cellular morphology and intracellular cyclic AMP content of Y1 adrenal tumor cells exposed to pLT or LT-like toxin. Monolayers of Y1 cells were exposed for the times indicated to purified pLT (2 ng/ml) or to partially purified LT-like toxin (4 μg/ml, without trypsin treatment). Rounding of the cells was scored as cytotoxicity on a scale of 0 to 4, and duplicate samples were collected for assay of intracellular cyclic AMP. All samples contained the cyclic AMP phosphodiesterase inhibitor l-methyl-3-isobutylxanthine (MIX) at 0.05 M. Symbols: LT-like toxin (o—o), pLT (•—•), MIX control (□—□).

antigenic subgroups of heat-labile enterotoxin. This antigenic heterogeneity is associated with differences among the heat-labile enterotoxins in other properties such as the isoelectric points and the electrophoretic mobilities of their subunits and fragments.

We have also identified an LT-like toxin produced by several strains of *E. coli* that does not cross-react immunologically with CT, pLT, hLT1, or hLT2. The LT-like toxin resembles the classical LTs in several biologic activities and activates adenylate cyclase in Y1 adrenal cells. In contrast, the LT-like toxin differs from the classical LTs in its behavior during purification and its isoelectric point. We have purified the LT-like toxin approximately 940-fold, but it has not yet been purified to homogeneity.

Research in our laboratory on heat-labile enterotoxins of *E. coli* has been supported in part by grant number 5 R22 AI-14107 from the National Institute of Allergy and Infectious Diseases, DHHS, United States Government. We thank Drs. Peter Echeverria, Werner Maas, Moyra McConnell, and Richard Finkelstein for providing bacterial strains and Dr. Samuel Formal for testing samples of LT-like toxin for secretory activity in rabbit ileal loops. Irmgard Dinger provided secretarial assistance.

134

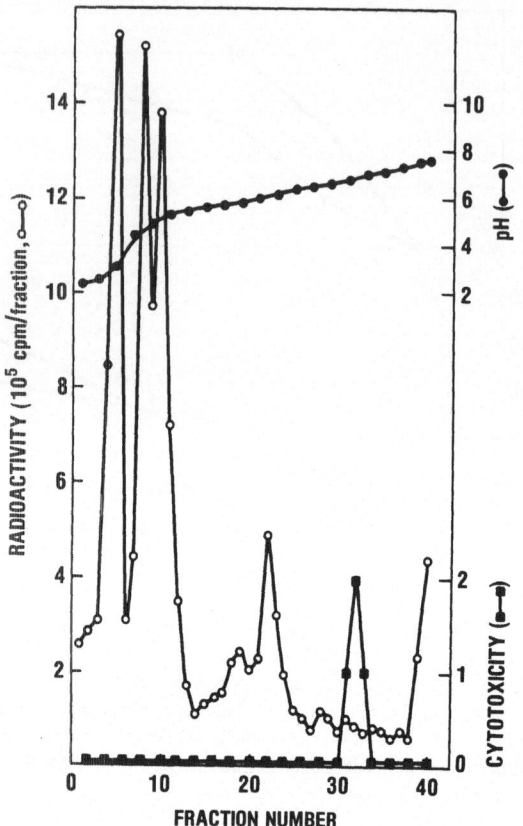

Fig. 6. Isoelectric focussing of LT-like toxin. The partially purified LT-like toxin was radiolabeled with ^{125}I, and samples of the (^{125}I)-labeled toxin were mixed with 2.4 μg amounts of unlabeled LT-like toxin and analyzed by analytical isoelectric focussing (pH 5-8). Each cylindrical gel was sliced into 40 equal fractions, and each fraction was analyzed by scintillation counting for total radioactivity and by Y1 adrenal cell assays for LT-like toxic activity that could be eluted from the gel. Data from a representative experiment are shown.

REFERENCES

1. Finkelstein, R. A., and J. J. LoSpalluto. 1969. Pathogenesis of experimental cholera. Preparation and isolation of choleragen and choleragenoid. J. Exp. Med. **130**: 185–202.

2. Field, M., J. S. Fordtran, and S. G. Schultz (eds.). 1980. Secretory diarrhea. American Physiological Society, Bethesda, MD.

3. Smith, H. W., and S. Halls. 1967. Studies on *Escherichia coli* enterotoxin. J. Path. Bacteriol. **93**: 531–543.

4. Gyles, C. L., and D. A. Barnum. 1969. Heat-labile enterotoxin from strains of *Escherichia coli* enteropathogenic for pigs. J. Infect. Dis. **120**: 419–426.

5. Finkelstein, R. A. 1976. Progress in the study of cholera and related enterotoxins. pp. 54–58, *In* Bernheimer, A.W. (ed.), Mechanisms in bacterial toxinology, John Wiley and Sons, N.Y.

6. Smith, H. W., and S. Halls, 1968. The transmissible nature of the genetic factor in *Escherichia coli* that controls enterotoxin production. J. Gen. Microbiol. **52**: 319–334.

7. Dallas, W. S., D. M. Gill, and S. Falkow. 1979. Cistrons encoding *Escherichia coli* heat-labile toxin. J. Bacteriol. **139**: 850–858.

8. Yamamoto, T., and T. Yokota. 1981. *Escherichia coli* heat-labile enterotoxin genes are flanked by repeated deoxyribonucleic acid sequences. J. Bacteriol. **145**: 850–860.

9. Clements, J. D., and R. A. Finkelstein. 1979. Isolation and characterization of homogeneous heat-labile enterotoxins with high specific activity from *Escherichia coli* cultures. Infect. Immun. **24**: 760–769.

10. Kunkel, S. L., and D. C. Robertson. 1979. Purification and chemical characterization of the heat-labile enterotoxin produced by enterotoxigenic *Escherichia coli*. Infect. Immun. **25**: 586–596.

11. Holmes, R. K., M. G. Bramucci, and E. M. Twiddy. 1980. Genetic and biochemical studies of heat-labile enterotoxin of *Escherichia coli*, pp. 17–201. In Proceedings of the Fifteenth Joint Conference on Cholera. NIH Publication 80-2003. National Institutes of Health, Bethesda, MD.

12. Bramucci, M. G., and R. K. Holmes. 1978. Radial passive immune hemolysis assay for detection of heat-labile enterotoxin produced by individual colonies of *Escherichia coli* or *Vibrio cholerae*. J. Clin. Microbiol. **8**: 252–255.

13. Holmes, R. K., M. G. Bramucci, and E. M. Twiddy. 1979. Genetics of toxinogenesis in *Vibrio cholerae* and *Escherichia coli*, pp. 165–177. *In* I. Hertman, A. Shafferman, A. Cohen, and S. R. Smith (eds.), Extrachromosomal Inheritance in Bacteria. Contributions to Microbiology and Immunology, Vol. 6, S. Karger, Basel.

14. Bramucci, M. G., E. M. Twiddy, W. B. Baine, and R. K. Holmes. 1981. Isolation and characterization of hypertoxinogenic (*htx*) mutants of *Escherichia coli* KL320(pCG86). Infect. Immun. **32**: 1034–1044.

15. Neill, R. J., and R. K. Holmes. 1983. Expression of plasmid genes encoding *Escherichia coli* heat-labile enterotoxin in bacterial strains with different genetic backgrounds, p 201–206. *In* S. Kuwahara and N. F. Pierce, ed., Advances in Research on Cholera and Related Diarrheas. KTK Scientific Publishers, Tokyo.

16. Holmes, R. K., E. M. Twiddy, and M. G. Bramucci. 1983. Antigenic heterogeneity among heat-labile enterotoxins from *Escherichia coli*, p 293–300. *In* S. Kuwahara and N. F. Pierce, ed., Advances in Research on Cholera and Related Diarrheas. KTK Scientific Publishers, Tokyo.

17. Mekalanos, J. J., R. J. Collier, and W. R. Romig. 1978. Purification of cholera toxin and its subunits: new methods of preparation and use of hypertoxinogenic mutants. Infect. Immun. **20**: 552–558.

18. Maneval, D. R., Jr., R. R. Colwell, S. W. Joseph, R. Grays, and S. T. Donta. 1980. A tissue culture method for the detection of bacterial enterotoxins. J. Tissue Culture Methods **6**: 85–90.

19. Mekalanos, J. J., R. J. Collier, and W. R. Romig. 1979. Enzymatic activity of cholera toxin. I. New methods of assay and the mechanism of ADP-ribosyltransfer. J. Biol. Chem. **254**: 5849–5854.

20. Honda, T., T. Tsuji, Y. Takeda, and T. Miwatani. 1981. Immunological non-identity of heat-labile enterotoxins from human and porcine enteropathogenic *Escherichia coli*. Infect. Immun. **34**: 337–340.

21. Cryz, S. J., Jr., S. L. Welkos, and R. K. Holmes. 1980. Immunochemical studies of diphtherial toxin and related nontoxic mutant proteins. Infect. Immun. **30**: 835–846.

22. Silva, M. L. M., W. K. Maas, and C. L. Gyles. 1978. Isolation and characterization of enterotoxin-deficient mutants of *Escherichia coli*. Proc. Natl. Acad. Sci. U.S.A. **75**: 1384–1388.

23. McConnell, M. M., H. R. Smith, G. A. Willshaw, S. M. Scotland, and B. Rowe. 1980. Plasmids coding for heat-labile enterotoxin production isolated from *Escherichia coli* 078: Comparison of properties. J. Bacteriol. **143**: 158–167.

24. Finkelstein, R. A., M. L. Vasil, J. R. Jones, R. A. Anderson, and T. Barnard. 1976. Clinical cholera caused by enterotoxigenic *Escherichia coli*. J. Clin. Microbiol. **3**: 382–384.

Bacterial Diarrheal Diseases, eds., Y. Takeda, T. Miwatani, 137–143.

HETEROGENEITY OF ENTEROTOXINS OF *VIBRIO CHOLERAE* AND ENTEROTOXIGENIC *ESCHERICHIA COLI*

Yoshifumi Takeda, Takeshi Honda, Takao Tsuji, Koichiro Yamamoto and Toshio Miwatani

Department of Bacteriology and Serology, Research Institute for Microbial Diseases, Osaka University, 3-1 Yamada-oka, Suita, Osaka 565, Japan

The molecular structure of heat-labile enterotoxin (LT) of enterotoxigenic *Escherichia coli* is similar to that of cholera enterotoxin (CT). Dallas and Falkow[1] showed that LT synthesized by minicells containing Ent plasmid DNA was composed of two distinct proteins with molecular weights of 25,500 and 11,500 daltons, values similar to those of the A and B subunits of CT. Clements and Finkelstein[2] demonstrated more directly that the subunit structure of purified LT was very similar to that of CT; that is LT consisted of two subunits, A and B, with molecular weights of 28,000 and 11,500, respectively. Moreover, similarities in the amino acid sequences of the A and B subunits of CT and LT were reported by Spicer *et al.*[3] and Dallas and Falkow[4], respectively.

The immunological similarity of LT and CT is also well established. Gyles and Barnum[5] first reported the immunological kinship of CT and LT, by showing cross neutralization of the ability of cell lysates to cause fluid accumulation in rabbit ileal loops. Gyles[6] confirmed the partial identity of CT and LT by the Ouchterlony double gel diffusion test. Subsequently, Clements and Finkelstein[7, 8] demonstrated the immunological cross-reactivity of LT with the A and B subunits of CT.

All the above experiments were carried out with LT produced by a strain of porcine enterotoxigenic *E. coli*. Kunkel and Robertson[9] have suggested, however, that there are molecular and immunological differences between LT's from human and porcine enterotoxigenic *E. coli*. In this paper, we report molecular and immunological heterogeneity of CT and LT from human strains (LT$_h$) and that from porcine strains (LT$_p$) of enterotoxigenic *E. coli*.

Molecular heterogeneity of CT, LT$_h$ and LT$_p$

Experiments to compare some physicochemical properties of CT, LT$_h$ and LT$_p$ revealed the molecular heterogeneity of these 3 enterotoxins. The ionic charges of CT, LT$_h$ and LT$_p$ were studied by polyacrylamide gel disc electrophoresis. As

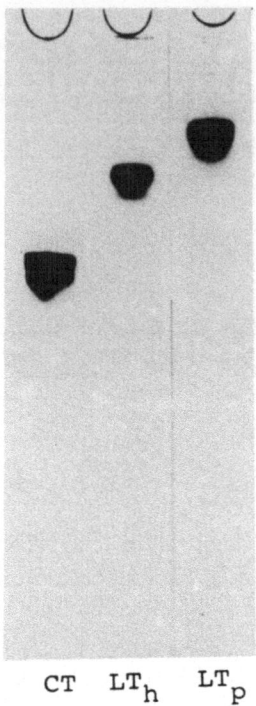

CT   LT$_h$ LT$_p$

Fig. 1. Polyacrylamide gel disc electrophoresis of CT, LT$_h$ and LT$_p$.

shown in Fig. 1, CT purified as described by Ohtomo *et al.*[10] and LT$_h$ and LT$_p$ purified as described previously[11] migrated to different positions, indicating that they differed in ionic charges. After LT$_h$ and LT$_p$ had been treated with trypsin, they migrated slightly faster than the untreated toxins, but they still differed in mobility. The isoelectric points of the 3 toxins were different: CT, 6.80; LT$_h$, 7.50; and LT$_p$, 8.10 (Fig. 2).

SDS-polyacrylamide slab gel electrophoresis showed that LT$_h$ and LT$_p$ also differed in size. As seen in Fig. 3, the B subunit of LT$_h$ migrated slower than those of CT and LT$_p$, which migrated to almost the same position. When CT and trypsin treated LT$_h$ and LT$_p$ were treated with dithiothreitol before analysis, the A$_1$ fragments of these toxins migrated to almost the same position, whereas the B subunit of LT$_h$ migrated slower than that of CT or LT$_p$. These results suggest that the sizes of the B subunits of CT, LT$_h$ and LT$_p$ have the following relationship: LT$_h$ > LT$_p$ = CT. Although the mobilities of the A subunits and A$_1$ fragments of CT, LT$_h$ and LT$_p$ were indistinguishable in preceeding experiments, careful examination showed a slight difference in their mobilities. When LT$_h$ and LT$_p$ were treated with trypsin and subjected to electrophoresis after dithiothreitol treatment, the A subunit gave two bands attributable to the A$_1$ and A$_2$ fragments. As shown in Fig. 4, the mobility of fragment A$_1$ of LT$_p$ was slightly less than that of CT or LT$_h$, the latter two migrating to almost the same position. The

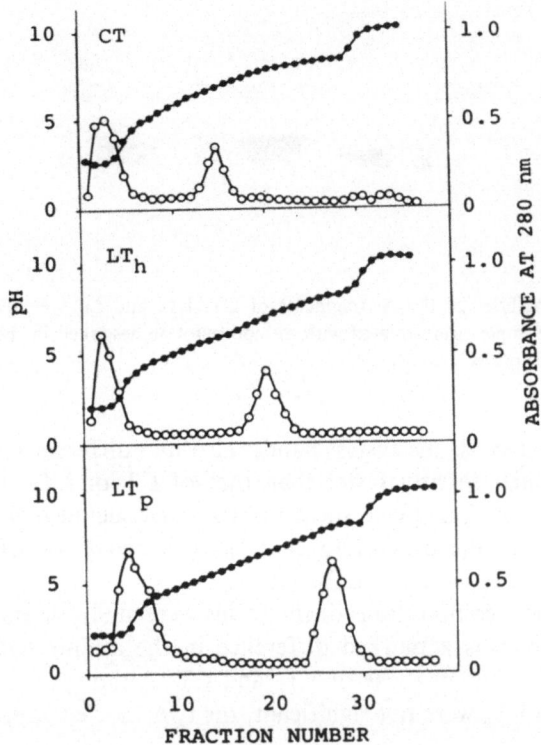

Fig. 2. Isoelectric focusing of CT, LT$_h$ and LT$_p$. •, pH; ○, absorbance at 280 nm.

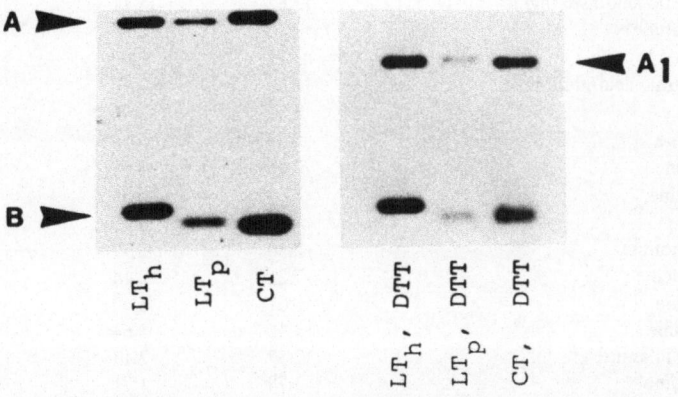

Fig. 3. SDS-polyacrylamide slab gel electrophoresis of CT, LT$_h$ and LT$_p$. Samples were heated at 100°C for 2 minutes in the absence or presence of 10 mM dithiothreitol and subjected to electrophoresis.

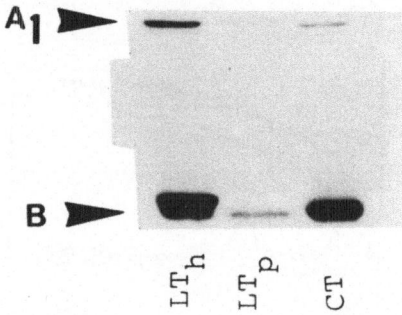

Fig. 4. Different mobilities of the A_1 fragments of CT, LT_h and LT_p on SDS-polyacrylamide slab gel electrophoresis. Samples were treated with dithiothreitol as described in the legend of Fig. 3 and subjected to electrophoresis.

bands of fragment A_2's, the fastest bands, also had different mobilities: fragment A_2 of LT_p migrated slightly faster than that of CT or LT_h, which migrated to almost the same position. From these results it is concluded that the sizes of the A_1 fragments are in the order $LT_p > LT_h = CT$ and those of the A_2 fragment are in the order $LT_h = CT > LT_p$.

The amino acid compositions of the toxins were analyzed and results are shown in Table 1. There was a marked difference in the amino acid compositions of LT_h and CT as well as in those of LT_p and CT. Although in general differences between LT_h and LT_p were not significant, the two showed appreciable differences

Table 1. Amino acid composition of CT, LT_h and LT_p.

Amino acid	Concentration (%)		
	CT	LT_h	LT_p
Aspartic acid/asparagine	11.62	11.11	11.12
Threonine	7.70	8.36	9.24
Serine	5.72	8.09	7.54
Glutamic acid/glutamine	11.73	12.45	12.61
Proline	4.32	3.76	3.76
Glycine	5.55	5.16	5.04
Alanine	9.36	5.78	5.23
Cysteine	1.57	1.55	1.52
Valine	4.02	3.65	3.63
Methionine	2.30	2.77	3.02
Isoleucine	7.21	9.14	9.10
Leucine	6.07	5.40	5.41
Tyrosine	4.36	5.64	5.42
Phenylalanine	2.57	2.17	2.23
Histidine	3.78	1.71	1.47
Lysine	6.75	6.61	7.08
Arginine	4.20	5.47	5.53
Tryptophan	1.17	1.17	1.05

in their contents of several amino acids, such as threonine, serine alanine, methionine and lysine.

Immunological heterogeneity of CT, LT_h and LT_p

To examine the immunological relation of CT, LT_h and LT_p, we carried out Ouchterlony double-gel diffusion tests with various combinations of these 3 toxins and antisera. Results showed that the precipitin line between LT_p and anti-LT_h, like that between CT and anti-LT_h, formed a spur (Fig. 5-1 and 5-3). They also showed that the precipitin line between LT_h and anti-LT_p and that between CT and anti-LT_p formed a spur (Fig. 5-5 and 5-6). These results indicate the existence of a common antigenic determinant between LT_h and LT_p that does not exist in CT. Similarly the spur formation between the precipitin line between LT_h and anti-CT and that between LT_p and anti-CT (Fig. 5-7 and 5-8) indicates the existence of a common antigenic determinant between CT and LT_h that does not exist in LT_p. Furthermore the spur formation between the precipitin line between LT_h and anti-LT_h and that between LT_p and anti-LT_h (Fig. 5-1 and 5-2) indicates the existence of an antigenic determinant in LT_h that does not exist in LT_p. Spur formation between the precipitin line between LT_h and anti-LT_h and that between CT and anti-LT (Fig. 5-2 and 5-3) indicates the existence of an antigenic determinant in LT_h that does not exist in CT. Similarly, spur formation between the precipitin line between CT and anti-CT and that between LT_p and anti-CT (Fig. 5-7 and 5-9) indicates the existence of an antigenic determinant in CT that does not exist in LT_p. Spur formation between the precipitin line between CT and anti-

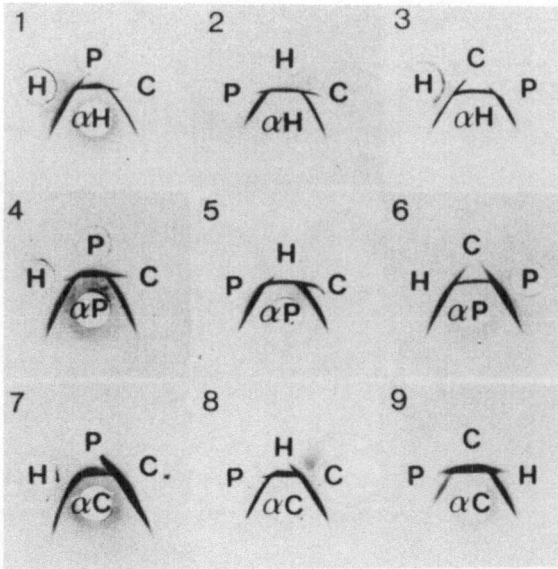

Fig. 5. Ouchterlony double-gel diffusion test of CT, LT_h and LT_p against anti-CT, anti-LT_h and anti-LT_p. c, CT; H, LT_h; P, LT_p; αC; anti-CT; αH, anti-LT_h; αP, anti-LT_p.

CT and that between LT_h and anti-CT (Fig. 5-8 and 5-9) indicates the existence of an antigenic determinant in CT that does not exist in LT_h. Also, spur formation between the precipitin line between LT_h and anti-LT_p and that between LT_p and anti-LT_p (Fig. 5-4 and 5-5) indicates the existence of an antigenic determinant in LT_p that does not exist in LT_h. Spur formation between the precipitin line between LT_p and anti-LT_p and that between CT and anti-LT_p (Fig. 5-4 and 5-6) indicates the existence of an antigenic determinant in LT_p that does not exist in CT.

These results indicate the immunological heterogeneity of CT, LT_h and LT_p and also demonstrate the existence of unique antigenic determinants that shared antigenic determinants of each toxin. However, the results in Fig. 5 do not suggest the existence of a common antigenic determinant between CT and LT_p that does not exist in LT_h. Further studies by using immunoaffinity column chromatography with purified antisera as described[12] will elucidate the immunological relatedness of these 3 toxins.

Since the results described above were obtained with LT_h and LT_p purified from a single strain of each human and porcine origin, it was necessary to determine whether other strains of human *E. coli* and porcine *E. coli*, respectively,

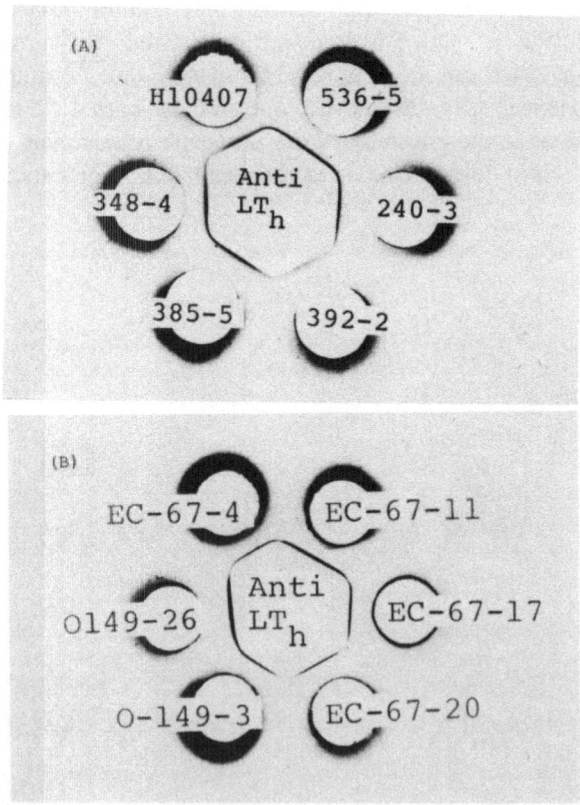

Fig. 6. Double gel diffusion test of crude LT preparations of various strains of human *E. coli* (A) and porcine *E. coli* (B).

produce immunologically identical LT's. For this we prepared crude LT's from several human and porcine *E. coli* and examined them by the double-gel diffusion test. As shown in Fig. 6A, the LT's from all the human *E. coli* strains tested, which were randomly selected, gave pricipitin lines that fused, indicating that they were identical. All the porcine *E. coli* strains were also found to produce immunologically identical LT's, as shown in Fig. 6B.

REFERENCES

1. Dallas, W. S., and S. Falkow. 1979. The molecular nature of heat-labile enterotoxin (LT) of *Escherichia coli*. Nature (London) **277**: 406–407.
2. Clements, J. D., and R. A. Finkelstein. 1979. Isolation and characterization of homogeneous heat-labile enterotoxins with high specific activity from *Escherichia coli* cultures. Infect. Immun. **24**: 760–769.
3. Spicer, E. K., W. M. Kavanaugh, W. S. Dallas, S. Falkow, W. H. Konigove, and D. E. Schafer. 1981. Sequence homologies between A subunits of *Escherichia coli* and *Vibrio cholerae* enterotoxins. Proc. Natl. Acad. Sci. U.S.A. **78**: 50–54.
4. Dallas, W. S., and S. Falkow. 1980. Amino acid sequence homology between cholera toxin and *Escherichia coli* heat-labile toxin. Nature (London) **288**: 499–501.
5. Gyles, C. L., and D. A. Barnum. 1969. A heat-labile enterotoxin from strains of *Escherichia coli* enteropathogenic for pigs. J. Infect. Dis. **120**: 419–426.
6. Gyles, C. L. 1974. Immunological study of the heat-labile enterotoxins of *Escherichia coli* and *Vibrio cholerae*. Infect. Immun. **9**: 564–570.
7. Clements, J. D., and R. A. Finkelstein. 1978. Immunological cross-reactivity between a heat-labile enterotoxin(s) of *Escherichia coli* and subunits of *Vibrio cholerae* enterotoxin. Infect. Immun. **21**: 1036–1039.
8. Clements, J. D., and R. A. Finkelstein. 1978. Demonstration of shared and unique immunological determinants in enterotoxins from *Vibrio cholerae* and *Escherichia coli*. Infect. Immun. **22**: 709–713.
9. Kunkel, S. L., and D. C. Robertson. 1979. Purification and chemical characterization of the heat-labile enterotoxin produced by enterotoxigenic *Escherichia coli*. Infect. Immun. **25**: 586–596.
10. Ohtomo, N., T. Muraoka, H. Inoue, H. Sasaoka, and H. Takahashi. 1974. Preparation of cholera toxin and immunization studies with cholera toxoid, pp. 132–142. In Proceedings of the 9th Joint Conference of the U.S.-Japan Cooperative Medical Science Program, Cholera Panel. National Institutes of Health, Bethesda, Md.
11. Takeda, Y., T. Honda, S. Taga, and T. Miwatani. 1981. In vitro formation of hybrid toxins between subunits of *Escherichia coli* heat-labile enterotoxin and those of cholera enterotoxin. Infect. Immun. **34**: 341–346.
12. Honda, T., Y. Takeda, and T. Miwatani. 1981. Isolation of special antibodies which react only with homologous enterotoxins from *Vibrio cholerae* and enterotoxigenic *Escherichia coli*. Infect. Immun. **34**: 333–336.

Bacterial Diarrheal Diseases, eds., Y. Takeda, T. Miwatani, 145–152.
Copyright © 1985 by KTK Scientific Publishers, Tokyo.

INTERNALIZATION OF CHOLERA TOXIN SUBUNITS INTO MOUSE THYMUS CELLS

Yutaka Zinnaka, Sumiaki Tsuru, Mayumi Oguchi, Nobuya Ohtomo* and Toyoharu Muraoka*

*Department of Bacteriology, National Defense Medical College, Tokorozawa, Saitama 359 and *the Chemo-Sero-Therapeutic Research Institute, Kumamoto 860, Japan*

It has been established that the cholera toxin (CT) molecule consists of two subunits: the B subunit (SB) is responsible for binding to receptors on the surface of the target cell, and the A subunit (SA) is responsible for biological activity, that is, activation of adenylate cyclase[see reviews 3, 7, 16, 25]. Models have been proposed for the internalization of CT or its subunits into the cell[2, 8], in which SA penetrates the cell membrane through a hydrophilic channel constructed by SB's extending into the lipid bilayer after binding to the receptor. From such models, it is readily conceivable that SA disappears from the surface of the cell sometime after adsorption, but that SB remains on the surface provided it is not endocytosed or dissociated from the receptor.

This paper describes experiments on the mode of internalization of CT subunits into mouse thymus cells as revealed by fluorescence-activated cell sorting and immune electron microscopy with specific antibodies against each subunit. The results suggest that not only SA but also SB penetrate the cell membrane after attachment of the whole toxin molecule to the cell surface.

Thymus cells were harvested from 5-week-old ddN mice, and 10^7 cells were suspended in 0.1 ml of CT solution (1 μg/ml) at room temperature for 10 min. Then cells were washed to remove unbound CT, resuspended in RPMI-1640 medium and incubated at 37°C under 5% CO_2 in air. AT an appropriate time, the cells were labeled with either fluorescein isothiocyanate (FITC)-conjugated rabbit anti-SA or -SB immunoglobulin (0.5 mg protein/ml) to detect the subunits. All the preparations were analyzed with a fluorescence-activated cell sorter (FACS II, Bacton Dickinson Electronics Lab., Mountain View, Calif.) to determine the rate of binding of each subunit[23].

More than 90% of the cells were labeled with either anti-subunit antibody immediately after CT treatment, but both the number of labeled cells and the relative intensity of fluorescence decreased with time and reached the control level after 4 h, irrespective of the kind of subunit. Fig. 1 shows the fluorescence profiles of CT-treated cells stained with anti-SB, which were not distinguishable from those stained with anti-SA (not shown). Scatter profiles of the same cell population

146

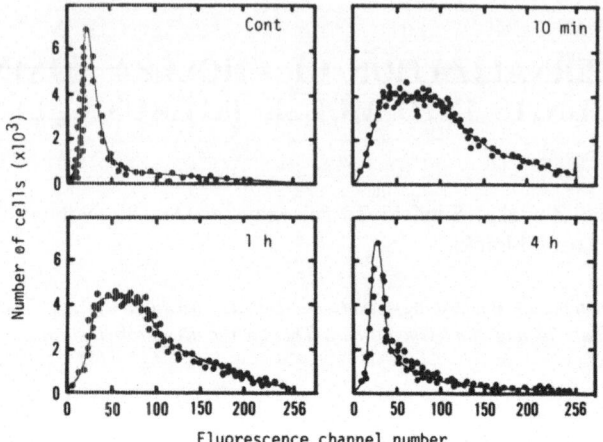

Fig. 1. Fluorescence distribution of CT-treated mouse thymus cells labeled with FITC-conjugated anti-SB rabbit serum. Cells were incubated at 37°C before labeling. Uper left: control cells without CT treatment (FITC-conjugated rabbit anti-SB only); upper right: SB-binding 10 min after CT treatment; lower left: SB-binding 1 h after CT treatment; lower right: SB-binding 4 h after CT treatment.

are shown in Fig. 2. Similar experiments were repeated except that the whole procedure was carried out at 4°C. The results obtained were the same as those shown in these figures[24].

Decrease in fluorescence may reflect either dissociation of the subunit(s) from the cell membrane or its incorporation into the cell. For examination of these possibilities, portions of the cells were treated with each of the anti-subunit rabbit

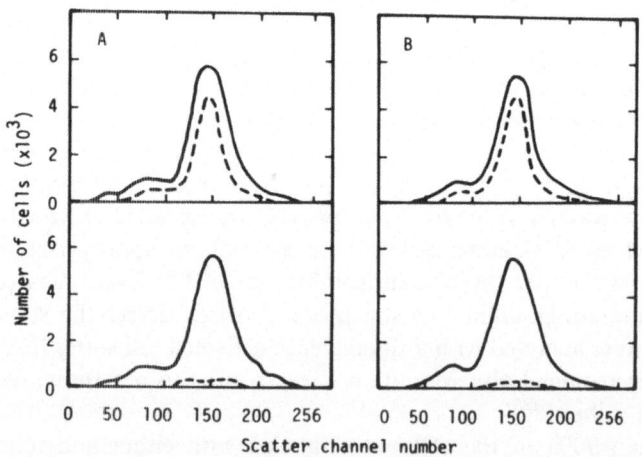

Fig. 2. Scatter profiles of CT-treated cells labeled with FITC-conjugatd anti-subunit antisera. (A) Anti-SA binding 10 min (upper) and 4 h (lower) after CT treatment. (B) Anti-SB binding 10 min (upper) and 4h (lower) after CT treatment. Solid line: scatter distribution of total cells; broken line: scatter distribution of fluorescent cells, *i. e.*, the cells with each subunit on the surface. Cells were incubated at 37°C before labeling.

immunoglobulins immediately after adsorption of the toxin, and then stained with FITC-conjugated anti-rabbit IgG at various times for FACS analysis. As shown in Fig. 3, no decrease in the percentage of fluorescent cells was observed. Since there is probably no interaction between these antibodies and the cell membrane, it is likely that the two subunits do not dissociate from the cell surface. It is also clear that the CT-antibody complex on the cell surface is not endocytosed.

Next we examined whether the toxin subunits are present inside the cell by treating cells with a critical concentration of saponin (0.1 mg/ml, for 15 min in an ice bath) before labeling with specific antibody[24]. This technique has been used to increase the permeability of the cell membrane to allow uniform entry of macromolecular tracers into cell compartments[18, 19, 20]. Ninety percent of the total cells treated with saponin immediately after adsorption of CT were stained with FITC-conjugated anti-SB. Undoubtedly, this positive fluorescence was due to toxin molecules on the cell surface. As shown in Fig. 4, after 4 h of incubation at 37°C, when the toxin molecule had already disappeared from the cell surface, fluorescence was still associated with cells treated with saponin, although the value had decreased about 50%. This specific fluorescence could also be detected after incubation at 4°C. Another experiment with FITC-conjugated anti-SA gave similar results. These results clearly show the presence of the toxin molecule within the cell. The light-scattering pattern of the saponin-treated cells was shifted to the left from the normal position, indicating decrease in scattering. This may be attributable to morphological change due to increased permeation. The small peak remaining in the position of that of normal cells may be due to cells that were not affected by saponin treatment. Scanning electron micrographs showed that these cells still retained their normal shape, although their surface was flattened (Fig. 5).

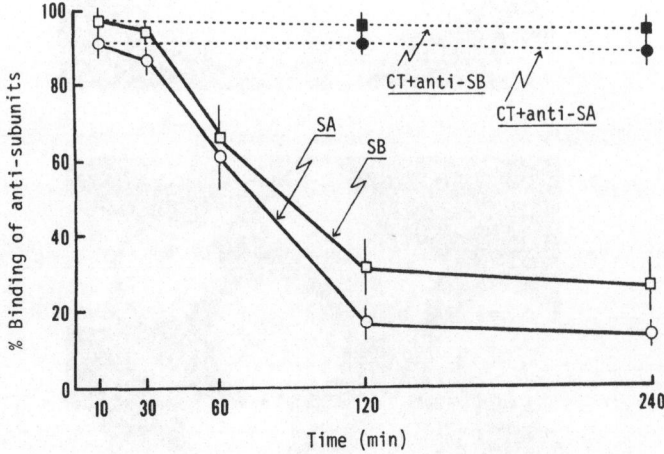

Fig. 3. Binding of anti-subunits to mouse thymus cells treatd with CT at various times. Cells were labeled indirectly with each anti-subunit rabbit antiserum and FITC-conjugated anti-rabbit IgG goat serum. Solid lines: cells were incubated at 37°C after CT treatment before anti-subunit serum was applied. Broken lines: cells were treated with anti-subunit serum immediately after CT treatment and fluorescence-labeled after incubation.

148

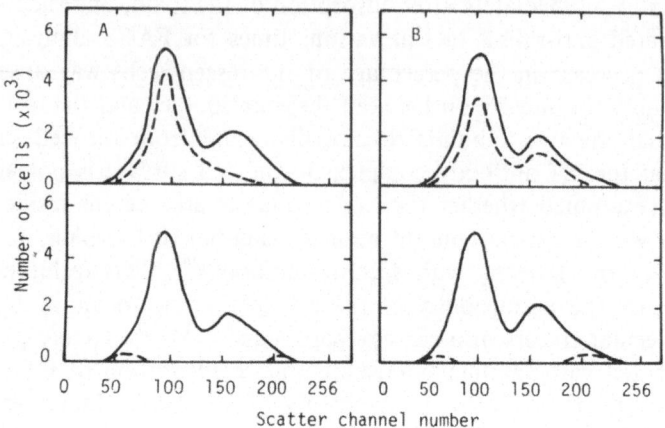

Fig. 4. Scatter profiles of saponin-treated cells. Cells were treated with saponin before labeling after CT treatment and incubation for 4 h. (A) Anti-SA binding; (B) anti-SB binding. Lower panels represent the profiles of control cells treated with only saponin and each FITC-conjugated anti-subunit serum. Compare these profiles with those shown in Fig. 2.

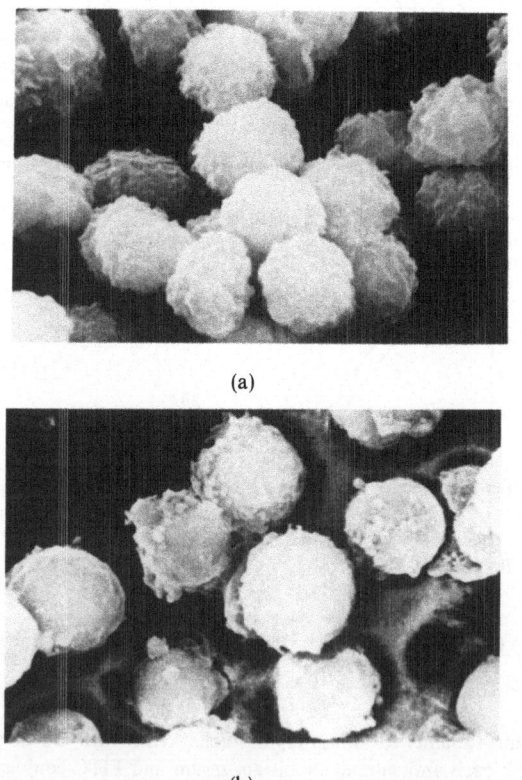

(a)

(b)

Fig. 5. Scanning electron micrographs of mouse thymus cells. (A) Cells treated with CT only. (B) Cells treatd with CT and saponin. Magnification: × 3,600.

It was a possibility that SB was incorporated into the cell membrane itself, which would also result in decrease in its immunofluorescence and reappearance of fluorescence after saponin treatment. To examine this possibility, we prepared the membrane fraction[12] from cells treated with CT and then with saponin after incubation at 4°C. This fraction was stained with FITC-conjugated anti-SB antibody and analyzed by FACS in the same way as intact thymus cells. About 90% of the membranes showed fluorescence with anti-SB when stained 10 min after CT treatment, but the percentage of fluorescent membranes decreased with time to about 5% after 4 h of incubation[24]. These results indicate that SB was not associated with the membrane at this time, but was present in the cytoplasm.

To demonstrate more directly the cytological localization of the subunits, the cells were examined by immune electron microscopy with horseradish peroxidase (HRP)-conjugated antibody as a marker. For detection of each subunit inside the cell, permeabilization of cells with saponin was used to allow the antibody to enter the cell[18], instead of the frozen section technique, because the latter technique is not readily applicable to free cells. Details of our procedure will be published elsewhere.

Fig. 6-A shows a control cell treated only with saponin and then two (specific and HRP-conjugated anti-rabbit IgG) antibodies successively. Perforation of the surface membrane and loss of soluble constituents seems to have taken place, but only a few weak deposits of HRP granules (stained with diaminobenzidine) are seen in the specimen. In contrast, in the cell treated with CT and processed for detection of the subunits, HRP granules are clearly seen. Fig. 6-B shows the localization of SA in a cell incubated for 2 h at 4°C after CT treatment. Numerous HRP granules are seen in the cytoplasm as well as on the cell membrane. In cells processed immediately after adsorption of CT, HRP granules were found mainly on the cell surface (picture not shown).

Stain on the location of SB gave similar results. The positive staining shown in Fig. 6-C indicates the presence of SB in the cytoplasm of a cell incubated for 2 h after CT treatment. Some stain still remains on the cell surface of this cell, but most HRP granules are within the cell and are uniformly distributed. To the question whether these granules were associated with the Golgi region, as reported for HRP-linked CT[10], HRP itself[5], and peptide hormones[4], we could not find any association of CT subunits with the Golgi region in these cells.

Intracellular cyclic AMP was measured in CT-treated cells to determine the relation between the entrance of SA into cells and the activation of adenylate cyclase. There was no increase of intracellular cyclic AMP in cells treated with CT and incubated at 4°C. However, when the temperature of incubation was shifted to 37°C, a normal cyclic AMP response took place with the usual lag period (data not shown).

It is believed that the biologically active component, or SA, of CT is internalized into cells as follows: After binding to the GM_1 ganglioside on the cell membrane, the SB molecule changes its conformation, and enters the lipid bilayer. Here several molecules of B peptide construct a hydrophilic channel with or without participation of membrane protein, and this allows the active peptide A_1 to enter the cell[2, 8, 13, 15]. The presence of "down-regulation", or decrease in the number

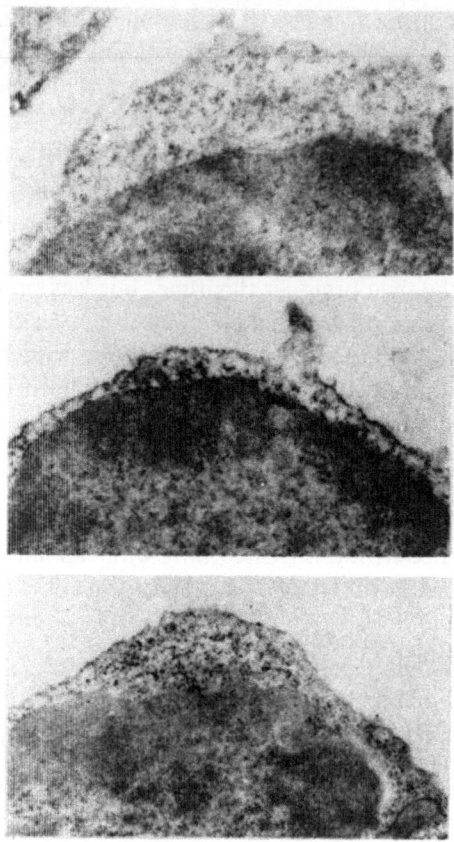

Fig. 6. HRP-labeling of CT-treated mouse thymus cells. Cells were treatd with saponin before labeling with anti-subunit rabbit serum and HRP-conjugated anti-rabbit IgG goat serum. Specimens were then processed with diaminobenzidine. No contrast staining with uranyl or lead salt was performed. Magnification; × 18,000. (A) Control cell (no CT treatment) processed with asnti-SA. Perforation of the cell membrane and leakage of some cytoplstmic constituents, but only a few weak deposits of HRP granules are observed. (B) SA-labeling of a cell incubatd for 2 h at 4°C after CT treatment. (C) SB-labeling of a cell incubated for 2 h at 4°C after CT treatment. Most HRP granules are in the cytoplasm, although some positive deposits are still present on the surface.

of receptors after the adsorption of CT, has been suggested by some workers[14, 17]. However, "down-regulation" is the result of the endocytotic process, and it is evident that endocytosis itself is not important for entry of the active component, because in this case, toxin molecules are still in the same topological position as they were before endocytosed.

The present results clearly indicate that both SA amd SB enter the cell after adsorption, irrespective of the temperature. Since the rate of endocytosis is usually very low at low temperature[21], it is reasonable to conclude that SB is also internalized into the cell by a mechanism other than endocytosis, at least at low temperature, although endocytosis, or "down-regulation", may take place at higher temperature. In fact, there was some evidence for the endocytotic process, because in some specimens small intracytoplasmic vesicles associated with HRP granules were observed.

Hansson et al.[6] examined the structural localization of CT in mouse thymus cells, and observed the presence of cap formation and of pinocytosed toxin after incubation for 30 min at 37°C, but they found that the toxin remained dispersed on the cell surface below 18°C. Their results are not inconsistent with the present observation, since they did not report the effect of prolonged incubation at low temperature or try to detect the subunits within the cell. Joseph et al.[10] stated that HRP-linked CT and SB were endocytosed by murine neuroblastoma cells, and that the endocytosed complex remained in the region near the Golgi apparatus. Since HRP itself is used as a marker of fluid-phase pinocytosis[22], and the behavior of the HRP-toxin complex may not represent that of the native toxin or its subunits, their results are also not inconsistent with ours. Holmgren and Lönnroth[9] stated that only about 1% of the cell-bound CT was found in the cytosol of mouse thymus cells. There is no satisfactory explanation for the difference between their results and outs at present.

Our data on the accumulation of cyclic AMP in mouse thymus cells are consistent with those of Lönnroth and Lönnroth[11]. It is interesting that although entry of the toxin molecule into the cell took place irrespective of the temperature, accumulation of cyclic AMP did not take place at lower temperature, but the normal response occurred with the usual time lag after shift of the temperature to 37°C. From this observation, we can say that the time lag in activation of adenylate cyclase may not represent the time required for penetration of toxin molecule into the cell, as stated by Fishman[1], but probably represents the time required for activation of the enzymatic process inside the cell.

This research was supported by a grant from the U.S.-Japan Cooperative Medical Science Program, Cholera Panel. The authors thank Akemi Takade and Yayoi Ichiki for help in electron microscopy.

REFERENCES

1. Fishman, P. H. 1980. Mechanism of action of cholera toxin: Studies on the lag period. J. Membrane Biol. **54**: 61–72.
2. Gill, D. M. 1976. The arrangement of subunits in cholera toxin. Biochemistry **15**: 1242–1248.
3. Gill, D. M. 1978. Seven toxic peptides that cross cell membranes. pp. 291–332. In Jeljaszewicz, J., and T. Wadström (eds.), Bacterial toxins and cell membrane. Academic Press, London, New York and San Francisco.
4. Gordon, P., L.-L. Carpentier, P. Freychert, and L. Orci. 1980. Internalization of polypeptide hormones. Diabetologia **18**: 263–274.
5. Goud, G., J.-C. Antoine, N. K. Gonatas, A. Stieber, and S. Avrameas. 1981. A comparative study of fluid-phase and adsorptive endocytosis of horseradish peroxidase in lymphoid cells. Exp. Cell. Res. **132**: 375–386.
6. Hansson, H. A., J. Holmgren, and L. Svennerholm. 1977. Ultrastructural localization of cell membrane ganglioside by cholera toxin. Proc. Natl. Acad. Sci. U.S.A. **74**: 3782–3786.
7. Holmgren J. 1978. Cholera toxin and the cell membrane. pp. 333–366. In Jeljaszewicz, J. and T. Wadström (eds.), Bacterial toxins and cell membrane. Academic Press, London, New York and San Francisco.

8. Holmgren, J., H. Elwing, P. Fredman, Ö. Strannegard, and L. Svennerholm. 1980. Gangliosides as receptors for bacterial toxins and Sendai virus. Adv. Exp. Med. Biol. 125: 453–470.

9. Holmgren, J., and I. Lönnroth. 1976. Cholera toxin and the adenylate cyclase activating signal. J. Infect. Dis. 133: supplement, 64–74.

10. Joseph, K. C., S. U. Kim, A. Stieber, and N. K. Gonatas. 1978. Endocytosis of cholera toxin into neuronal GERL. Proc. Natl. Acad. Sci. U.S.A. 75: 2815–2819.

11. Lönnroth, I., and C. Lönnroth. 1977. Interaction of cholera toxin and its subunits with lymphocytes, the effects on intracellular cAMP. Exp. Cell Res. 104: 15–24.

12. Misra, D. N., C. T. Ladoulis, L. W. Estes, and T. J. Gill, III. 1975. Biochemical and enzymatic characterization of thymic and splenic lymphocyte plasma membranes from inbred rats. Biochemistry 14: 3014–3024.

13. Moss, J., P. H. Fishman, R. L. Richards, C. R. Alving, M. Vaughan, and R. O'Brady. 1976. Choleragen-mediated release trapped glucose from liposomes containing ganglioside GM_1. Proc. Natl. Acad. Sci. U.S.A. 73: 3480–3488.

14. Moss, J., R. H. Fishman, and P. A. Watkins. 1980. In vivo degradation of ^{125}I-choleragen by normal human fibroblasts. pp. 279–288. In Proc. 15th Joint Conf. on Cholera, U.S.-Japan Cooperative Medical Science Program, NIH Publication no. 80-2003.

15. Moss, J., R. L. Richards, C. R. Alving, and P. H. Fishman. 1977. Effect of the A and B protomers of choleragen on release of trapped glucose from liposomes containing or lacking ganglioside GM_1. J. Biol. Chem. 252: 797–798.

16. Moss, J., and M. Vaughan. 1979. Activation of adenylate cyclase by choleragen. Ann. Rev. Biochem. 48: 581–600.

17. Oh'hara, I., and N. Ohsawa. 1982. The effect of cholera toxin on the HCG receptor in rat's testis. pp. 94–99. In Proc. 16th Joint Conf. on Cholera, U.S.-Japan Cooperative Medical Science Program, Japanese Cholera Panel, Toho University, Tokyo.

18. Ohtsuki, I., R. M. Manzi, G. E. Palade, and J. D. Jamieson. 1978. Entry of macromolecular tracers into cells fixed with low concentrations of aldehydes. Biol. Cellul. 31: 119–126.

19. Seeman, P. 1967. Transient holes in the erythrocyte membrane during hypotonic hemolysis and stable holes in the membrane after lysis by saponin and lysolecithin. J. Cell Biol. 32: 55–70.

20. Seeman, P., D. Cheng, and G. H. Iles. 1973. Structure of membrane holes in osmotic and saponin hemolysis. J. Cell Biol. 56: 519–527.

21. Silverstein, S. C., R. M. Steinman, and Z. A. Cohn. 1977. Endocytosis. Ann. Rev. Biochem. 46: 669–722.

22. Steinman, R. M., S. E. Brodie, and Z. A. Cohn. 1976. Membrane flow during pinocytosis, a stereologic analysis. J. Cell Biol. 68: 665–687.

23. Tsuru, S., M. Matsuguchi, N. Ohtomo, Y. Zinnaka, and K. Takeya. 1982. Entrance of cholera enterotoxin subunits into cells. J. Gen. Microbiol. 128: 497–502.

24. Tsuru, S., Y. Zinnaka, and K. Nomoto. 1981. Decrease in cholera toxin-binding T cells in aged mice and human volunteers. Int. Archs Allergy Appl. Immun. 64: 217–221.

25. Vaughan, M., and J. Moss. 1978. Mechanism of action of choleragen. J. Supramol. Struct. 8: 473–488.

Bacterial Diarrheal Diseases, eds., Y. Takeda, T. Miwatani, 153–160.

MECHANISM OF ACTION OF CHOLERAGEN: EFFECT OF TOXIN ON BINDING OF GUANYL NUCLEOTIDES

J. Moss, D. L. Burns, and M. Vaughan

Laboratory of Cellular Metabolism, National Heart, Lung, and Blood Institute, National Institutes of Health, Bethesda, Maryland 20205, U.S.A.

Choleragen (cholera toxin), the enterotoxin produced by *Vibrio cholerae* which is in large part responsible for the symptomatology of cholera, exerts its effects on cells through the activation of adenylate cyclase, resulting in an increase in intracellular cAMP[1-3]. Adenylate cyclase, a membrane-bound, multisubunit system, consists of at least three components: a specific hormone receptor, a guanyl nucleotide-binding protein referred to as G/F, and a catalytic unit[4, 5]. The hormone receptors are necessary for the binding of specific agonists to the cell membrane and are responsible, for example, for the effect of certain prostaglandins and peptide hormones on intracellular cAMP[4]; the catalytic unit is responsible for the conversion of ATP to cAMP[6, 7], and G/F is necessary for the coupling of receptor and catalytic unit as well as for the activation of catalytic unit by guanyl nucleotides[4, 5].

As first shown by Rodbell and co-workers[4, 8] hormonal activation of adenylate cyclase requires GTP (or a suitable analog). Cyclase activation by choleragen results from the NAD-dependent ADP-ribosylation of G/F catalyzed by the A_1 peptide of the toxin[9]. The participation of G/F in toxin-mediated effects on adenylate cyclase is supported by the observations that GTP plays a critical role in the toxin-dependent activation. GTP is required to observe optimal ADP-ribosylation of G/F, for stabilization of the activated enzyme, and for expression of the catalytic function of the activated enzyme[10-13]. It is generally believed that the cyclase is active when GTP is bound to G/F; hydrolysis of this bound GTP by an intrinsic GTPase produces an inactive cyclase ·GDP complex[14]. It has been suggested that choleragen enhances cyclase activity by inhibiting the specific GTPase activity, thereby preserving the active GTP· cyclase complex[15].

We investigated the possibility that choleragen might activate adenylate cyclase activity by another mechanism. It is known that isoproterenol, a β-adrenergic agonist that stimulates adenylate cyclase, enhances release of [^{3}H]GDP from turkey erythrocyte membranes that had previously bound [^{3}H]GTP in the presence of a β-adrenergic agonist[16]. Although [^{3}H]GTP was present during binding, the guanyl nucleotide released by isoproterenol in the second incubation appeared to be predominantly [³H]GDP[16, 17]. The conversion of [³H]GTP to [³H]GDP was attributed to the intrinsic GTPase associated with the adenylate cyclase complex[16]. Release of bound [³H]GDP by isoproterenol would clear the guanyl nucleotide-binding site, thereby facilitating GTP binding and resultant activation of the cyclase.

Effect of [³²P]ADP-ribosylation by toxin on release of specifically bound guanyl nucleotides from turkey erythrocyte membranes

To investigate the possibility that activation of adenylate cyclase by choleragen might result from enhanced release of guanyl nucleotides from G/F secondary to the toxin-catalyzed [³²P]ADP-ribosylation of this protein, membranes were specifically loaded with guanyl nucleotides by exposure to [³H]GTP and isoproterenol. They were then incubated with choleragen with or without NAD, and release of labeled nucleotides was determined. Release was enhanced by incubation of membranes with choleragen plus NAD but not by toxin or NAD alone or by toxin plus NADP (Table 1)[18]. In the presence of NAD, toxin catalyzes the ADP-ribosylation of G/F, resulting in the activation of adenylate cyclase; in the absence of NAD, toxin does not activate the cyclase[2]. NADP, which cannot substitute for NAD as a substrate for choleragen[19, 20], also could not replace NAD in the toxin-catalyzed reaction which leads to enhanced release of guanyl nucleotides by turkey erythrocyte membranes (Table 1). In addition, the increased release of guanyl nucleotides from the toxin-modified erythrocyte membranes was not apparently a secondary phenomenon resulting from activation of adenylate cyclase leading to an increase in cAMP; the addition of cAMP directly to the assay medium did not increase the rate of release of guanyl nucleotides (Table 2). Since the toxin-stimulated release would presumably proceed through a mechanism different from that of a β-adrenergic agonist, the rate of release of guanyl nucleotides from erythrocyte membranes by toxin and NAD was compared to that observed with isoproterenol (Fig. 1). Isoproterenol-stimulated release was considerably more rapid than that induced by toxin and NAD (Fig. 1). The maximal amounts of guanyl nucleotide released by the two treatments were, however,

Table 1. Effects of choleragen and pyridine nucleotides on release of guanyl nucleotides from turkey erythrocyte membranes

Membranes were incubated with additions as indicated for 60 min and guanyl nucleotide release was determined as previously described (18). At the beginning of the incubation, bound nucleotide was 0.82 pmol/mg protein. Data are the means ($\pm$S.E.) of values from three assays in a representative experiment. (Data reprinted from ref. 18.)

Additions	Nucleotide released
	(pmol/mg protein/hr)
None	0.33 ± 0.017
Choleragen, 250 μg/ml	0.32 ± 0.016
NAD, 2 mM	0.33 ± 0.004
NAD plus choleragen	0.45 ± 0.014
NADP, 2 mM	0.32 ± 0.017
NADP plus choleragen	0.33 ± 0.006

Table 2. Effect of cAMP on guanyl nucleotide release from turkey erythrocyte membranes
Membranes were incubated for 60 min as described (18) for assay of guanyl nucleotide release with
the addition of 2 mM NAD and, where indicated, 50 μM isoproterenol, 0.5 mM cAMP, and/or
choleragen, 250 μg/ml (activated by incubation at a concentration of 1 mg/ml for 10 min at 30°C in
50 mM glycine buffer, pH 8, containing 20 mM dithiothreitol). At the beginning of the 1-hr
incubation, bound nucleotide was 0.71 pmol/mg of protein. Data are reported as in Table 1.

Additions	Nucleotide released	Effect of isoproterenol
	(pmol/mg protein/hr)	
None	0.38 ± 0.018	+0.12
Isoproterenol	0.50 ± 0.021	
cAMP	0.37 ± 0.005	+0.12
cAMP, isoproterenol	0.49 ± 0.018	
Choleragen	0.45 ± 0.022	+0.03
Choleragen, isoproterenol	0.48 ± 0.020	

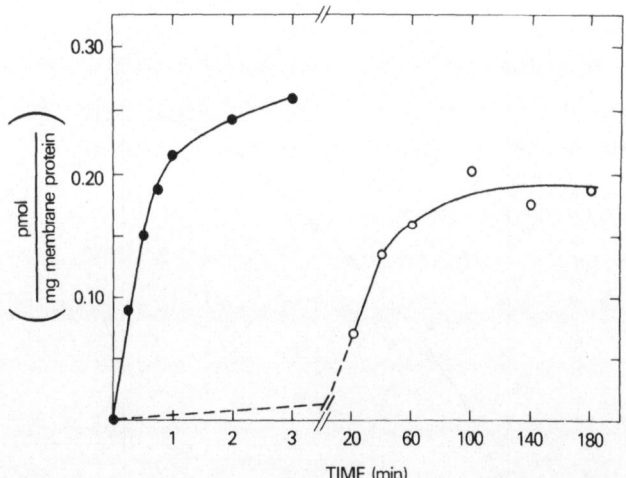

Fig. 1. Time course isoproternol-stimulated and choleragen-stimulated release of guanyl nucleotides.
Turkey erythrocyte membranes [³H]GTP were prepepared and incubated at 37°C in the presence of 2
mM NAD as described previously[18]. in one exproment, samples were incubated with or without 50 μM
isoproterenol and in another with or without choleragen, 250 μg/ml (activated as described in the
lengend to Table 2). At the indicated times, release of [³H] guanyl nucleotides was assayed[18]. The incre-
ment in nucleotide release induced by isoroternol (●) or choleragen (○) is shown. Release in the absence
of additions was 0.16 pmol/mg of protein/3 min in the experiment in which isoproternol-stimulated
rease was measured and 1.00 pmol/mg of protein/3 hr when choleragen-stimulated release was
measured. (From Ref. 18.)

Table 3.   Effect of choleragen on isoproterenol-stimulated release of guanyl nucleotides from turkey
erythrocyte membranes

Samples of membranes (0.5 mg of protein/ml) that had not been subjected to the final 1-hr
incubation and subsequent wash after "loading" with GTP (18) were incubated at 37°C for 1 hr in
the medium used for assay of nucleotide release containing 0.2 mM NAD with or without
choleragen, 250 μg/ml (activated as described in the legend to Table 2). Release was not
determined, however. Membranes were collected by centrifugation (5 min, 17,000 × g), washed
with cold buffer, sedimented again, and finally suspended in nine volumes of buffer. Samples were
then incubated for 8 min in buffer containing 4 mM MgCl$_2$, 1 mM dithiothreitol, and 0.5 mM
GTP without or with 50 μM isoproterenol (total volume 0.4 ml), and nucleotide released during
this period was determined. At the beginning of this incubation, nucleotide bound to membranes
not incubated with choleragen was 1.02 pmol/mg protein and that bound to membranes incubated
with the toxin was 0.91 pmol/mg protein. Data are reported as in Table 1. (Data reprinted from ref.
18.)

Membranes incubated with	Addition during release	Nucleotide released	Effect of isoproterenol
		(pmol/mg protein/8 min)	
NAD	None	0.13 ± 0.024	+0.12
	Isoproterenol	0.25 ± 0.017	
NAD plus choleragen	None	0.12 ± 0.008	+0.02
	Isoproterenol	0.14 ± 0.010	

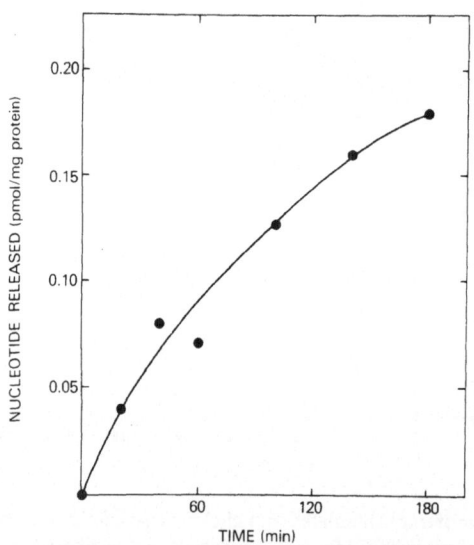

Fig. 2. Time course of choleragen-stimulated release of guanyl nucleotides. Membranes were loaded
with [³H]GTP[18]. Samples (0.11 mg of membrane protein) were incubated in buffer containing 20
mM thymidine, 4 mM GTP, 50 μM NAD, 0.3 mM App(NH)p and 0.35 mM Gpp(NH)p either with
or without activated choleragen (250 μg/ml) at 37°C for various times (total volume 0.1 ml). Release
was terminated by addition of 1.6 ml ice-cold buffer and assayed as previously described[18]. The
difference in the amount of guanyl nucleotide released from membranes incubated with and without
choleragen is plotted. Release from the latter in 3 hr was 0.87 pmol/mg of protein; bound nucleotide
before incubation was 1.09 pmol/mg of protein.

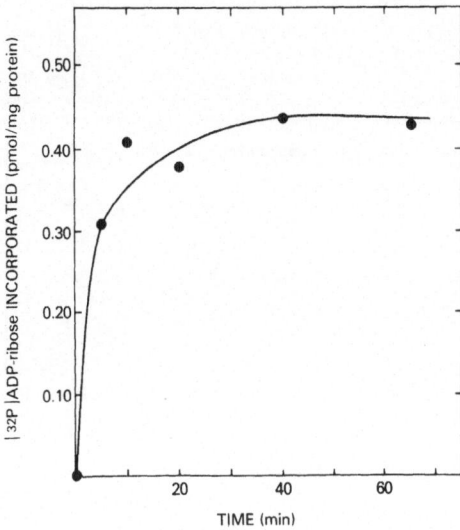

Fig. 3. Time course of choleragen-stimulated ADP-ribosylation of 42,000 dalton protein. Membranes were prepared as in Fig. 2 except that these were loaded with nonradioactive GTP and, during incubation either with or without activated choleragen, NAD was replaced by [^{32}P]NAD (1500 cpm/pmol). At the indicated times after addition of toxin, ADP-ribosylation was terminated by the addition of 2 ml of 10% trichloroacetic acid. Precipitate was sedimented for 5 min at 17,000 × g and subsequently prepared for sodium dodecyl sulfate-gel electrophoresis. Incorporation of ^{32}P into the 42,000 dalton subunit of G/F was determined quantitatively by cutting gels into 1-mM slices and measuring the radioactivity which migrated as a protein having that molecular weight. Radioactivity incorporated in the absence of toxin (0.68 pmol/mg of protein in 1 hr) was subtracted from that found in the presence of choleragen to obtain a value for toxin-stimulated incorporation.

similar (Fig. 1, Table 2). These data are consistent with the hypothesis that both toxin and isoproterenol specifically release guanyl nucleotide from the same membrane sites. In fact, when turkey erythrocyte membranes were loaded with guanyl nucleotides and then incubated with toxin and NAD, isoproterenol no longer enhanced release (Table 3).

As the critical event in adenylate cyclase activation in all probability is the toxin-catalyzed ADP-ribosylation of G/F, the rate of release of guanyl nucleotides was compared to the rate of ADP-ribosylation of G/F (Figs. 2 and 3)[21]. The release of guanyl nucleotide required more than 1 hr (Fig. 2). In contrast, ADP-ribosylation of G/F was essentially complete within 10 min (Fig. 3). It appears that the release of guanyl nucleotides is slow relative to the rate of [^{32}P]ADP-ribosylation of G/F.

Identification of guanyl nucleotide-binding protein as G/F factor

Since multiple guanyl nucleotide-binding proteins are present in avian erythrocyte membranes[22], an attempt was made to identify the protein responsible for binding the fraction of guanyl nucleotide that was released in response to isoproterenol or choleragen. Erythrocyte membranes were loaded with [^{3}H]GTP and then treated with toxin plus NAD or the β-adrenergic agonist; membrane

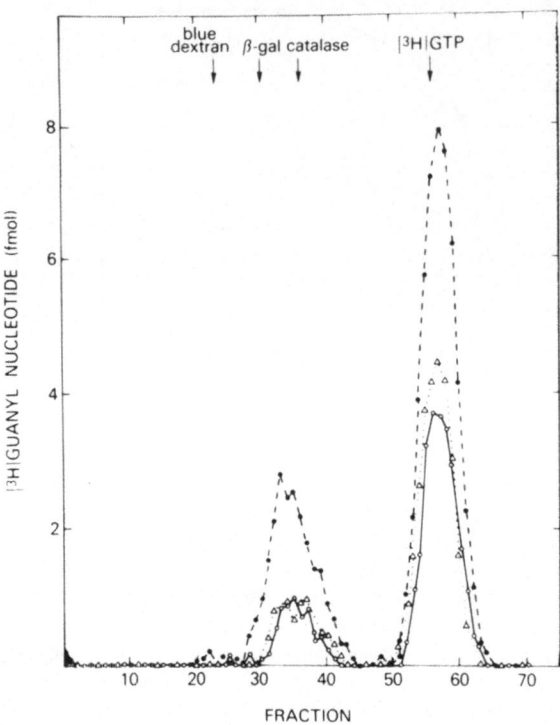

Fig. 4. Chromatography of solubilized membrane proteins on Ultrogel AcA 34. Membranes were incubated with 0.1 mM GTP and subsequently washed three times before loading with radiolabeled GTP in an attempt to decrease "nonspecific" binding of the latter. Loading of membranes with [³H]GTP (20,000 cpm/pmol) was performed as previously described[18]. Membranes were then incubated at 37°C for 1 hr in buffer containing 50 μM NAD and 0.1 mM Gpp(NH)p either with or without activated choleragen, 250 μg/ml. To further decrease "nonspecific" binding, membranes were washed and then incubated for 1 hr at 37°C in buffer containing 50 mM KCl, 30 mM MgCl₂, 0.05 mM EGTA, 0.1 mM App(NH)p, 0.5 mM GTP, 0.5 mM phosphoenolpyruvate, and pyruvate kinase, 37 units/ml. After repeating this process, membranes were incubated for 1 hr at 37°C in buffer containing 0.15 mM Gpp(NH)p, 0.5 mM GTP, 0.6 mM dithiothreitol with or without isoproterenol, 50 μM. Membranes were sedimented, washed once, sedimented and suspended in buffer (6 mg of protein/ml; total volume = 0.6 ml) and subsequently solubilized at 0°C in solutions containing 1% Lubrol PX, 35 mM Tris-HCl (pH 7.5), 0.1 mM MgCl₂, 0.1 mM EDTA, and 1 mM dithiothreitol (2.5 mg of protein/ml). After 15 min on ice and centrifugation at 100,000 × g for 30 min, a sample of the supernatant (280 μg of protein) was transferred to a column (0.8 cm × 43 cm) of Ultrogel AcA 34 eluted with 50 mM Tris-HCl (pH 7.5) containing 0.5% Lubrol PX, 0.1 mM EDTA, 0.1 mM MgCl₂, and 1 mM dithiothreitol. Radioactivity in fractions from untreated membranes (---), membranes treated with choleragen (—) membranes treated with isoproterenol (···) is shown. Positions of calibration standards (blue dextran, β-galactosidase, catalase and [³H]GTP) are indicated.

proteins solubilized with Lubrol PX were separated by gel filtration on Ultrogel AcA 34 columns. This procedure revealed a peak of guanyl nucleotide-binding activity that was clearly larger in solubilized preparations from untreated membranes than it was from toxin- or isoproterenol-treated membranes (Fig. 4). To identify this guanyl nucleotide-binding activity further, membranes that had been incubated with [^{32}P]NAD and toxin were solubilized in Lubrol PX and the extracted proteins were chromatographed on an Ultrogel AcA 34 column. The [^{32}P]ADP-ribosylated proteins in the peak of guanyl nucleotide-binding activity were analyzed by sodium dodecyl sulfate-polyacrylamide gel electrophoresis. The [^{32}P]ADP-ribosylated 42,000 dalton peptide of G/F chromatographed as a protein of the same size as the protein that released guanyl nucleotides upon incubation with isoproterenol or choleragen (data not shown). These data are consistent with the proposal that the GTP-binding protein, which specifically binds guanyl nucleotides under the assay conditions employed, is G/F. Both choleragen and isoproterenol by different mechanisms, one dependent on ADP-ribosylation[2] and one resulting from interaction of the agonist with the β-adrenergic receptor[23], enhance release of bound guanyl nucleotide from G/F[16, 18, 24]. In both cases, the released guanyl nucleotide is predominantly [^{3}H]GDP (data not shown).

Model for the role of guanyl nucleotides in the activation of adenylate cyclase

It is currently believed that adenylate cyclase is active as a cyclase·GTP complex. Inactivation of the complex occurs when an intrinsic GTPase converts cyclase·GTP to cyclase·GDP[15]. Reactivation of the cyclase·GDP results from release of GDP, freeing the guanyl nucleotide-binding site to once more bind GTP. Cassel and Selinger[15] proposed that choleragen acts in part by preserving the cyclase·GTP complex through inhibition of the activity of a specific intrinsic GTPase. The present studies demonstrate that choleragen may also activate adenylate cyclase by enhancing release of GDP from G/F. Assuming that inactivation of adenylate cyclase results from formation of cyclase·GDP from cyclase·GTP and that the rate-limiting step in reactivation is release of GDP from the inactive cyclase·GDP complex, choleragen may stimulate adenylate cyclase, in part, by accelerating release of guanyl nucleotides. In view of the prior observations that β-adrenergic agonists, which also activate adenylate cyclase, enhance release of guanyl nucleotide, albeit by a receptor-linked rather than by an ADP-ribosylation mechanism, there would appear to be precedent for activation resulting from removal of an inhibitory ligand.

We thank Mrs. D. Marie Sherwood for expert secretarial assistance.

REFERENCES

1. Finkelstein, R. A. 1973. Cholera. CRC Crit. Rev. Microbiol. **2**: 553–623.
2. Moss, J., and M. Vaughan. 1979. Activation of adenylate cyclase by choleragen. Ann. Rev. Biochem. **48**: 581–600.
3. Holmgren, J. 1981. Actions of cholera toxin and the prevention and treatment of cholera. Nature **292**: 413–417.
4. Rodbell, M. 1980. The role of hormone receptors and GTP-regulatory proteins in membrane

transduction. Nature **284**: 17–22.

5. Ross, E. M., and A. G. Gilman. 1980. Biochemical properties of hormone-sensitive adenylate cyclase. Ann. Rev. Biochem. **49**: 533–564.

6. Strittmatter, S., and E. J. Neer. 1980. Properties of the separated catalytic and regulatory units of brain adenylate cyclase. Proc. Natl. Acad. Sci. U.S.A. **77**: 6344–6348.

7. Ross, E. M. 1981. Physical separation of the catalytic and regulatory proteins of hepatic adenylate cyclase. J. Biol. Chem. **256**: 1949–1953.

8. Rodbell, M., L. Birnbaumer, S. L. Pohl, and H. M. J. Krans. 1971. The glucagon-sensitive adenylate cyclase system in plasma membrane of rat liver. V. The obligatory role of guanyl nucleotides in glucagon action. J. Biol. Chem. **246**: 1877–1882.

9. Moss, J., and M. Vaughan. 1981. Mechanism of action of choleragen and *E. coli* heat-labile enterotoxin: Activation of adenylate cyclase by ADP-ribosylation. Mol. Cell. Biochem. **37**: 75–90.

10. Enomoto, K., and D. M. Gill. 1980. Cholera toxin activation of adenylate cyclase. J. Biol. Chem. **255**: 1252–1258.

11. Moss, J., and M. Vaughan. 1977. Choleragen activation of solubilized adenylate cyclase: Requirement for GTP and protein activator for demonstration of enzymatic activity. Proc. Natl. Acad. Sci. U.S.A. **74**: 4396–4400.

12. Lin, M. C., A. F. Welton, and M. F. Berman. 1978. Essential role of GTP in the expression of adenylate cyclase activity after cholera toxin treatment. J. Cyclic Nucleotide Res. **4**: 159–168.

13. Nakaya, S., J. Moss, and M. Vaughan. 1980. Effects of nucleotide triphosphates on choleragen-activated brain adenylate cyclase. Biochemistry **19**: 4871–4874.

14. Cassel, D., and Z. Selinger. 1976. Catecholamine-stimulated GTPase activity in turkey erythrocyte membranes. Biochem. Biophys. Acta **452**: 538–551.

15. Cassel, D., and Z. Selinger. 1977. Mechanism of adenylate cyclase activation by cholera toxin: Inhibition of GTP hydrolysis at the regulatory site. Proc. Natl. Acad. Sci. U.S.A. **74**: 3307–3311.

16. Cassel, D., and Z. Selinger. 1978. Mechanism of adenylate cyclase activation through the β-adrenergic receptor: Catecholamine-induced displacement of bound GDP by GTP. Proc. Natl. Acad. Sci. U.S.A. **75**: 4155–4159.

17. Pike. L. J., and R. J. Lefkowitz. 1981. Correlation of β-adrenergic receptor-stimulated [³H]GDP release and adenylate cyclase activation. J. Biol. Chem. **256**: 2207–2212.

18. Burns, D. L., J. Moss, and M. Vaughan. 1982. Choleragen-stimulated release of guanyl nucleotides from turkey erythrocyte membranes. J. Biol. Chem. **257**: 32–34.

19. Moss, J., J. C. Osborne, Jr., P. H. Fishman, H. B. Brewer, Jr., M. Vaughan, and R. O. Brady. 1977. Effect of gangliosides and substrate analogues on the hydrolysis of nicotinamide adenine dinucleotide by choleragen. Proc. Natl. Acad. Sci. U.S.A. **74**: 74–78.

20. Gill, D. M. 1975. Involvement of nicotinamide adenine dinucleotide in the action of cholera toxin *in vitro*. Proc. Natl. Acad. Sci. U.S.A. **72**: 2064–2068.

21. Burns, D. L., J. Moss, and M. Vaughan. 1982. Choleragen accelerates release of guanyl nucleotides from the GTP-binding protein of adenylate cyclase. Fed. Proc. **41**: 5075.

22. Pfeuffer, T. 1977. GTP-binding proteins in membranes and the control of adenylate cyclase activity. J. Biol. Chem. **252**: 7224–7234.

23. Maguire, M. E., E. M. Ross, and A. G. Gilman. 1977. β-adrenergic receptor: Ligand binding properties and the interaction with adenyl cyclase. Adv. Cyclic Nucleotide Res. **8**: 1–83.

24. Cassel, D., and Z. Selinger. 1977. Catecholamine-induced release of [³H]Gpp(NH)p from turkey erythrocyte adenylate cyclase. J. Cyclic Nucleotide Res. **3**: 11–22.

Bacterial Diarrheal Diseases, eds., Y. Takeda, T. Miwatani, 161–168.

CHOLERA TOXIN AS A MITOTIC STIMULATOR OF EPIDERMAL CELLS *IN VITRO* AND *IN VIVO*

T. Kuroki

Department of Cancer Cell Research, Institute of Medical Science, University of Tokyo, Shirokanedai, Minato-ku, Tokyo-108, Japan

In our laboratory we have long been interested in the cellular and molecular mechanisms of chemical carcinogenesis in tissue culture systems for transformation, mutation and differentiation *in vitro*. We have recently started a project using human epidermal keratinocytes for this purpose, because of the importance of epithelial cells, especially human epithelial cells, in chemical carcinogenesis. In parallel with studies on benzo(a)pyrene metabolism in these cells[1, 2], we also examined suitable conditions for cultivation of epidermal cells for efficient utilization of limited amounts of materials. As reported by Green[3], we found that cholera toxin (CT) markedly stimulates growth of epidermal cells *in vitro*. We extended this finding by showing that CT induces epidermal hyperplasia *in vivo* by two successive synchronous divisions[4]. Here I would like to summarize our observations on epidermal cells. These observations seem significant in understanding not only the mode of action of CT but also the kinetics of cell proliferation.

Stimulation of in vitro growth of epidermal cells by CT

Human epidermal keratinocytes were isolated from dermatome-sectioned skin, obtained as discarded material during plastic surgery as described elsewhere[1, 2]. In primary cultures, CT at a concentration of 1 nM decreased the initial cell loss during the first 4 days: in the absence of CT the number of cells plated decreased to one-quarter on day 4 but in its presence the initial decrease was only 50%. However, CT had no significant effect on the growth rate during exponential growth or on the saturation density in the stationary phase. Colonial growth of these cells in secondary cultures was stimulated by CT, when cells were plated on top of lethally irradiated C3H10T1/2 cells as a feeder layer (Fig. 1). The plating efficiency was increased dose-dependently by CT and 1 nM CT caused two-fold increase in colony formation. CT also stimulated growth of cells after frozen stock of skin specimens. Thus, the stimulatory effect of CT on the epidermal cells seemed to be more pronounced when growth was limited. Epidermal growth factor (EGF) also stimulated growth of cells synergistically with CT.

The responses to CT of a variety of cells, including epidermal keratinocytes

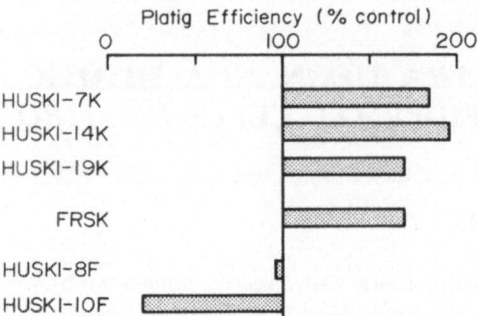

Fig. 1. Effect of CT on colony formation of epidermal and dermal cells. The plating efficiency in the absence of CT is taken as 100%. HUSKI-7K, -14K and -19K: human epidermal keratinocytes, FRSK: rat epidermal keratinocytes, HUSKI-8 and -10F: human dermal fibroblasts.

and dermal fibroblasts, were examined. As summarized in Fig. 1, CT specifically stimulated the growth of epidermal keratinocytes, both human (HUSKI-7K, -14K and -19K) and rat (FRSK). It is interesting that dermal fibroblasts, a counterpart of epidermal cells in skin tissue, were not stimulated, but rather inhibited (HUSKI-10F) or not affected by the toxin (HUSKI-8F).

The mechanism of action of CT was investigated with respect to the receptor of the toxin and induction of intracellular cyclic AMP. GMl ganglioside, the membrane receptor of the toxin, was isolatd from human epidermal and dermal cells by the method of Ledeen et al.[5]. CT caused marked increase in the level of intracellular cyclic AMP. As seen in Fig. 2, induction in epidermal cells was maximal 10 h after addition of CT, being 1280 pmoles per mg protein, or 340-fold the control level. It is interesting that cyclic AMP was also induced in dermal fibroblasts, irrespective of their growth response to CT. These results suggest that elevation of the cyclic AMP level may act as a mitotic signal in epidermal cells, while in dermal fibroblasts its level is not necessarily related to cell proliferation.

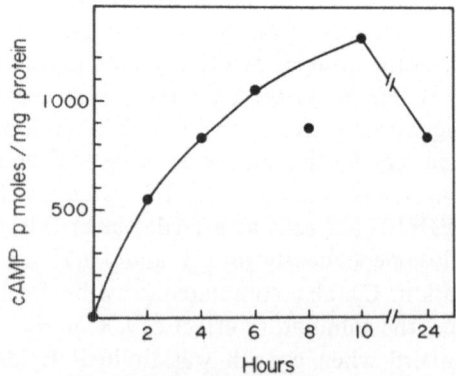

Fig. 2. Induction of cyclic AMP in epidermal keratinocytes by CT at a concentration of 1 nM.

Induction of synchronous divisions of epidermal cells in vivo by CT

During these *in vitro* studies, we noticed the report of Craig, published in 1965[6], that intracutaneous injection of CT into guinea pigs or rabbits evoked an acute reaction that was followed by a residual induration palpable for 6 to 7 days. Based on our observation that CT specifically stimulates growth of epidermal cells, we thought that this induration might be due to epidermal hyperplasia produced by CT, and this was, in fact, found to be the case.

Intracutaneous injection of CT at doses of more than 0.2 ng evoked an acute reaction at the site of injection, which was characterized by formation of a round blister and followed by residual induration of the skin for about 7 days, as described by Craig[6]. Histologically, the most prominent features of the skin lesion were edematous change of the dermis and subcutaneous tissues and mitotic stimulation of the epidermis. The edematous reaction is primarily due to increased permeability of capillaries, as shown by intravenous injection of pontamine sky blue, which evoked blueing at the site of skin lesion. The most striking observation was that CT stimulatd mitosis of basal cells of the epidermis and as a consequence produced epidermal hyperplasia. As seen in Fig. 3B and C, abundant mitotic figures were seen in demecolcine-treated epidermis 24 and 48 h after injection of 1 ng of CT. Epidermal hyperplasia reached a maximum on day 4 with formation of 8 to 12 cell layers (Fig. 3D), or 4- to 6-fold increase over normal or PBS-treated skin, which consists of two cell layers (Fig. 3A). This hyperplasia was induced by CT at doses of more than 0.2 ng.

The time course of events was investigated by measurement of mitotic cells 3 h after demecolcine-injection, DNA synthesizing cells 1 h after [^{3}H]-thymidine injection and the thickness of the epidermis. As shown in Fig. 4A, the mitotic index of basal cells increased from 18 h after the injection, reaching a first peak at 24 h and a second peak at 48 h. DNA synthesizing cells, determined by autoradiography as [^{3}H]-thymidine-incorporating cells, also showed two sharp peaks at 24 and 48 h after the injection (Fig. 4B). These indices returned to the normal range after 3 days. As a result of cell divisions, the thickness of the interfollicular epidermis had increased 4- to 6-fold on day 4 and then returned to normal on day 7 (Fig. 4C). This rapid recovery from epidermal hyperplasia seemed to be due to terminal differentiation of stimulated cells, as seen in the time course of change in thickness of the stratum granulosum and stratum corneum (Fig. 4D). This sequence of events indicates that CT induced two successive synchronous divisions of the epidermis and produced temporary hyperplasia without affecting epidermal differentiation.

These two synchronous divisions can be achieved either by division of the same cells twice successively or by division of different cells in the first and second divisions. The first possibility was supported by an experiment in which cells were pulse labelled with [^{3}H]-thymidine in the first division and chased for labelled mitosis by autoradiography.

The above experiments were performed by intracutaneous injection of 0.1 ml of CT solution into the skin of the back of mice. This was rather difficult because the skin is thin (Fig. 3A) and a skin reaction is produced in only a small

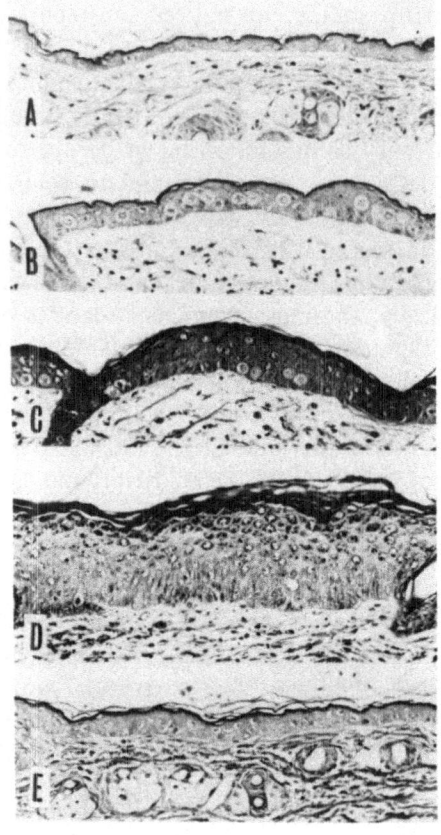

Fig. 3. Histological changes in mouse skin induced by intracutaneous injection of 1.0 ng of CT. A: control skin 24 h after PBS injection, B-E: Hyperplasia 24 h (B), 48 (C), 4 days (D) and 7 days (E) after CT injection. Mitoses were arrested by treatment with demecolcine for 3 h.

area; i.e. lesions of about 7 to 12 mm diameter were formed by 1 and 10 ng CT, respectively. We, therefore, improved this method by use of tongue forceps (ring-shaped, 20 mm in internal diameter) according to the method of Ishikawa *et al.*[7]. The skin of the back of mice under anesthesia with avertin was clamped in a double fold with tongue forceps for 1 h and 0.5 ml of CT solution was injected subcutaneously into the clamped area (Fig. 5). This method is much easier than intracutaneous injection and gives satisfactory results with high reproducibility. Painting the back of mice with CT evoked no response with up to 50 μg of CT per 3.0 cm², because the surface of the skin is protected by the stratum corneum and does not allow penetration of hydrophilic compounds such as CT.

Intact molecules of CT are required for inducton of epidermal hyperplasia. Preincubation of CT with anti-CT antibody at dilutions of up to 1 : 1250 for 60 min at 4°C abolished formation of blisters and induction of hyperplasia. Injection of the A or B unit of CT alone at doses of up to 320 ng evoked no skin

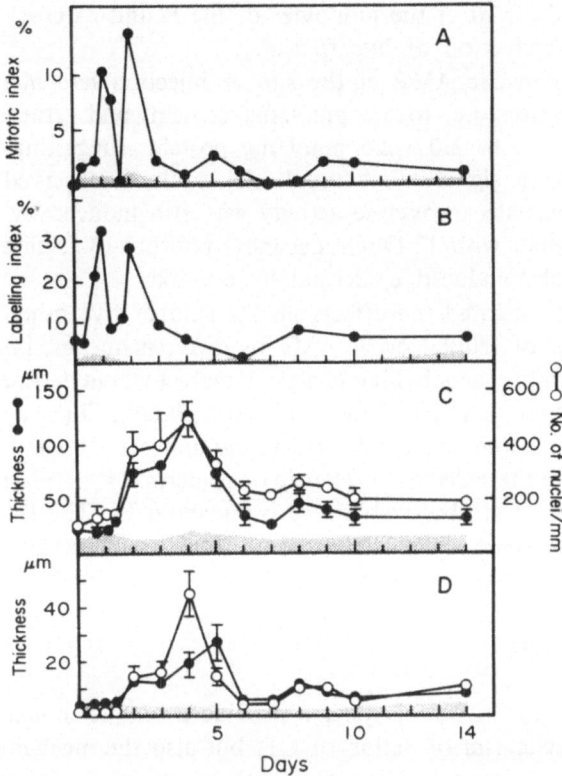

Fig. 4. Time-course of events induced by injection of 1.0 ng of CT into the dorsal skin of mice. The mice were killed between 4 to 6 p.m. to avoid the complication of possible circadian variation of the epidermal cell cycle. Demecolcine (2 μg/g of body weight) and [³H] thymidine (2 μCi/g of body weight) were injected intraperitoneally 3 h and 1 h, respectively, before the mice were killed. A: mitotic index (%) of basal cells, B: labeling index (%) of basal cells, C: thickness of the epidermis (o) and number of nuclei per 1-mm basement membrane (o), D:thickness of stratum corneum (•) and stratum granulosum (o). The shaded area in panels A, B, C, and D shows values for the controls treatd with phosphate buffer.

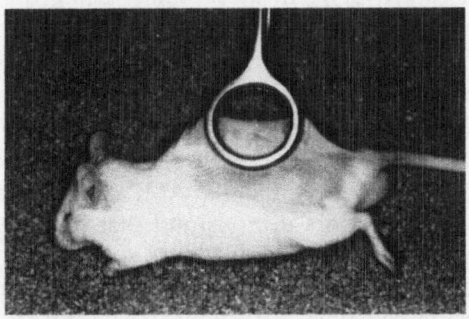

Fig. 5. Clamping of the skin with ring-shaped tongue forceps under anesthesia for injection of CT.

reaction at the site of injection. Preincubation of CT with GMl ganglioside at a molar ratio of 1 : 10 of the monomer of the B unit to GM1 ganglioside completely blocked induction of hyperplasia.

The level of cyclic AMP at the site of injection had increased two-fold 2 h after the injection, i.e. to 5.3 pmol/mg protein, and returned to the normal level after 6 h, i.e. to 2.0 - 2.5 pmol/mg protein, suggesting that cyclic AMP may act as a mitotic signal in epidermal cells *in vivo* as observed in those cultured *in vitro*. Ornithine decarboxylase activity was also induced by CT but to much a lesser extent than with 12-*O*-tetradecanoyl phorbol-13-acetate (TPA), a tumor promoter that also induced epidermal hyperplasia.

We then investigated the effects on the skin of five other agents known to increase the level of cellular cyclic AMP by different means, i.e., dibutyryl cyclic AMP (1 μg - 1 mg), theophylline (1 μg - 1 mg), 3-isobutyl-1-methylxanthine (0.1 - 100 μg), isoproterenol (1 μg - 1 mg) and prostaglandin El (10 ng - 10 μg), injected intracutaneously at the doses indicated in parentheses. However, these chemicals did not produce either edematous change or epidermal hyperplasia, although slight increse of mitosis was observed with prostaglandin El. The level of cyclic AMP after injection of these chemicals might be insufficient to trigger cell division of epidermal cells.

Concluding remarks

The present experimental systems provide a unique model for investigating not only the mechanism of action of CT, but also the mechanism of control of cell divisions *in vivo* and *in vitro*. Our preliminary results suggested that CT induces incresed permeability and epidermal hyperplasia by different mechanisms. Elucidation of these mechanisms would be of value in understanding the pathogenesis of diarrhea in chorera patients.

It is most surprising that there has been no previous report on CT-induced epidermal hyperplasia, because intracutaneous injection of CT has been used for quantitation of CT since the report of Craig in 1965[6]. CT induces much greater epidermal hyperplasia than TPA, suggesting that it could be used as a tumor promoter in two-stage skin carcinogenesis in mouse skin.

The possible implication of cyclic nucleotides in the regulation of cell division is a subject of much controversy. In most studies using fibroblastic cells, an increase in cellular cyclic AMP has been thought to result in inhibition of cell division, mainly based on the following three observations[8]. First, elevation of the intracellular level of cyclic AMP by various means results in inhibition of multiplication of various culturd cells. Second the intracellular level of cyclic AMP is low in growing fibroblasts in culture but increases as the cells cease division. Third, transformed cells have a low level of cyclic AMP and this is independent of the cell cycle. However, recent studies demonstratd that cyclic AMP plays a positive role in cell proliferation in certain cell types, as summarized in Table 1. A common feature of these cells is their epithelial or endothelial nature, suggesting that CT stimulates a specific cell type. CT should be useful in cell biology, e.g. in investigating the role of cyclic AMP in regulation of cell proliferation.

Table 1. Cells of which growth was stimulated by CT or other means to increase the intracellular level of cyclic AMP

Species	Cells	Use of CT	Rererences
Mouse	3T3 cells	yes	9, 10, 11
	Lymphocytes	no	12
	Melanoma cells (A variant)	no	13
	Epidermal keratinocytes	yes	14
Rat	Schwann cells	yes	15
	Liver epithelial cells	no	16
	Pancreatic islet cells	yes	17
	Epidermal keratinocytes	yes	unpublished data
Human	Vascular endothelial cells	yes	18
	Mammary epithelial cells	yes	19
	Epidermal keratinocytes	yes	3

Almost all synchronous divisions of cells have been achieved using cultured cells *in vitro* and only a few cases of synchronous cells *in vivo* have been reported, including salivary cells induced by isoproterenol and epidermal cells induced by TPA and ionophore A23187. CT is unique in that it induces two synchronous divisions. Possible association of various agents with the cell cycle can be investigated in the present system.

REFERENCES

1. Kuroki, T., N. Nemoto, and Y. Kitano. 1980. Metabolism of benzo(a)pyrene in human epidermal keratinocytes in culture. Carcinogenesis 1: 559–565.
2. Kuroki, T, J. Hosomi, K. Munakata, T. Onizuka, M. Terauchi, and N. Nemoto. 1982. Metabolism of benzo(a)pyrene in epidermal keratinocytes and dermal fibroblasts of humans and mice with reference to variations among species, individuals and cell types. Cancer Res. 42: 1859–1965.
3. Green, H. 1978. Cyclic AMP in relation to proliferation of the epidermal cells: A new view. Cell 15: 801–811.
4. Kuroki, T. 1981. Induction by cholera toxin of synchronous divisions *in vivo* in the epidermis resulting in hyperplasia. Proc. Natl. Acad. Sci U.S.A. 78: 6958–6962.
5. Ledeen, R. W., R. K. Yu, and L. F. Eng. 1973. Gangliosides of human myelin: Sialosylgalactosylceramide (G7) as a major component. J. Neurochem. 21: 829–839.
6. Craig, J. P. 1965. A permeability factor (toxin) found in cholera stools and culture filtrates and its neutralization by convalescent cholera sera. Nature 207: 614–616.
7. Ishikawa, T., K. Kodama, F. Ide, and S. Takayama. 1982. Demonstration of *in vivo* DNA repair synthesis in mouse skin exposed to various chemical carcinogens. cancer Res. 42: 5216–5221.
8. Pastan, I. H., G. S. Johnson, and W. B. Anderson. 1975. Role of cyclic nucleotides in growth control. Ann. Rev. Biochem. 44: 591–522.
9. Pruss, R. M., and H. R. Herschman. 1979. Cholera toxin stimulates division of 3T3 cells. J. Cell. Physiol. 98: 469–474.
10. Rozengurt, E., A. Legg, G. Strang, and N. Courtenay-Luck. 1981. Cyclic AMP: A mitogenic signal for Swiss 3T3 cells. Proc. Natl. Acad. Sci. U.S.A. 78: 4392–4396.
11. Schor, S., and E. Rozengurt. 1981. Enhancement by purine nucleosides and nucleotides of serum-induced DNA synthesis in quiescent 3T3 cells. J. Cell. Physiol. 81: 339–346.
12. Wang, T., J. R. Sheppard, and J. E. Foker. 1978. Rise and fall of cyclic AMP required for onset of lymphocyte DNA synthesis. Science. 201: 155–157.

13. Pawelek, J., R. Halaban, and G. Christle. 1975. Melanoma cells which require cyclic AMP for growth. Nature **258**: 539–540.

14. Marcelo, C. L. 1979. Differential effects of cAMP and cGMP on *in vitro* epidermal cell growth. Exp. Cell Res. **120**: 201–210.

15. Raff, M. C., A. Hornby-Smith, and J. P. Brockes. 1978. Cyclic AMP as a mitogenic signal for cultured rat Schwann cells. Nature **273**: 672–673.

16. Boynton, A. L., and J. F. Whitfield. 1979. The cyclic AMP-dependent initiation of DNA synthesis by T51B rat liver epithelioid cells. J. Cell. Physiol. **101**: 139–148.

17. Rabinovitch, A., B. Blondel, T. Murray, and D. H. Mintz. 1980. Cyclic adenosine-3',5'-monophosphate stimulats islet B cell replication in neonatal rat pancreatic monolayer cultures. J. Clin. Invest. **66**: 1065–1071.

18. Davison, P. M., and M. A. Karasek. 1981. Human dermal microvascular endothelial cells in vitro: Effect of cyclic AMP on cellular morphology and proliferation rate. J. Cell. Physiol. **106**: 253–258.

19. Taylor-paradimitriou, J., P. Purkis, and I. S. Fentiman. 1980. Cholera toxin and analogues of cyclic AMP stimulate the growth of cultured human mammary epithelial cells. J. Cell. Physiol. **102**: 317–321.

Bacterial Diarrheal Diseases, eds., Y. Takeda, T. Miwatani, 169–174.
Copyright © 1985 by KTK Scientific Publishers, Tokyo.

SECRETORY IMMUNITY TO VIBRIO CHOLERAE BACTERIA AND CHOLERA TOXIN: PROSPECTS FOR AN IMPROVED CHOLERA VACCINE

A-M Svennerholm, M. Jertborn, L. Gothefors, A. Karim, D. Sack and J. Holmgren

Department of Medical Microbiology, University of Göteborg, Guldhedsgatan 10, S-413 46 Göteborg, Sweden and International Centre for Diarrhoeal Disease Research, Bangladesh, G P O Box 128, Dhaka-2, Bangladesh

Evidence of protective immunity in cholera

While all age groups have been susceptible to cholera when it has spread into new areas, cholera is predominantly a disease of childhood in endemic areas. Studies in Bangladesh have shown a close inverse relationship between attack rate of cholera and age and also with serum (vibriocidal) antibody titers. This kind of epidemiologic pattern is characteristic of infections which evoke immunity following either disease or inapparent infection. There is also epidemiologic data from endemic areas which indicates that second attacks of cholera within a year or two are extremely rare (1, 2, R Glass *et al.*, to be published).

The most covincing evidence that cholera evokes protective immunity has come from volunteer studies. Recovery from disease, induced by perorally administered cholera vibrios, is associated with solid resistance for at least 3 years to rechallenge with either homologous or heterologus vibrio serotypes[3]. This protection not only prevents the clinical manifestations of disease, but also reduces multiplication of vibrios in the bowel so that organisms cannot be found in stool cultures.

Nature of protective immunity

Studies of convalescents have shown that clinical cholera evokes a significant vibriochidal as well as enterotoxin-neutralizing antibody response in serum[1]. The vibriocidal antibodies are mainly directed against the cell wall lipopolysaccharide (LPS) of *Vibrio cholerae*. Studies in animals have clearly shown that both the anti-LPS and the anti-toxin antibodies can protect against experimental cholera, and furthermore, that the two types of antibodies, when present in the gut, give synergistic protective cooperation[4]. The identification of these two protective antibodies does not exclude the possible importance of additional protective antibody specificities, directed for instance against flagellar or outer membrane protein (e.g. hemagglutinin) antigens.

Although the protective specificities of antibodies appear in serum after cholera infection it is unlikely that the serum antibodies per se have more than a marginal protective role[5]. The cholera vibrios do not invade the intestinal tissue but remain in the lumen or are reversibly attached to the epithelium. Also the pathogenic enterotoxin is confined to the lining intestinal epithelium. Only antibodies present in the gut lumen, in the mucus layer or on the epithelial surface can thus protect against development of disease, mainly by counteracting colonization and multiplication of the vibrios and/or preventing binding of enterotoxin to the intestinal epithelium. While very high concentrations of serum antibodies by way of diffusion into the intestine may contribute to protection, it is likely that the main protective role is played by secretory IgA antibodies produced locally in the gut[5]. Recent studies have shown that natural cholera infection evokes local formation of secretory IgA antibodies against both *V. cholerae* LPS and enterotoxin[6]. The associated serum antibody levels seem to represent a combination of IgA and, possibly, IgM "spill-over" from the intestinal synthesis, and IgG and IgM antibodies formed by lymph nodes and spleen in response to immunogenic fragments of bacteria and toxin absorbed from the gut.

Recent studies in animals have yielded new knowledge about the local immune response to cholera antigens. An important finding has been the identification of a mucosal immunologic memory which may persist for a much longer period than the IgA response in itself[7]. It is presently unknown whether the long-lasting immunity after clinical cholera infection is due to the persistence of a protective antibody synthesis or to an immunologic memory which responds so efficiently to renewed antigen contact that it turns into a protective IgA antibody response, which aborts the new infection before it has given rise to clinical symptoms.

Implications for the design of cholera vaccines

In contrast to clinical cholera disease the parenteral whole-cell cholera vaccines (WCV) give only partial immunity for <6 months. The WCV probably fail both because they lack any toxin-derived antigen and because the injection route may be relatively inefficient in stimulating local immunity in the gut mucosa[5].

Purified cholera B subunit is a logical "toxoid" immunogen against cholera, especially for oral immunization. It is a strong protective immunogen against experimental cholera in rabbits when given either alone or in combination with somatic antigens[8]. It was recently tested for its ability to stimulate mucosal immunity in humans; a single oral administration stimulated a marked local secretory IgA antibody response in 80% of the recipients[9].

With regard to the somatic antigen component in an improved oral cholera vaccine El Tor cholera vibrios, grown and killed so that not only LPS but also more delicate antigens such as hemagglutinin are preserved, is the most readily available alternative.

Genetic methods may also supply *V. cholerae* strains which selectively lack the gene for the "toxic" A subunit. By retaining the ability to colonize the intestine and produce immunogenic B subunit, such strains could be useful as live oral cholera vaccines. It must be borne in mind, however, that any living vaccine of this sort will require thorough testing for stability and lack of side-effects before it can be used in humans. In that respect it is disappointing that the first such *V. cholerae* strain (Texas Star)[10], produced diarrhoea (although usually very mild) in about 20% of recipient American volunteers in spite of producing no detectable holotoxin when grown *in vitro*.

Mucosal immunogenicity in humans of an oral, combined B subunit - whole cell vaccine

With these aspects in mind we have recently undertaken a study in Bangladeshi volunteers which was designed to answer several important questions about gut mucosal antibody formation and immunologic memory to vaccine candidate cholera antigens: 1) Will a combination of B subunit and whole-cell vaccine (B + WCV) stimulate mucosal antitoxic as well as antibacterial antibody formation? 2) Is the response comparable to that attained by clinical cholera infection? 3) How does the immunologic memory for a mucosal response to immunization compare between naturally-exposed volunteers, the same volunteers after a single immunization, and convalescents after clinical cholera?

Three groups (I-III) with eight healthy women in each were given two peroral (PO) or two IM immunizations with combined vaccine 28 days apart and one group (nine persons) of cholera convalescents a single PO vaccination in the doses indicated in Table 1. Intestinal lavage specimens were collected as previously described[6,9] on day 0, 3, 9 and 28 after each immunization or 9 and 28 days after onset of disease. Antitoxin and antibacterial antibodies in the lavages were measured by means of the ELISA using purified cholera toxin (CT) and lipopolysaccharide (LPS) respectively as solid phase antigens[11]. Total IgA was determined by means of a very sensitive immunobead ELISA method[12] to permit expression of all titres in relation to total Ig. Preliminary data from these analyses are now available.

It was found that a single PO administration of 2.5 mg of B subunit (group I) induced a significant IgA antitoxin increase with the same frequency (88%) as did the clinical infection (89%), (Table 2). Also the magnitude and the duration

Table 1.   Immunization protocol for combined cholera B subunit-whole cell vaccine

Immunization group	Immunization						
	Initial			Second			
	Route	B-sub (mg)	WCV (vibrios)	Route	B-sub (mg)	WCV (vibrios)	
Cholera convalescents	Clinical cholera			PO	0.5	5×10^{10}	
I	PO	2.5	5×10^{10}	PO	—"—	—"—	
II	PO	0.5	5×10^{10}	PO	—"—	—"—	
III	IM	0.15	6×10^9	IM	0.15	6×10^9	

of the responses were similar after the two types of immunization (Fig. 1). A secondary immunization with 0.5 mg of B subunit was equally effective in inducing an antitoxin antibody response irrespective of whether it followed a high PO dose of B subunit or "priming" due to cholera infection. The magnitude of the secondary responses only slightly exceeded those obtained by the initial immunization (Fig. 1). When the lower dose of B subunit (0.5 mg) was given throughout (group II) the immunization had to be repeated to induce a significant titre increase in most of the women (Table 2). Also a single or two IM injections (group III) induced significant antitoxin IgA titre rises in most instances, 67% and 57% respectively, but the duration of the response after the initial immunization was significantly shorter after the IM than the PO route (Fig. 1).

With regard to the antibacterial antibody response, clinical cholera induced a substantial IgA titre rise to *V. cholerae* LPS in intestinal lavage (Fig. 2) in 8/9 of the women. A single PO or IM vaccination with WCV induced an anti-LPS titre increase in several instances (Table 2) but the response was much smaller than after the clinical infection (Fig. 2). Two PO administrations of WCV, on the other hand, induced IgA anti-LPS responses comparable to those evoked by the clinical infection in 12/13 of the women (see Fig. 2, and combined groups I + II in Table 2). Not only the magnitude but also the duration were superior to the results after the conventional 2-dose parenteral immunization regimen (Fig. 2).

With regard to memory induction, a single PO immunization with combined vaccine was apparently equally effective as clinical cholera in preparing the intestine for a local IgA antibody response to restimulation by cholera antigens. Thus, the second PO immunization with combined vaccine (group I) resulted in antitoxin as well as antibacterial antibody responses of similar magnitude to those achieved in the cholera convalescents after vaccination (Figs. 1 and 2). Furthermore, in both groups these responses were seen within three days, which is earlier than the detectable response to a single immunization (Figs. 1 and 2).

CONCLUSIONS

Locally-produced IgA antibodies are of prime importance for protective im-

Table 2. Frequency of antitoxin (anti-CT) and antibacterial (anti-LPS) responses in intestinal IgA among cholera convalescents and vaccine recipients

Immunization group	Responders to:			
	Initial immunization		Second immunization	
	anti-CT	anti-LPS	anti-CT	anti-LPS
Cholera convalescents	8/9*	8/9	7/9	8/9
I PO + PO	7/8	4/6	8/8	5/6
II PO + PO	3/8	4/8	5/7	7/7
III IM + IM	6/9	5/9	4/7	4/6

*Number of volunteers with a > 2-fold rise in ELISA IgA antibody/total IgA in intestinal lavage in relation to day 0

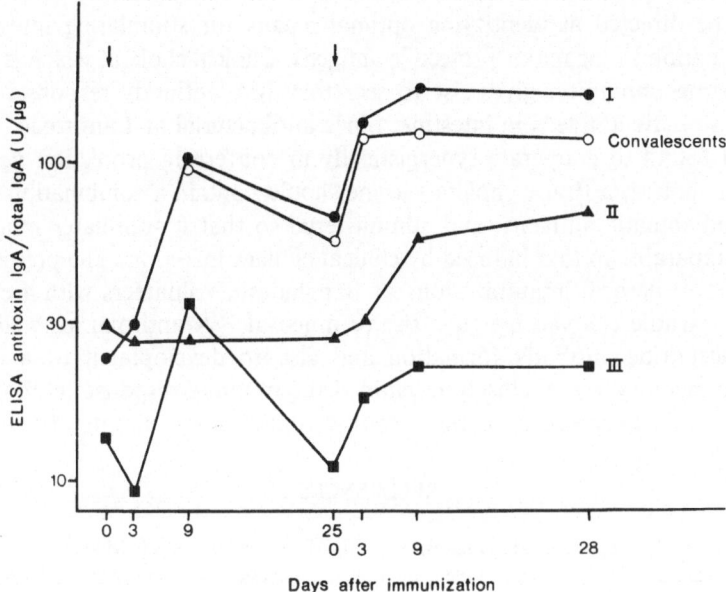

Fig. 1. The IgA antitoxin antibody response in intestinal lavage after clinical cholera infection and after one or two immunizations with combined B subunit - WCV. Geometric means of IgA antitoxin titres per total amount of IgA are shown. For immunization groups see Table 1. (↓) day of immunization.

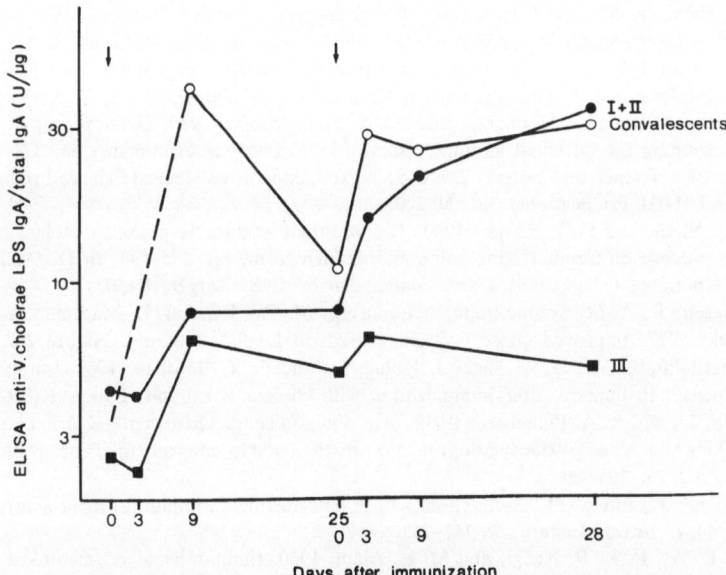

Fig. 2. The IgA antibody response to *V. cholerae* LPS in intestine after clinical cholera infection and after PO (•) or IM (■) administration of combined vaccine. Geometric means of IgA anti-LPS titres per total amount of IgA are shown. (↓) day of immunization.

munity against noninvasive enteric infections. The immunization efforts should therefore be directed at identifying optimal means for stimulating intestinal antibody formation to the major protective antigens. Clinical cholera, which is followed by longlasting immunity, gives rise to secretory IgA antibody responses to toxin as well as somatic antigens in intestine. Since antibacterial and antitoxic immunity have been found to cooperate synergistically in conferring protection against experimental cholera, a future cholera vaccine should contain a combination of toxin-derived and somatic antigens, and administered so that it stimulates mucosal immunity comparable to that induced by clinical cholera infection. The present results show that two peroral immunizations of Bangladeshi volunteers with a combined B subunit - whole cell vaccine gave rise to mucosal IgA antitoxin as well as anti-lipopolysaccharide antibody formation and also to development of a local immunologic memory which closely resembled the immune response in cholera convalescents and was superior to the response obtained by parenteral vaccination.

REFERENCES

1. Glass, R. I., S. Becker, I. M. Hug, B. J. Stoll, M. V. Kahn, M. H. Merson, J. W. Lee and R. E. Black. 1982. Endemic cholera in rural Bangladesh 1966–1980. Am. J. Epidemiol. **116**: 959–970.

2. Merson, M. H., R. E. Black, M. Kahn, and I. Huq. 1980. Epidemiology of cholera and enterotoxigenic *Escherichia coli* diarrhea, pp. 34–45. *In* Ö. Ouchterlony and J. Holmgren (ed.), Cholera and related diarrheas. S. Karger, Basel.

3. Levine, M. M., R. E. Black, M.-L. Clements, D. R. Nalin, L. Cisneros, and R. A. Finkelstein. 1981. Volunteer studies in development of vaccines against cholera and enterotoxigenic *Escherichia coli*, pp. 444–459. *In* T. Holme *et al.* (ed.), Acute enteric infections in children. Elsevier, Amsterdam.

4. Svennerholm, A.-M., and J. Holmgren. 1976. Synergistic protective effect in rabbits of immunization with *Vibrio cholerae* lipopolysaccharide and toxin/toxoid. Infect. Immun. **13**: 735–740.

5. Svennerholm, A.-M. 1980. Nature of protective cholera immunity, pp. 171–184. *In* Ö. Ouchterlony and J. Holmgren (ed.), Cholera and related diarrheas. S. Karger, Basel.

6. Sack, D., A. Islam, J. Holmgren, and A.-M. Svennerholm. 1980. Development of methods for determining the intestinal immune response to *V. cholerae* in humans, pp. 423–439. *In* 15th Joint Conference on Cholera. The U.S.-Japan Cooperative Medical Science Program, Cholera Panel, NIH Publications, No. 80-2003.

7. Pierce, N. F., and F. T. Koster. 1980. The intestinal immune response to cholera toxin/toxoid: Dependence on immunization route and antigen form, pp. 185–194. *In* Ö. Ouchterlony and J. Holmgren (ed.), Cholera and related diarrheas. S. Karger, Basel.

8. Holmgren, J., A.-M. Svennerholm, I. Lönnroth, M. Fall-Persson, B. Markman, and H. Lundbäck. 1977. Improved cholera vaccine based on L-subunit toxoid. Nature **269**: 602–604.

9. Svennerholm, A.-M., D. A. Sack, J. Holmgren, and P. K. Bardhan. 1982. Intestinal antibody responses in humans after immunization with cholera B subunit. Lancet *I* (8267): 305–308.

10. Honda, T., and R. A. Finkelstein. 1979. Selection and characteristics of a *Vibrio cholerae* mutant lacking the A (ADP ribosylating) portion of the cholera enterotoxin. Proc. Natn. Acad. Sci. U.S.A., **76**: 2052–2056.

11. Holmgren, J., and A.-M. Svennerholm. 1973. Enzyme-linked immunosorbent assays for cholera serology. Infect. Immun. **7**: 757–763.

12. Sack, D. A., P. K. B. Neogi, and M. K. Alam. 1980. Immunobead enzyme-linked immunosorbent assay for quantitation of immunoglobulin A in human secretions and serum. Infect. Immun. **29**: 281–283.

Bacterial Diarrheal Diseases, eds., Y. Takeda, T. Miwatani, 175–189.
Copyright © 1985 by KTK Scientific Publishers, Tokyo.

MOLECULAR HETEROGENEITY OF *VIBRIO CHOLERAE* NON-O1 ENTEROTOXINS

K. Yamamoto[1], Y. Takeda[1], T. Miwatani[1], and J. P. Craig[2]

Department of Bacteriology and Serology, Research Institute for Microbial Diseases, Osaka University, 3-1, Yamada-oka, Suita, Osaka 565, Japan[1]*, and Department of Microbiology and Immunology, State University of New York, Downstate Medical Center, Brooklyn, New York, U.S.A.*[2]

Vibrio cholerae non-O1 strains are now recognized as causative agents of diarrheal disease[1-9]. Some cases of diarrhea due to non-O1 vibrios have been reported to be very similar to cholera, and production of cholera-like enterotoxin by some strains of non-O1 vibrios has been suggested. Zinnaka and Carpenter[10] and Ohashi and his coworkers[11] independently reported that some strains of non-O1 vibrios produced an active substance which was biologically similar to cholera toxin. However, a high degree of purification of the enterotoxin produced by non-O1 vibrios has not been reported. We recently reported[12] that a strain of non-O1 vibrio, serovar 0344, isolatd from fresh water in Louisiana, produces an enterotoxin which is biologically similar to cholera toxin and we demonstrated that the toxin was immunologically identical to cholera toxin in the Ouchterlony immunodiffusion test.

In this paper, we report the purification of the enterotoxin from this strain of non-O1 vibrio and conclude that the purified toxin could not be distinguished from cholera toxin in biological and immunolocal properties or in molecular structure. We also report here, however, that the enterotoxin purified from a strain of non-O1 vibrio isolated from a diarrhea patient was biologically and immunologically similar, but *not identical* to cholera toxin in its molecular structure.

Partial purification of E8498 non-O1 enterotoxin

Table 1 summarizes the procedure used for the purification of the toxin. This method is essentially based on that reported for cholera toxin[13-15]. A lincomycin-resistant strain[16] of *Vibrio cholerae* E8498 isolated from fresh water in Lousiana in 1978 was used. This strain was kindly supplied by Dr. Paul Blake, Centers for Disease Control, Atlanta, Georgia, U.S.A. The strain was inoculated into Roux flasks containing 150 ml of Casamino acids-Yeast extract medium supplemented with glucose and 300 μg/ml lincomycin and incubated in the resting state for 48 hrs at 30°C. The cultures were pooled and centrifuged. The pH of the culture supernatant was adjusted to 5.0 with hydrochloric acid. 0.1% aluminum hydrox-

Table 1.　Purification procedure

V. cholerae E8498Lin^r, non-01
48-hr stationary culture with
300 μg/ml lincomycin
↓
Culture supernatant
↓
Al (OH)$_3$ absorption at pH 5.0
↓
Washing
↓
Elution with TEAN buffer,* pH 8.5
↓
50% Sat. AmSO$_4$ precipitation
↓
Column chromatography

---

*50 mM Tris-HCl buffer containing 3 mM NaN$_3$, 1 mM EDTA and 0.2 N NaCl.

ide powder was added to the supernatant and the mixture was stirred 6 hrs and allowed to stand for 18 hrs. After centrifugation, the precipitate was washed several times with 0.01M ammonium formate, then eluted with TEAN buffer, pH 8.5. This elution procedure was repeated six times and the supernatants were pooled. The pooled eluates were concentration by 50% saturation with solid ammonium sulfate. The precipitate was dissolved in TEAN buffer pH 8.5 and this preparation was used for further purification.

Purification of E8498 non-O1 enterotoxin by column chromatography

This partially purified toxin was applied to a column of Sephadex G-100 equilibrated with TEAN buffer, pH 7.8. As shown in Fig. 1, one major protein peak was found and the toxin as monitored by passive immune hemolysis (PIH) using purified cholera antitoxin, was eluted after the major protein peak. The active fractions (toxin antigen) were pooled and concentrated by Amicon PM10 membrane.

The Sephadex G-100 eluate was applied to a Bio-Gel A-5m column and three peaks of protein were obtained as shown in Fig. 2. The immunological activity was found in the third peak. The active fractions were concentrated and applied to a Sephadex G-75 column. The results are shown in Fig. 3. Two peaks of toxin antigen as determined by PIH were obtained by gel filtration on Sephadex G-75. The first peak was eluted simultaneously with the absorbance peak at 280 nm. Since vascular permeability activity was found only in the first peak it was considered likely that the second antigen peak might be a choleragenoid–like substance[13]. The first peak was concentrated and rechromatographed on the same column (Fig. 4). The protein peak corresponded well with the peak of toxin antigen. The antigen-containing fractions were concentrated and used as purified E8498 toxin for further studies. The steps used in the purification of E8498 toxin are summarized in Table 2.

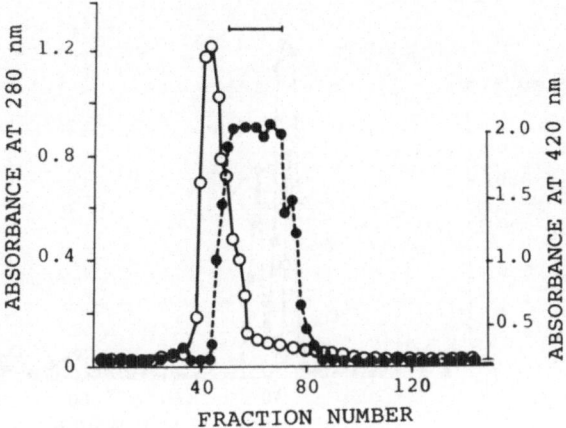

Fig. 1. Sephadex G-100 column chromatogram of E8498 enterotoxin. Toxin partially purified by Al(OH)$_3$ was applied to the column. ○, A$_{280}$; •, hemolysis by PIH(A$_{420}$); —, pooled active fractions.

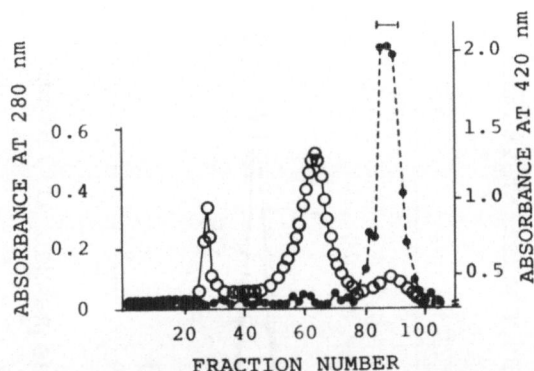

Fig. 2. Bio-Gel A-5m column chromatogram of E8498 enterotoxin. Sample prepared by Sephadex G-100 (Fig. 1) was applied to the column. ○, A$_{280}$; •, hemolysis by PIH(A$_{420}$); —, pooled active fractions.

Polyacrylamide gel disc electrophoresis

The homogeneity of the purified toxin was examined on conventional polyacrylamide gel disc electrophoresis (Fig. 5). The purified non-O1 toxin gave a single disc and identical mobility to that of purified O1 cholera toxin. The reference cholera toxin used in these studies was purified from *Vibrio cholerae* 569B[14] and was provided by Dr. N. Ohtomo.

Biological and immunological activities

We then carried out studies to determine whether or not E8498 toxin has biological and immunological properties similar to those of 569B toxin. The effect

178

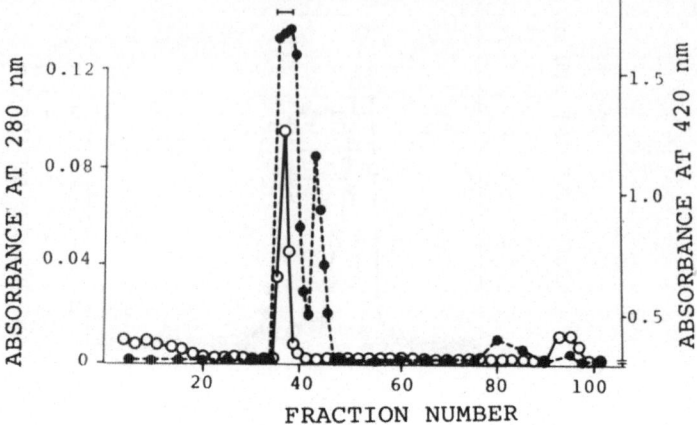

Fig. 3. Sephadex G-75 column chromatogram of E8498 enterotoxin. Sample prepared by Bio-Gel A-5m (Fig. 2) was applied. ○, A_{280}; •, hemolysis by PIH(A_{420}); —, pooled active fractions.

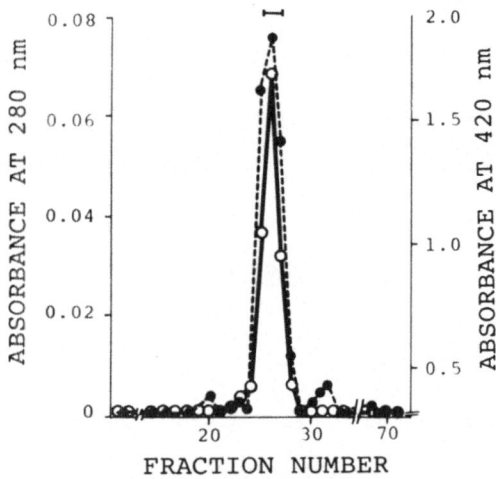

Fig. 4. Sephadex G-75 column chromatogram of E8498 enterotoxin. Sample prepared by sephadex G-75 (Fig. 3) was rechromatographed. ○, A_{280}, •, hemolysis by PIH(A_{420}); —, pooled active fractions.

on Chinese hamster ovary cells[17] was examined. Dose-response curves are shown in Fig. 6. 50% of the CHO cells became elongated when about 1.3 ng/ml of non-O1 toxin was added to the medium whereas about 4.2 ng/ml of cholera toxin were needed to give equal activity.

Non-O1 toxin caused accumulation of clear fluid in adult mouse ligated intestinal loops[18]. Fig. 7 shows that the weight per length ratio of 140 mg/cm, which is about half of the mean maximal intensity, was produced by about 70-80

Table 2. Purification of enterotoxin from *V. cholerae* E8498, 0344

Fraction	Total volume (ml)	Total Protein (mg)	Total PF activity (BD$_4$)	Specific activity (BD$_4$/mg)	Relative activity	Yield of PF activity (%)
Partially purified enterotoxin	26	385	5.6×10^8	1.5×10^6	1	100
Sephadex G-100 column eluate	9.3	42	1.2×10^8	2.6×10^6	1.7	21
Bio-gel A-5M column eluate	2.0	4.0	1.0×10^8	2.5×10^7	17	18
1st Sephadex G-75 column eluate	1.0	2.8	9.9×10^7	3.5×10^7	23	18
2nd Sephadex G-75 column eluate	1.2	0.68	6.4×10^7	9.4×10^7	63	11

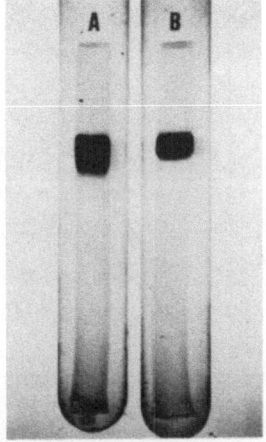

Fig. 5. Polyacrylamide gel disc electrophoresis of 569B and E8498 enterotoxins. A, 569B toxin; B, purified E8498 enterotoxin; 100 μg of each toxin was applied.

ng of both 569B and E8498 toxin, indicating that enterotoxic potencies were about the same for both toxins.

E8498 toxin also caused increased vascular permeability in rabbit skin[12, 19, 20]. Dose-response curves, with and without cholera antitoxin, are shown in Fig. 8. E8498 toxin contained 94 million BD$_4$/mg and 569B toxin, 98 million. Thus one BD$_4$ of 569B toxin was 10.2 pg and one BD$_4$ of E8498 to toxin was 10.6 pg. Limit of blueing (Lb) titrations[21] are shown on the right in Fig. 8. Graded doses of toxin were mixed with equal volumes of standard cholera antitoxin at a concentration of 1 antitoxin unit per ml. One Lb of 569B toxin was 56.8 ng and one Lb of E8498 toxin was 57.8 ng. These results show that not only was the specific PF activity the same for both toxins, but also the amount of antitoxin needed for neutralization was identical.

180

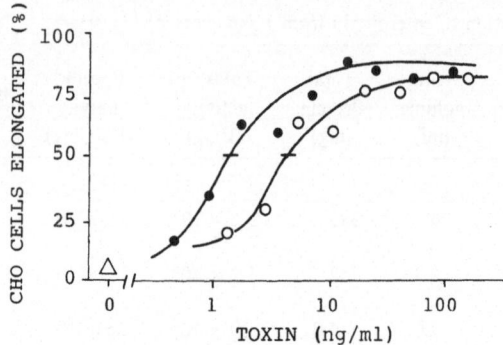

Fig. 6. Dose-response curve of morphological change in Chinese hamster ovary (CHO) cells by purified E8498 enterotoxin and 569B toxin. ○, 569B toxin; •, purified E8498 enterotoxin. Each toxin was added to the culture medium of CHO cells at the final concentration indicated and percentages of elongated cells were enumerated after 18 h incubation. Each point indicates a mean of 8 determinations.

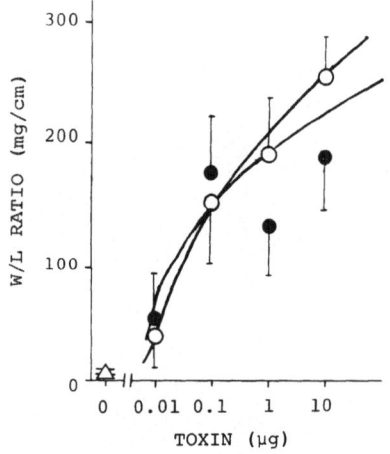

Fig. 7. Fluid accumulation in mouse intestinal loops by E8498 and 569B toxins. 569B toxin (○) or E8498 toxin (•) were inoculated into ligated small intestinal loops of adult mice. Each value represents mean ± one standard error of five determinations.

In passive immune hemolysis[22] both toxins showed very similar dose-response curves, where 6.6 ng of E8498 toxin, and 9.5 ng of 569B toxin produced hemolysis of 50% of red blood cells in this system. Fig. 9 shows that purified E8498 toxin is very similar to 569B toxin not only in biological activities but also in antigenic content. Thus, we can say that specific biological and immunological activities of both toxins were very similar considering the possible experimental errors of these systems. The comparisons of specific activities of E8498 and 569B toxins are summarized in Table 3.

181

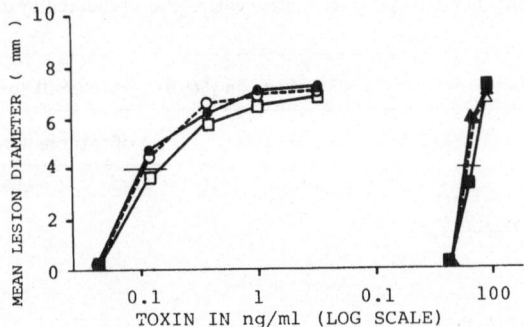

Fig. 8. Dose-response curves of PF activity of 569B, E8498 and S7 enterotoxins. BD₄ (•, ○, □) and Lb (▲, △, ■) of 569B toxin (•, ▲), E8498 toxin (○, △) and S7 toxin (□, ■) were determined for each curve. Each value represents the mean blueing lesion diameter (mm) observed 1 hr after iv injection of blue dye given 24 h after intracetaneous injection of toxin. The description of S7 toxin appears later in the text.

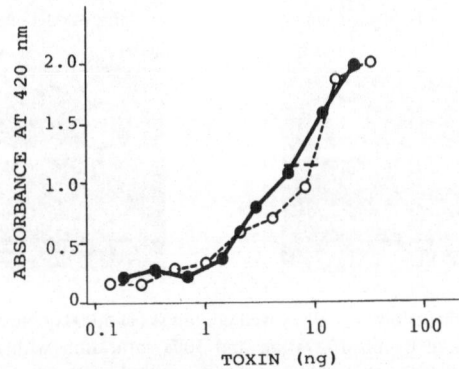

Fig. 9. Dose response curves of E8498 and 569B toxins by PIH. ○, 569B toxin; •, E8498 toxin.

Immunodiffusion test

More evidence that both toxins were immunologically identical was obtained by Ouchterlony immunodiffusion test[23] using anticholera toxin and anti-purified E8498 non-O1 toxin as shown in Fig. 10. Each serum gave an identical single precipitation line against all three antigens with no spurs, indicating that purified and crude E8498 toxins are immunologically identical and are both identical to 569B toxin.

Analysis of molecular structure by SDS-PAGE

In order to analyze molecular structure of this non-O1 toxin, sodium dodecyl sulfate polyacrylamide gel electrophoresis (SDS-PAGE) was carried out. As shown in Fig. 11, in column 2, E8498 toxin gave two bands showing mobility identical

Table 3. Biological and immunological activities of enterotoxins produced by 01 and non-01 strains of *V. cholerae*

Assay	01 toxin (569B)	Non-01 toxin (E8498,0344)
	ng of toxin required	
CHO cell assay (Amount causing 50% elogation, Final concentration in the medium, per ml)	4.2	1.3
Mouse intestinal loop test (Mount producing W/L = 140 mg/cm)	70–80	
Rabbit skin test		
BD$_4$	0.0102	0.0106
Lb	56.8	57.8
Passive immune hemolysis (Amount causing 50% hemolysis)	9.5	6.6

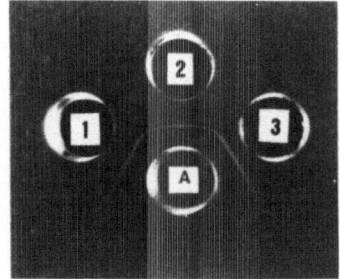 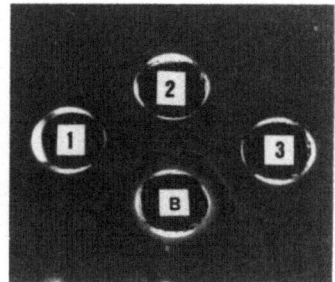

Fig. 10. Agar gel immunodiffusion test. Each well contains: (1) 5,000x concentrated *V. cholerae* E8498 culture supernatant prepared by ultrafiltration and 50% saturation with ammonium sulfate[12], (2) purified E8498 toxin, (3) 569B toxin, (A) anti-569B antitoxin (B) anti-E8498 antitoxin.

to each of the A and B of 569B toxin, which are shown in the left column. When the samples were reduced by dithrothreitol (DTT), the larger subunit of E8498 toxin, which was coincident with subunit A of 569B toxin, split into two bands, A$_1$ and A$_2$, as shown in column 4. The four columns on the right serve as references.

These patterns suggest that E8498 toxin is composed of the same A and B subunits as 569B toxin. That is, the biologically active A subunit appears to be composed of a single molecule each of A$_1$ and A$_2$, which are linked by a disulfide bond[24, 25] and the A subunit complex is noncovalently bound to the aggregate of B subunits[26-28] as is now well-established for 569B toxin.

Since the toxin produced by E8498, an environmental strain, has the same specific biologic activity as 569B toxin, it clearly provides this organism with the potential for being a causative agent of diarrhea. The amount of toxin produced in vitro by E8498 is relatively small, but no less than that synthesized in vitro by many known virulent O1 strains of *V. cholerae* of the el tor biotype[29]. Since,

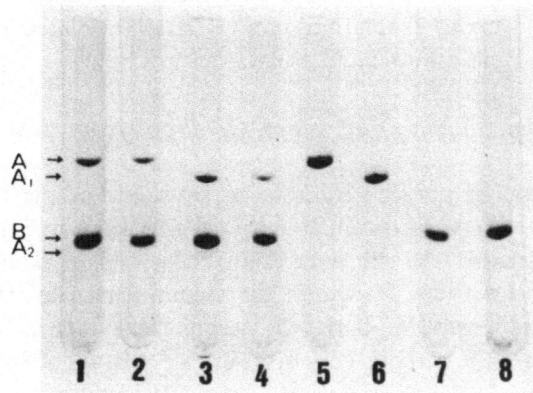

Fig. 11. SDS-PAGE of E8498 enterotoxin. Columns 1 and 3, 569B toxin; columns 2 and 4, purified E8498 toxin; columns 5 and 6, subunit A of 569B toxin; columns 7 and 8, subunit B of 569B toxin; columns 2, 4, 6 and 8, reduced with DTT.

however, other factors of virulence, in addition to the enterotoxin, are no doubt required to produce diarrhea in humans, the actual enteropathogenic potential of this non-O1 strain can be demonstrated only by oral challenge in volunteers.

Immunodiffusion test of enterotoxins from V. cholerae non-O1 strains from patients with diarrhea

Toxins produced by several other non-O1 strains were then examined by the Ouchterlony immunodiffusion test (Fig. 12). Strain S7 was isolated from a diarrhea patient in the Sudan in 1968 by Dr. Y. Zinnaka. Strain 62058 was isolated from a patient in Bangladesh and provided by Dr. I. Huq; strain WBDV-101E₁ was isolated from a patient in Thailand and provided by Dr. P. Echeverria.

As shown in Fig. 12, the toxin preparations in the peripheral wells gave single

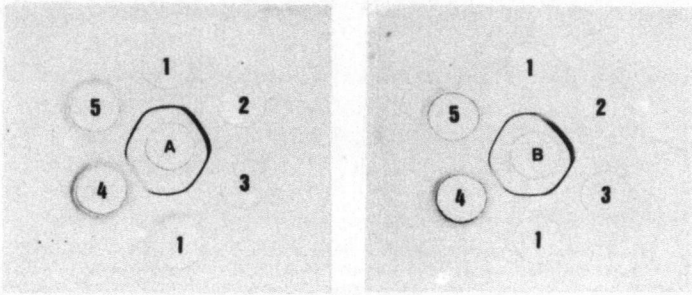

Fig. 12. Agar gel immunodiffusion test of enterotoxins from *V. cholerae* non-O1 strains from patients with diarrhea. Well 1, 569B toxin; well 2, purified E8498 toxin; well 3, partially purified S7 toxin; well 4, partially purified WBDV-101E₁ toxin; well 5, partially purified 62058 toxin; well A, anti-569B antitoxin; well B, anti-purified E8498 anti-toxin.

lines against both anti-569B antitoxin and anti-E8498 antitoxin. These findings suggested that the toxins from four non-O1 strains isolated from patients were immunologically identical to 569B toxin.

Purification of enterotoxin from a non-O1 strain from a human patient

We then prepared purified enterotoxin from one of the patient strains, S7. Fig. 13 shows the last purification step by gel filtration on Sephadex G-75. Two peaks of absorbance at 280 nm were found. The first peak has both biological and immunological activity. However, the second peak was immunologically active but biologically inactive. Thus, the second peak looked like choleragenoid. The first peak had PF activity very similar to 569B and E8498 toxins (Fig. 8). The Lb doses of S7, 569B, and E8498 toxins were also very similar.

Immunodiffusion test of S7 toxin

In Ouchterlony double immunodiffusion test, 569B, E8498 and S7 toxins gave single lines against anti-569B antitoxin, anti-E8498 antitoxin and anti-S7 antitoxin (Fig. 14).

PAGE studies of S7 toxin

When purified S7 toxin was analyzed on SDS-disc gel electrophoresis it showed a molecular pattern similar to that of 569B toxin (Fig. 15). This finding at first suggested that S7 and 569B toxins were identical. However, when conventional disc electrophoresis was carried out. S7 toxin migrated faster than 569B or E8498 toxins as shown in Fig. 16. That is, the relative mobility (R_f) of S7 toxin was about 0.38 whereas those of 569B and E8498 toxins were about 0.27. This finding agrees with the earlier finding of Zinnaka and Fukuyoshi[30] concern-

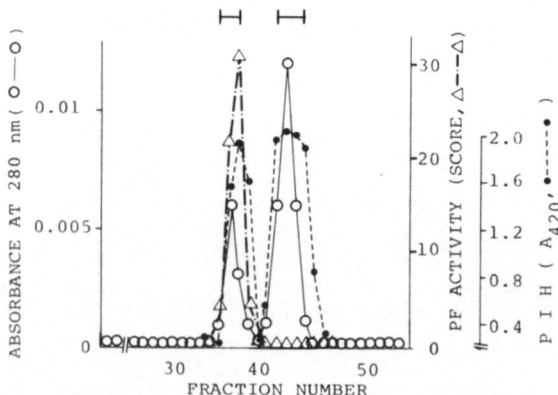

Fig. 13. Sephadex G-75 column chromatogram of S7 enterotoxin. Sample was prepared by column chromatography on Sephadex G-100 and Bio-Gel A-5m. ○, A_{280}; •, hemolysis by PIH(A_{420}); △, PF activity (Scores of blue lesions[12]).

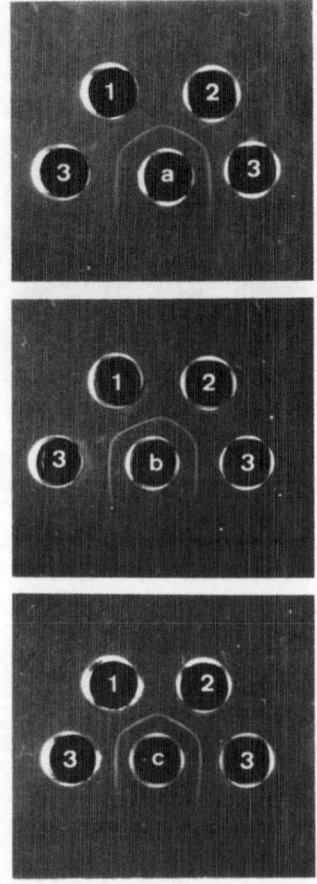

Fig. 14. Agar gel immunodiffusion test of 569B, E8498 and S7 toxins. (a) anti-569B antitoxin (b) anti-E8498 antitoxin (c) anti-S7 antitoxin (1) 569B toxin (2) E8498 toxin (3) S7 toxin.

ing an enterotoxin produced by strain S2, a strain which was isolated from the same epidemic as S7 in the Sudan.

SDS slab gel electrophoresis

Since this difference suggested differences in molecular size, we attempted to determine the molecular weight of each subunit of S7, using SDS-slab gel electrophoresis (Fig. 17). Subunit B of S7 was slightly smaller than that of 569B and E8498 toxins. This difference is probably less than 1,000 daltons judging from the molecular weight calibration curve (not shown). We then obtained further evidence that the molecular compositions of S7 and 569B toxins are not identical (Fig. 18). Mild treatment with 0.1% SDS for 30 min at 37°C before electrophoresis would be expected to yield aggregated subunit B. Unexpectedly the aggregated subunit B of S7 toxin was much larger than those of 569B and E8498 toxins.

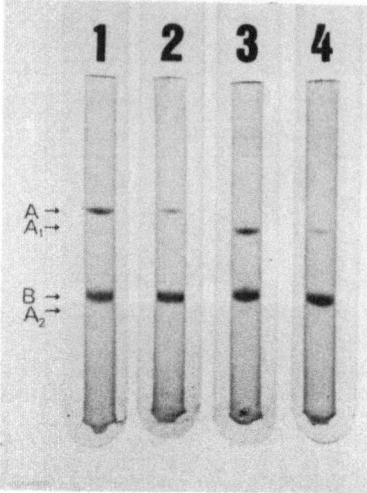

Fig. 15. SDS-disc PAGE of S7 toxin. Columns 1 and 3, 569B toxin; columns 2 and 4, purified S7 toxin; columns 3 and 4, reduced by DTT.

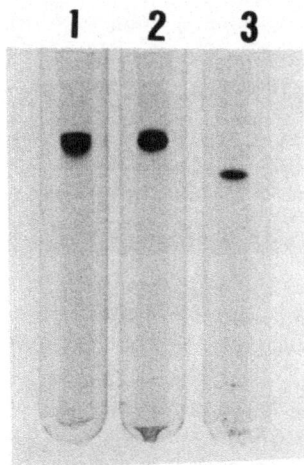

Fig. 16. Conventional PAGE of 569B, E8498 and S7 toxins. (1) 569B toxin (2) E8498 toxin (3) S7 toxin; 100 μg of each toxin was applied.

Moreover the choleragenoid-like substance of S7, called S7-oid in Fig. 13, was of identical molecular size to the aggregated subunit B of S7 toxin as shown in column 4 of the slab gel (Fig. 18). Therefore, if the molecular weight of each B subunit of S7 toxin is less than that of 569B toxin (Fig. 17), and if the aggregate of the B subunits is larger than that of cholera toxin (Fig. 18), then the number of B subunits in S7 toxin is greater than that of 569B toxin.

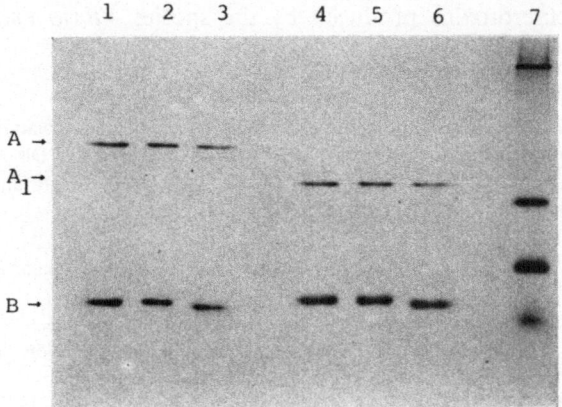

Fig. 17. SDS-slab PAGE of 569B, E8498 and S7 toxins. (1, 4) 569B toxin; (2, 5) E8498 toxin; (3, 6) S7 toxin; (7) protein markers; (4, 5, 6) reduced by DTT. Each sample was boiled for 3 min with 0.1% SDS before electrophoresis.

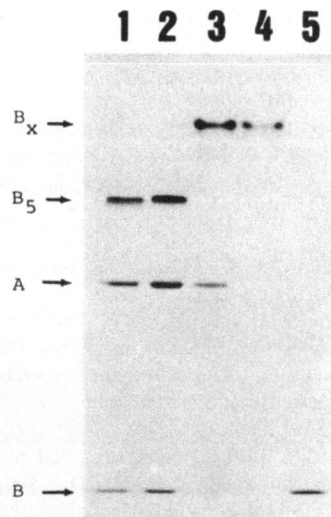

Fig. 18. SDS-slab PAGE of unboiled 569B, E8498 and S7 toxin. Each sample except column 5 was incubated for 30 min at 37 C with 0.1% SDS. Column 5 was boiled for 3 min with 0.1% SDS. (1) 569B toxin, (2) E8498 toxin, (3) S7 toxin, (4, 5) choleragenoid substance (S7-oid) of S7 toxin (second peak of Fig. 13).

SUMMARY

Preliminary findings described in this paper suggest that some non-O1 strains may produce a toxin which is identical to the toxin produced by the O1 strain, 569B, whereas other non-O1 stains produce a toxin with minor differences in B subunit size and number. We think this is the first demonstration of molecular differences in enterotoxins produced by the species *Vibrio cholerae*.

REFERENCES

1. Aldová, E., K. Laznickova, E. Stepankova, and J. Lietava. 1968. Isolation of non-agglutinable vibrios from an enteritis outbreak in Czechoslovakia. J. Infect. Dis. **118**: 25–31.
2. Bhattacharya, S., A. K. Bose, and A. K. Ghosh. 1971. Permeability and enterotoxic factors of non-agglutinable vibrios, *Vibrio alkaligenes* and *Vibrio parahaemolyticus*. Appl. Microbiol. **22**: 1159–1161.
3. Blake, P. A., R. E. Weaver and D. G. Hollis. 1980. Dseases of humans (other than cholera) caused by vibrios. Ann. Rev. Microbiol. **34**: 341–367.
4. Finkelstein, R. A. 1973. Cholera, Crit. Rev. Microbiol. **2**: 553–623.
5. Goodner, K., H. L. Smith, Jr., K. A. Monsur, and I. Huq. 1966. Non-cholera vibrios in diarrheal diseases of East Pakistan. East Pakistan Med. J. **10**: 1–9.
6. Hughes, J. M., D. G. Hollis, E. J. Gangarosa, and R. E. Weiner. 1978. Non-cholera vibrio infections in the United States. Amer. Int. Med. **88**: 602–606.
7. Kaper, J. B., S. L. Moseley, and S. Falkow. 1981. Molecular characterization of environmental and nontoxigenic strains of *Vibrio cholerae*. Infect. Immun. **32**: 661–667.
8. MacIntyre, O. R., J. C. Feeley, W. B. Greenough, III, A. S. Benenson, S. I. Hassan, and A. Saad. 1966. Diarrhea caused by non-cholera vibrios. Amer. J. Trop. Med. Hyg. **14**: 412–418.
9. Singh, S. J. and S. C. Sanyal. 1978. Enterotoxicity of the so-called NAG vibrio. Ann. Soc. Belg. Med. Trop. **58**: 133–140.
10. Zinnaka, Y. and C. C. J. Carpenter. 1972. An enterotoxin produced by non-cholera vibrios. Johns Hopkins Med. J. **131**: 403–411.
11. Ohashi, M., T. Shimada, and H. Fukumi. 1972. *In vitro* production of enterotoxin and hemorrhagic principle by *Vibrio cholerae*, NAG, Jpn. J. Med. Sci. Biol. **25**: 179–194.
12. Craig, J. P., K. Yamamoto, Y. Takeda, and T. Miwatani. 1981. Production of cholera-like enterotoxin by a *Vibrio cholerae* non-O1 strain isolated from the environment. Infect. Immun. **34**: 90–97.
13. Finkelstein, R. A. and LoSpalluto, J. J. 1972. Production of highly purified choleragen and choleragenoid. J. Infect. Dis. **141**: 64–70.
14. Ohtomo, N., T. Muraoka, H. Inoue, H. Sasaoka and H. Takahashi. 1973. Preparation of cholera toxin and immunization studies with cholera toxoid, pp. 132–142, *In* Proceedings of the Ninth Joint Cholera Conference of the U.S.-Japan Cooperative Medical Science Program, Grand Canyon, Arizona, Department of State Publication No. 8762, U.S. Department of State, Washington, D.C.
15. Spyrides, G. J., and J. C. Feeley. 1970. Concentration and purification of cholera toxin by absorption on aluminum compound gels. J. Infect. Dis. Suppl. **121**: S96–S99.
16. Yamamoto, K., Y. Takeda, T. Miwatani, and J. P. Craig. 1981. Stimulation by lincomycin of production of cholera-like enterotoxin in *Vibrio cholerae* non-O1. FEMS Microbiol. Letters. **12**: 245–248.
17. Honda, T., M. Shimizu, Y. Takeda, and T. Miwatani. 1976. Isolation of a factor causing morphological changes of Chinese hamster ovary cells from the culture filtrate of *Vibrio parahaemolyticus*. Infect. Immun. **14**: 1028–1033.
18. Takeda, Y., T. Takeda, T. Yano, K. Yamamoto, and T. Miwatani. 1979. Purification and partial characterization of heat-stable enterotoxin of enterotoxigenic *Escherichia coli*. Infect. Immun. **25**: 978–985.
19. Craig, J. P. 1965. A permeability factor (toxin) found in cholera stool and culture filtrates and its neutralization by convalesent cholera sera. Nature (London) **207**: 614–616.
20. Craig, J. P. 1971. Cholera toxin. pp. 189–254, *In* Bacterial toxins vol. IIA Davis, S., Montie, T. and Ajl, S. J., (eds.), Academic Press, New York.
21. Craig, J. P. 1978. Toward the development of a standard reference cholera antitoxin. Report of Ad Hoc Committee of the US cholera Panel. Develop. Biol. Standard., **41**: 414–422.

22. Tsukamoto, T., Y. Kinoshita, S. Taga, Y. Takeda, and T. Miwatani. 1980. Value of passive immune hemolysis for detection of heat-labile enterotoxin produced by enterotoxigenic *Escherichia coli*. J. Clin. Microbiol., **12**: 768–771.

23. Ouchterlony, O. 1969. Antigen-antibody reactions in gels. Acta Pathol. Microbiol. Scand. **26**: 507–515.

24. Lai, C. Y., E. Mendez, and D. Chang. 1976. Chemistry of cholera toxin: the subunit structure. J. Infect. Dis. Suppl. **133**: S32–S30.

25. van Heyningen, S. 1976. The subunits of cholera toxin: structure, stoichiometry, and function. J. Infect. Dis. Suppl. **133**: S5–S13.

26. Cuatrecasas, P., I. Parikh, and M. D. Hollenberg. 1973. Affinity chromatography and structural analysis of *Vibrio cholerae* enterotoxin- Ganglioside agarose and the biological effects of ganglioside-containing soluble polymers. Biochemistry, **12**: 4253–4264.

27. Lönnroth, I., and J. Holmgren. 1973. Subunit structure of cholera toxin. J. Gen. Microbiol. **76**: 417–427.

28. Ohtomo, N., T. Muraoka, A. Tashiro, Y. Zinnaka and D. Amako. 1976. Size and structure of the cholera toxin molecule and its subunits. J. Infect. Dis. Suppl. **133**: S31–S40.

29. Craig, J. P. 1982. The vibrio diseases in 1982: an overview. Proceedings of this Symposium.

30. Zinnaka, Y. and S. Fukuyoshi. 1973. Further observations on the NAG vibrio toxin. pp. 61–81. *In* Proceedings of the Ninth Joint Cholera Conference of the U.S.-Japan Cooperative Medical Science Program, Grand Canyon, Arizona, Department of State Publication no 8762, U.S. Department of State, Washington, D.C.

Bacterial Diarrheal Diseases, eds., Y. Takeda, T. Miwatani, 191–199.
Copyright © 1985 by KTK Scientific Publishers, Tokyo.

MOLECULAR GENETIC STUDY ON THE PATHOGENICITY OF AN ENTEROTOXIGENIC *ESCHERICHIA COLI* STRAIN OF HUMAN ORIGIN

T. Yamamoto and T. Yokota

Department of Bacteriology, School of Medicine, Juntendo University, 2-1-1 Hongo, Buykyo-ku, Tokyo, Japan

An enterotoxigenic *Escherichia coli* strain H10407 (serotype O78:H11) was isolated from a patient with diarrhoea in Bangladesh. It has been demonstrated that *E. coli* H10407 causes diarrhoea by adhesion of bacterial cell-surface structures, named colonization factor antigen I (CFA/I), to epithelial cells of the small intestine and by production of enterotoxins named heat-labile toxin (LT) and heat-stable toxin (ST)[1, 2]. Three species of plasmids have been found in *E. coli* H10407[1-6]: a CFA/I- and ST-coding plasmid ($56-60 \times 10^6$ molecular weight), an LT-coding plasmid (42×10^6 molecular weight) and a cryptic plasmid ($3.7-3.8 \times 10^6$ molecular weight). To gain further information on the molecular nature of the plasmids and the genetic traits of the virulence in *E. coli* H10407, we isolated and characterized each species of plasmid. We found that *E. coli* H10407 carries at least four distinct species of plasmid: the CFA/I- and ST-coding plasmid found previously, an LT- and ST-coding plasmid, a self-transmissible plasmid and a small cryptic plasmid(s).

Isolation of E. coli H10407-plasmids

In previous experiments[7], we isolated an LT- and ST-coding plasmid (pJY11) from *E. coli* H10407, a strain originatd in the laboratory of D. G. Evans and kindly provided by H. Ohashi. Briefly, the experimental procedure was as follows: (i) RP4 carrying an ampicillin (Ap) transposon, Tn*l*, was introduced into *E. coli* H10407; (ii) the resultant Ap resistant *E. coli* H10407 strain was mated with *E. coli* 20SO, and Ap resistant, LT$^+$ (*E. coli* 20SO) transconjugants were selected and chosen (these clones all specified ST production as well); (III) Ap sensitive segregants (LT$^+$ and ST$^+$) were obtained spontaneously, and pJY11 was isolated from one such strain; and (IV) an Ap resistant self-transmissible plasmid (named pJY12) was isolated from another type of spontaneous segregant (Ap resistant, LT$^-$ and ST$^-$). These results indicate that *E. coli* H10407 carries a self-transmissible plasmid (named pTRAl) which can mobilize the LT- and ST-coding plasmid (pJY11) and the pJY12 is pTRAl:Tn*l*. To confirm these observations and to characterize the plasmids, we attempted to isolate intact plasmids carried by *E. coli* H10407.

For this, pJY12 was introduced into another *E. coli* H10407, originated in the laboratory of S. Donta and kindly provided by Y. Takeda, by bacterial mating (the transfer frequency was about 1×10^{-6} transconjugants per donor). The resultant Ap resistant transconjugant (designated as *E. coli* TY201) was again mated with *E. coli* 20SO, and Ap resistant *E. coli* 20SO clones were selected (the transfer frequency was about 1×10^{-2} transconjugants per donor). Next, these Ap resistant clones were tested for LT[7] or CFA/I[8] production; 1.3% of the clones were LT$^+$, and 60% were CFA/I$^+$. As expected, the LT$^+$ or CFA/I$^+$ clones tested all specified ST production as well, as determined in the suckling mouse test[7]. The LT- and ST-coding plasmid (named pJY11b) and CFA/I- and ST-coding plasmid (named pCSl) were isolated after spontaneous elimination of pJY12 from those clones.

For isolation of a self-transmissible plasmid (pTRAl), pMK1 (ColEl carrying a kanamycin, Km, transposon Tn5, 9) DNA was introduced into *E. coli* H10407, which was used for isolation of pJY11b or pCSl, by genetic transformation (50 μg of DNA gave five Km resistant transformants). The resultant transformant (named *E. coli* TY202) was mated with *E. coli* 20SO, and Km resistant *E. coli* 20SO clones were selected (transfer frequency, about 1×10^{-6} transconjugants per donor). pMK1 was then spontaneously climinatd from these clones, and a strain containing pTRAl was obtained. This pTRAl isolation method is based on the finding that pJY12 can mobilize the ColEl plasmid as well. The plasmids of *E. coli* H10407 thus confirmed are illustrated in Fig. 1.

Mobilization of pCSl and pJY11 by pTRAl in E. coli K12 strains

pJY12 (pTRAl:Tn/) was transferred at a frequency of 10^{-1} to 10^{-2} among *E. coli* K12 strains. In contrast, no conjugal transfer was observed with pCSl and pJY11 or even with genetically labeled derivatives. However, when *E. coli* 20SO cells carrying the three plasmids were constructd, transfer of pCSl and pJY11 was observed at frequencies of 65% and 3% of that of pTRAl transfer, respectively. Simultaneous transfer of the three plasmids (pCSl, pJY11 and pTRAl) was also demonstrated at a frequency of 1.5% of pTRAl transfer.

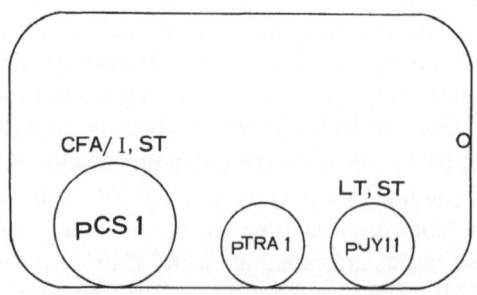

Fig. 1. Plasmids of E. coli H10407 (serotype 078:H11).

Characterization of plasmids

The molecular natures of the plasmids carried by *E. coli* 20SO were examined, and results are summarized in Table 1. pTRAl and pJY11 (or pJY11b) had the same molecular weight. pCSl DNA has a significantly different buoyant density (or G + C mol%) from other plasmids, or even the *E. coli* H10407 chromosome (1.710 g/cm³). This finding suggests different paths of evolution of the plasmids. Thus, pCSl may have originated in another species of bacterium than *E. coli* (H10407).

Recently, McConnell *et al.*[5] and Willshaw *et al.*[6] showed thast the "LT plasmid" (42 × 10⁶ molecular weight) isolated from *E. coli* H10407 specified T5 phage restriction as well. In confirmation of this observation, we found that both pJY11 and pJY11b manifested T5 and T6 phage restriction in addition to LT and ST production.

Agarose gel analysis and fragments containing the toxin gene

Although pTRAl was not distinguishable from pJY11 (or pJY11b) in molecular weight or base composition (Table l), the *Eco*RI and *Pst*I digestion patterns of the two plasmids were quite different. Two independent isolates, pJY11 and pJY11b, gave indistinguishable digestion patterns with restriction endonucleases *Pst*I (Fig. 2C), *Eco*RI, *Bam*HI, *Xba*I, *Xho*I, *Sal*I, *Hind*III, *Sma*I and *Hpa*I, indicating that pJY11 and pJY11b are the same plasmid. Thus, it is evident that the LT- and ST-coding plasmid (pJY11) exists in *E. coli* H10407.

Fragments of pCSl and pJY11 containing the toxin gene were identified by cloning these fragments into cloning vehicles such as pBR322 and pGA24; cloning analysis of the toxin genes of pJY11 has been described[7, 11, 12]. The ST⁺ *Eco*RI and *Pst*I fragments of pCSl and pJY11 were readily distinguishable from each other (Fig. 2), and further digestion of the purified ST⁺ *Pst*I fragments of pCSl and pJY11 with restriction endonucleases *Hinc*II, *Taq*I, *Mbo*II and *Hae*III showed significant heterogeneity of the two fragments.

Table 1. Molecular nature of *E. coli*-10407-derived plasmids

Plasmid	Molecular weight × 10⁶	(size in kb)	Boyant density g/cm³	(G + C mol%)	Plasmid copy number per chr.
pCS1	62	(94)	1.706	(47)	2.8
pTRA1	42	(64)	1.710	(51)	2.2
pJY11	42	(64)	1.710	(51)	3.6
pJY11b	42	(64)	1.710	(51)	3.5

The molecular weights of plasmids were determined by alkaline sucrose gradient analysis (10) and by agarose gel electrophoresis (7, 9). The bouyant density of plasmids was analyzed by neutral CsCl density gradient centrifugation (10).
The plasmid copy number in *E. coli* 20SO was determined by alkaline sucrose gradient analysis (10).

194

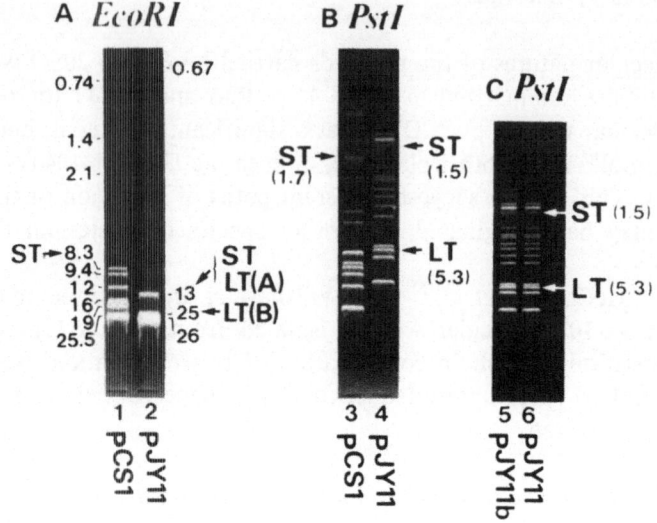

Fig. 2. Agarose gel analysis–identification of toxin gene-containing fragments.

Structure of the LT operon (toxA, B)

(i) *Location on pJY11.* The LT operon[12] straddles the two *Eco*RI fragments, E1 and E2, as shown in Fig. 3. The entire LT producing region was cloned as a 5.3 kb *Pst*I fragment (Pa-Pb) or as a 2.4 kb *Hind*III fragment (Ha-Hc). It was unambiguously shown that this LT operon is flanked by repeating DNA sequences, named β (0.75 kb in size): β1 and β3 in a reversed orientation or β1 and β2 in a direct orientation[11]. This suggests that the LT operon may be on

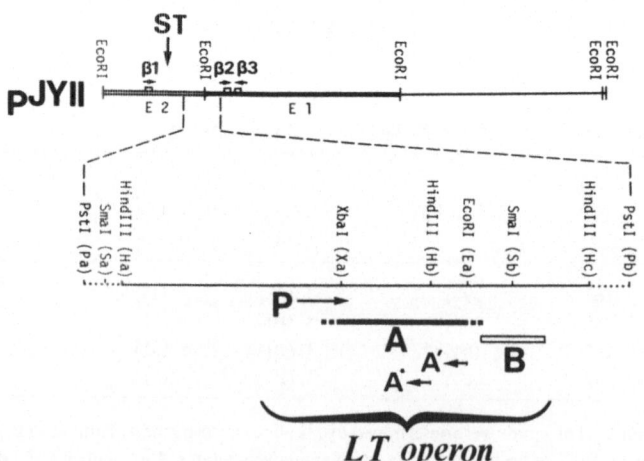

Fig. 3. Location of the LT operon (toxA, B) on pJY11.

a transposon. Interestingly, the ST gene is also located within this transposon-like structure.

(ii)   LT gene-products. pJYL2299 (a pBR322 recombinant plasmid carrying the entire LT region, Pa-Pb) was analyzed in *E. coli* minicells, by using antisera to cholera toxin subunit A or B[11]. Under these conditions, the β-lactamase gene (*bla*) of pBR322 is destroyed, and therefore β-lactamase (a major product of pBR322) is not produced. As shown in Fig. 4, only three major peptides were found: LT-A of 26,800-27,000 molecular weight, LT-Al (?) of 22,000 molecular weight and LT-B of 11,800-12,000 molecular weight. The LT-B is aparently larger than cholera toxin subunit B (11,590 molecular weight, 13).

(iii)   Toxoid-producing recombinant plasmids. By using *in vitro* recombination techniques, we succeeded in constructing recombinant plasmids that produce toxoids of LT[11, 12] such as LT-B and LT-A* (Table 2). Although deletion of a small carboxy terminal region of the *toxA* still resulted in the production of a biologically active peptide (e.g., LT-A' from pJY23 and pJY183, Fig. 3 and Table 2), a more truncated *toxA*, which lacks the last 0.25 kb, coded for a biologically inactive peptide, LT-A* (see pJY34b, Table 2 and Fig. 3). Recently, Spicer *et al.*[14] reported the locations of the LT-A1 and LT-A2 loci of a porcine *E. coli* LT operon. In confirming this observation, we demonstrated similar LT-A1 and LT-A2 loci in our human *E. coli* LT operon. Thus, it is evident that LT-A* lacks the LT-A2 moiety.

LT-B producing recombinant plasmids were constructed by inserting *toxB* in-

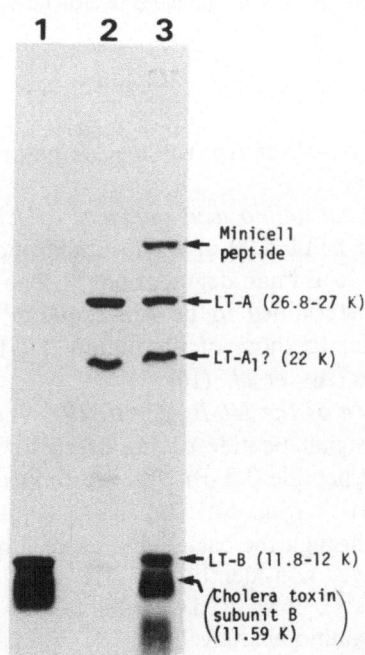

Fig. 4. Analysis of the LT operon-products in E. coli minicells.

Table 2. Recombinant plasmids carrying various regions of the LT operon

Group	Plasmid name	Cloned region	Cloning vehicle
LT producing plasmids	pJY137	E1, E2	pMK1
	pJY183	E1, E2	pMK1
	pJYL2299	Pa-Pb	pBR322
	pJY27	Ha-Hc	pACYC177
LT-A producing plasmid	pJY31	Sa-Sb	pACYC177
LT-A′ producing plasmid	pJY23	Pa-Ea	pBR322
LT-A* producing plasmid	pJY34b	Ha-Hb	pACYC177
LT-B producing plasmids	pJY24	Ea-Pb	pBR322
	pJY26	E1	pGA24
	pJY35	Ea-Hc	pGA24
	pJY37a	Hb-Hc	pACYC177

LT-A has a molecular weight of 26,800–27,000. LT-A′ has a molecular weight of 24,500 and shows LT activity in the presence of LT-B (pJY183 produces LT-A′ and LT-B).
LT-A* has a molecular weight of 17,000 and does not show LT activity even in the presence of LT-B. LT-A′ and LT-A* are also described in Fig. 3. LT-B has a molecular weight of 11,800–12,000, and the LT-B producing plasmids code for LT-B by using a promoter resident on a vactor. Abbreviations for restriction endonuclease cleavage sites are described in Fig. 3.

to the downstream region of the Ap, Km or Cm (chloramphenicol) resistance gene-operons on the vectors[12].

(iv) Amino-terminal amino acid sequence of LT-B. After it had been ^{14}C-labeled, the peptide of pJYL2299 of 11,800-12,000 molecular weight (Fig. 4) was purified, and subjectd to Edman degradation[15]. The amino acid sequence at the amino-terminus was determined to be Ala-Pro-Gln[16]. These first three amino acid residues are similar to those of the mature LT-B of porcine *E. coli*, which were reported by Clements *et al.* (16).

(v) DNA sequence of the LT-B gene (toxB). The amino-terminal coding sequence, covering the signal peptide of the precursor (preLT-B) and the amino-terminus of the mature peptide (LT-B), was determined[16] by the chemical method of Maxam and Gilbert[18] (Fig. 5). The signal sequence, which is supposed to play a role in passing through the bacterial inner membrane, consisted of 21 amino acid residues, and showed non-identity but extensive homology to that of the porcine *E. coli* LT-B gene[19]: it showed 97% homology at the nucleotide level and 90% homology at the amino acid level. So far, comparison of the amino-terminal coding sequences of mature LT-B human and porcine *E. coli* has shown only one single base change (and therefore one amino acid residue change). Thus, the

LT operons of human and porcine *E. coli* seem to be closely related, but not identical.

Recently, we found that LT subunit A and B genes (*toxA* and *toxB*) overlap.

(vi) Complementation of the LT genes. For production of LT, clustering of LT genes (*ToxA* and *ToxB*) is not essential. Two genes located separately on two compatible plasmids can also produce LT[11], as illustrated in Fig. 6. For example, a combination of pJY23 and pJY26 (Table 2) shows marked LT production.

Release of LT subunits by E. coli. Although a significant amount of LT synthesized in *E. coli* is cell-associated, a small portion (approximately 10%) is released into the culture supernatant. It was found, by using the recombinant plasmids listed in Table 2, that (i) LT-B is released into the culture supernatant in amounts equal to those of LT; (ii) in contrast, LT-A or its derivatives (LT-A' and LT-A*) cannot be released into the culture supernatant; (iii) introduction of LT-B into *E. coli* calls producing LT-A (or LT-A') restores the release of LT-A (or LT-A') into the culture supernatant; but (iv) LT-A* is not released into the culture super-

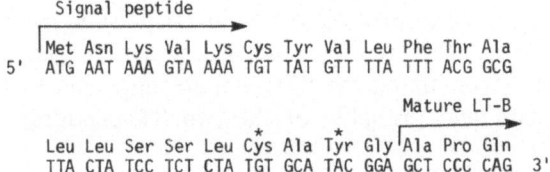

Fig. 5. Amino-terminal nucleotide sequence of the toxB.

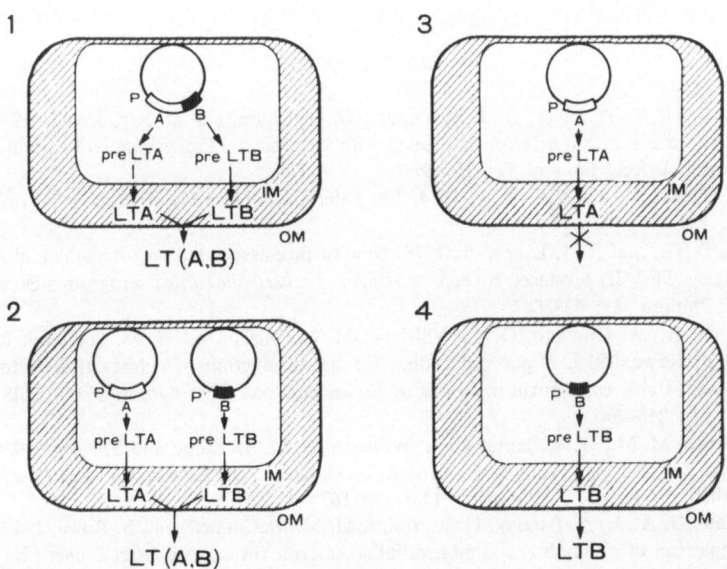

Fig. 6. A possible mechanism of the release of LT subunits across bacterial membranes.

natant even in the presence of LT-B[20]. We therefore speculate that the precursors of LT-A and LT-B (preLT-A and preLT-B) independently pass through the inner membrane, presumably owing to a signal peptide, but after that, the mature LT-A (or mature forms of LT-A derivatives) accumulates in the periplasmic space or within the outer membrane and require LT-B for their release into the culture supernatant (Fig. 6). We also speculate that LT-A* cannot interact with LT-B (presumably because it lacks the LT-A2 moiety) and, therefore, remains inside the cells.

Two STs. As described in the preceding section, *E. coli* H10407 produces two species of ST: one from pCSl and the other from pJY11. The two STs were both (i) detected in suckling mice, (ii) completely neutralized by antiserum to STa, (kindly provided by Y. Takeda), (iii) positive in a ligated loop test using 2-week-old piglets, but (iv) negative in the ligated loop test using 8-week-old piglets. These results indicate that the two STs are both STa's. However, the ST levels of pJY11 and pCSl, as detected in suckling mice, were quite different. pCS1 produced more than 10 times more ST than pJY11 did. A comparison of the ST levels of the cloned ST regions of pJY11 and pCS1 also gave similar results; in this experiment, pJYS101 (a pBR322 recombinant plasmid carrying the ST+ 1.5 kb *Pst*I fragment of pJY11, 7) and pJYS201 (a pBR322 recombinant plasmid carrying the ST+ 1.7 kb *Pst*I fragment of pCSl) were employed. These data, together with molecular analysis of fragments containing the ST gene, strongly suggest the heterogeneity of the two ST genes (and probably of the two ST peptides).

Experiments on amino acid sequencing and nucleotide sequencing were carried out in collaboration with M. Ryoji and A. Kaji (University of Pennsylvania) and T. Tamura and T. Takano (Keio University), respectively. We thank Y. Takeda for encouragement throughout the studies.

REFERENCES

1. Evans, D. G., R. P. Silver, D. J. Evans, Jr., D. G. Chase, and D. L. Gorbach. 1975. Plasmid-controlled colonization factor associated with virulence in *Escherichia coli* enterotoxigenic for humans. Infect. Immun. **12**: 656–667.
2. Glyes, C., M. So, and S. Falkow. 1974. The enterotoxin plasmids of *Escherichia coli*. J. Infect. Dis. **130**: 40–49.
3. Evans, D. G., and D. J. Evans, Jr. 1978. New surface-associated heat-labile colonization factor antigen (CFA/II) produced by enterotoxigenic *Escherichia coli* of serogroups O6 and O8. Infect. Immun. **21**: 638–647.
4. Smith, H. R., A. Cravioto, G. A. Willshaw, M. M. McConnell, S. M. Scotland, R. J. Gross, and B. Rowe. 1979. A plasmid coding for the production of colonization factor antigen I and heat-stable enterotoxin in strains of *Escherichia coli* of serogroup O78. FEMS Microbiol. Letts. **6**: 255–260.
5. McConnell, M. M., H. R. Smith, G. A. Willshaw, S. M. Scotland, and B. Rowe. 1980. Plasmids coding for heat-labile enterotoxin production isolated from *Escherichia coli* 078: a comparison of their properties. J. Bacteriol. **143**: 158–167.
6. Willshaw, G. A., E. A. Barclay, H. R. Smith, M. M. McConnell, and B. Rowe, 1980. Molecular comparison of plasmids encoding heat-labile enterotoxin isolated from *Escherichia coli* strains of human origin. J. Bacteriol. **143**: 168–175.
7. Yamamoto, T., and T. Yokota. 1980. Cloning of deoxyribonucleic acid regions encoding a heat-labile and heat-stable enterotoxin originating from an enterotoxigenic *Escherichia coli* strain

of human origin. J. Bacteriol. **143**: 652–660.

8. Evans, D. G., D. J. Evans, Jr., and W. Tjoa. 1977. Hemagglutination of human group A erythrocytes by enterotoxigenic *Escherichia coli* isolated from adults with diarrhea: correlation with colonization factor. Infect. Immun. **k8**: 330–337.

9. Yamamoto, T., and T. Yokota. 1980. Construction of a physical map of a kanamycin (Km) transposon, Tn5, and a comparison to another Km transposon, Tn903. Mol. Gen. Genet. **178**: 77–83.

10. Yamamoto, T., and T. Yokota. 1977. Host-dependent, theremosensitive replication of an R plasmid, pJY5, isolated from *Enterobacter cloacae*. J. Bacteriol. **132**: 923–930.

11. Yamamoto, T., and T. Yokota. 1981. *Escherichia coli* heat-labile enterotoxin genes are flanked by repeated deoxyribonucleic acid sequences. J. Bacteriol. **145**: 850–860.

12. Yamamoto, T., T. Yokota, and A. Kaji. 1981. Molecular organizaiton of heat-labile enterotoxin genes originating in *Escherichia coli* of human origin and construction of heat-labile toxoid-producing strains. J. Bacteriol. **148**: 983–987.

13. Kurosky, A., D. E. Markel, J. W. Peterson, and W. M. Fitch. 1977. Primary structure of cholera toxin β-chain: a glycoprotein hormone analog? Science **195**: 299–30l.

14. Spicer, E. K., W. M. Kavanaugh, W. S. Dallas, S. Falkow, W. H. Konigsberg, and D. E. Schafer. 1981. Sequence homologies between A subunits of *Escherichia coli* and *Vibrio cholerae* enterotoxins. Proc. Natl. Acad. Sci. U.S.A. **78**: 50–54.

15. Ryoji, M., and A. Kaji. 1982. High sensitivity amino acid sequence determination of radioactive proteins made *in vivo* or *in vitro*. Anal. Biochem., in press.

16. Yamamoto, T., T. Tamura, M. Ryoji, A. Kaji, T. Yokota, and T. Takano. 1982. Sequence analysis of the heat-labile enterotoxin subunit B gene originating in human enterotoxigenic *Escherichia coli*. J. Bacteriol. **152**: 506–509.

17. Clements, J. D., R. J. Yancey, and R. A. Finkelstein. 1980. Properties of homogeneous heat-labile enterotoxin from *Escherichia coli*. Infect. Immun. **29**: 91–97.

18. Maxam, A. M., and W. Gilbert. 1980. Sequencing end-labeled DNA with base-specific chemical cleavages. Methods Enzymol. **65**: 499–560.

19. Dallas, W. S., and S. Falkow. 1980. Amino acid sequence homology between cholera toxin and *Escherichia coli* heat-labile toxin. Nature (London) **288**: 499–501.

20. Yamamoto, T., and T. Yokota. 1982. Release of heat-labile enterotoxin subunits by *Escherichia coli*. J. Bacteriol. **150**: 1482–1484.

Recently we have determined the complete nucleotide sequence of the LT operon in *E. coli* H10407: Yamamoto, T. et al. 1984. J. Biol. Chem. **259**: 5037–5044; Yamamoto, T. et al. 1984. FEBS Lett. **169**: 241–246.

Bacterial Diarrheal Diseases, eds., Y. Takeda, T. Miwatani, 201–207.

INCREASED PRODUCTION OF HEAT-LABILE ENTEROTOXIN AS A RESULT OF TN3 INSERTION INTO A CHIMERIC R/ENT PLASMID

R. N. Picken, A. J. Mazaitis, R. Maas and W. K. Maas

New York University School of Medicine, New York, N. Y. 10016, U.S.A.

We are studying the genetics of enterotoxin synthesis in *Escherichia coli* and its control. For these studies we are using pCG86, a conjugative, naturally occurring recombinant plasmid that contains genes for heat-labile enterotoxin (LT), heat-stable enterotoxin (ST) and resistance to tetracycline, streptomycin/spectinomycin, sulfonamides and mercuric ions[1]. The presence of drug resistance genes in this plasmid has been advantageous in that it enabled us to develop a method for the enrichment and isolation of LT⁻ and ST⁻ mutants, for which there is no direct selection procedure available[2]. For further genetic studies we mapped the known genes in pCG86. This was done with the use of electron microscope heteroduplex analysis and self-annealing of isolated plasmid DNA molecules[3]. The physical map we obtained is shown in Fig. 1. To construct it, we used in addition to normal pCG86 molecules, 2 deletion mutants, one for tetracycline resistance (pWM2981) and one for LT and ST (pWM2982) and Tn5 insertion mutants in ST (pWM2983), LT (WM2984), mercury resistance (pWM2985) and streptomycin resistance (pWM2986). Tn5 contains a gene for kanamycin resistance.

For our mapping studies we isolated besides Tn5 insertion mutants also Tn3 insertion mutants. This transposon contains a gene for ampicillin resistance. We scored LT hyperproduction as a possible mutant trait and noticed that, in contrast to Tn5 insertion mutants, many of the Tn3 insertion mutants were hyperproducers of LT (Htx). The method we used to score LT hyperproduction was developed by Bramucci and Holmes[4] and involves the overlaying of blood agar plates with soft agar containing antibodies to LT or cholera toxin and complement. Htx colonies are surrounded by a clear halo, due to immune lysis of red blood cells as a result of LT secretion, whereas normal colonies have no or a very small halo, since they secrete very little LT.

As a source of Tn3 in our genetic experiments we used 2 miniplasmids, first Rsc13[5] and later the temperature-sensitive plasmid, pSC301–Tn3[6]. With both miniplasmids, Tn3 insertions into pCG86 were secreened by mating a strain containing a miniplasmid and pCG86 with a F⁻ recipient and selecting for streptomycin and ampicillin doubly resistant progeny. Rsc13 and pSC301–Tn3 are reported to be non-conjugative and non-mobilizable by conjugative plasmids.

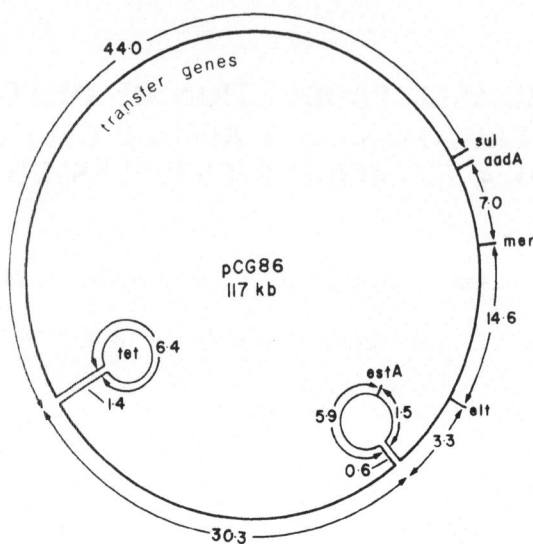

Fig. 1. Physical map of plasmid pCG86. The map was constructed from E. M. studies of self-annealed wild-type and deletion plasmid molecules and derivatives thereof with Tn5 insertions in the toxin and drug resistance genes and from heteroduplexes of these plasmids in different pairwise combinations. The regions flanked by inverted repeat sequences are shown as stem-loop structures. Numbers are distances in kilobases.

To learn more about the mechanism of LT hyperproduction we wanted to map the sites of Tn3 insertion in Htx mutants. We planned to do this by restriction enzyme analysis of pCG86 plasmids containing Tn3 insertions. With Htx mutants isolated with Rsc13 as a source of Tn3 we encountered difficulties, because we were unable to obtain strains that had no other plasmids besides pCG86–Tn3. We always found a miniplasmid to be present in the progeny strains selected for resistance to streptomycin and ampicillin, and attempts to eliminate these miniplasmids either by physical methods (sucrose gradients, agarose gel electrophoresis) or biological methods (transformation, transduction) were unsuccessful. We then switched to the use of pSC301–Tn3 as the source of Tn3. With this temperature-sensitive plasmid transpositions of Tn3 into another plasmid can be enriched by growing the cells containing the 2 plasmids at a non-permissive temperature (42°C) in the presence of streptomycin and ampicillin, prior to mating with a F⁻ recipient strain.

With pSC301–Tn3 as a source of Tn3 we used pWM2981 as the recipient plasmid and isolated 17 Htx mutants. These mutants contained a single plasmid and the Htx property was transmitted in matings with other strains together with the plasmid.

We found that the Htx mutants had a 4 to 8 fold increase in the level of resistance to streptomycin and ampicillin over non-Htx strains. A similar increase was found for LT production. This suggested that LT hyperproduction in due to an increase in plasmid copy number. The results of the mapping experiments described in the following sections support this notion.

Mapping of Tn3 insertions in Htx plasmids

Initially we used the restriction endonuclease *Bam*HI, since it has a single site within Tn3 and cuts it asymetrically. Plasmid DNA was isolated from the 17 Htx strains and from the parent strain carrying pWM2981, digested with *Bam*HI and analyzed by agarose gel electrophoresis. The fragment patterns of the 17 Htx plasmids were found to be only of 2 types and each type was clearly different from pWM2981. In each type one of the pWM2981 fragments disappeared and 2 new fragments appeared. The eliminated fragment of pWM2981 was the same in type 1 and type 2 Htx plasmids. Of the 17 Htx plasmids, 8 belonged to type 1 and 9 belonged to type 2. We conclude from these results that all 17 Tn3 insertions are in the same *Bam*HI fragment. Since the gel patterns within each type are identical, we assume that the Tn3 insertions in each type are in the same site or very close to each other. We therefore chose one representative of each type for further study, designated pWM36 for type 1 and pWM3 for type 2.

To find out how type 1 insertions differ from type 2 insertions, we measured the sizes of the newly arisen fragments in *Bam*HI digests of type 1 and type 2 plasmids. Since the size of Tn3 and the location of the *Bam*HI cutting site within this transposon are known, the possible insertion sites within the *Bam*HI fragment can be limited to 4 possible location in each type. If we assume that type 1 insertions differ from type 2 insertions in the orientation in which Tn3 is inserted, we find that the insertion sites in the 2 types are at the same location or nearly so. From results and considerations presented below this seems to be a reasonable assumption and we have come to the tentative conclusion that the difference between type 1 and type 2 is in the orientation of the inserted Tn3, the insertion sites being identical or very near each other.

A similar restriction enzyme analysis of pWM2981, pWM36 and pWM3 was carried out with *Pvu*I, which, like *Bam*HI cuts Tn3 once and asymetrically. The results obtained were entirely analogous to those obtained with *Bam*HI, in support of the notion of opposite orientation of Tn3 insertions in type 1a and type 2 plasmids.

To locate the position of the *Bam*HI and *Pvu*I fragments containing the Tn3 insertions in the map of pCG86, restriction enzyme analysis was carried out with a series of endonucleases, besides *Bam*Hi and *Pvu*I and plasmids 2981-2986 with mapped deletions or Tn5 insertions were used as guides. The enzymes used were *Xho*I, *Sal*I, *Kpn*I and *Bgl*II. Tn3 has one or more cutting sites for *Bam*HI and *Pvu*I, Tn5 for *Xho*I, *Sal*I, *Bam*HI and *Bgl*II. Without going into detail of the experiments, we are showing the results of these analyses in Fig. 2. As can be seen, we were able to construct a map for all the sites of these enzymes from the *aadA* gene to a region beyond the *estA* gene (Fig. 1). For convenience we have assigned kilobase (kb) coordinates to this map, starting with 0 at *aadA* and continuing in a clockwise direction. The site of the Tn3 insertions is at or near 14.4 kb and is within a 5.1 kb. *Bgl*II fragment, designated Rep. As will be shown below, this fragment contains genes for autonomous replication.

Before proceeding with the discussion of the Tn3 insertions in the Rep fragment, 2 features of Fig. 2 should be noted. L. A region of homology with another

204

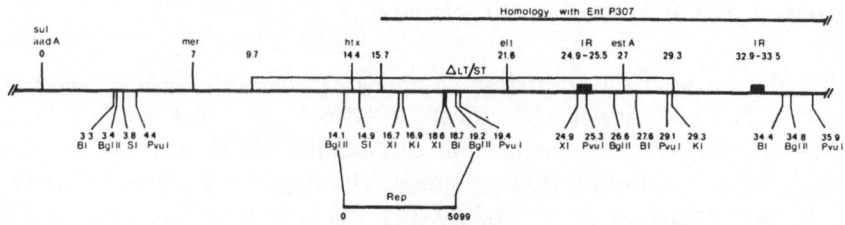

Fig. 2. Restriction enzyme map of a 36 kb region of pCG86. LT/ST shows the extent of the deletion in pWM2982. B1 = *Bam*HI, S1 = *Sal*I, X1 = *Xho*I, K1 = KpnI.

Ent plasmid, Ent p307 is indicated. This plasmid has extensive homology with pCG86, the region of complete homology actually extending to the "Tet" stem-loop structure (Fig. 1). Part of the Rep fragment is homologous with Ent p307. 2. A segment labelled ΔLT/ST deleted in pWM2982 is indicated. This deletion includes the Rep fragment and raises the question of how pWM2982 is able to replicate. This question will be considered at the end.

Relationship between Htx Tn3 insertions and replication of pCG86

Previously we had cloned the 5.1 kb *Bgl*II Rep fragment shown in Fig. 2, together with a 2.7 kb *Bgel*II fragment containing the gene for tetracycline resistance and had found that the resulting miniplasmid could replicate autonomously. We called this plasmid pWM5. Agarose gel patterns of *Bgl*II digests of pWM5 and several other plasmids are shown in Fig. 3. The pWM5 digest gives rise to 2 fragments of 5.1 kb and 2.7 kb. The 2.7 kb fragment is absent in the pWM2981 digest, as expected. The 5.1 kb fragment is present in all the Tn5 insertion mutants, in pWM2981, but not in pWM2982. The type 1 and type 2 plasmids do not contain the 5.1 kb fragment, but instead a 10.1 kb fragment, which presumably is composed of the 5.1 kb fragment and Tn3 (length = 4.9 kb).

The presence of a Tn3 insertion in the 5.1 kb Rep fragment in pWM36 and pWM3 suggested the possibility of cloning the corresponding Rep fragments from these plasmids, using ampicillin resistance as a marker for plasmid selection. This was done in the same manner as for pCG86: Plasmid DNA was digested to completion with *Bgl*II and the resulting fragments were ligated and transformed into *E. coli* strain C600, with selections for ampicillin resistance. Examination of plasmid DNA from ampicillin resistant colonies derived from both type 1 and type 2 plasmids showed that in each case a 10.1 kb plasmid had been formed possessing a single *Bgl*II site. One miniplasmid of each type was selected for further study, pWM14 from type 1 and pWM17 from type 2.

Further restriction enzyme analysis was then carried out on the Rep fragments, first of pWM5 and then on pWM14 and pWM17.

pWM5 was subjected to single, double and triple digestions with the enzymes *Bgl*II, *Sal*I, *Xho*I, *Bam*HI, *Eco*RI, *Hin*dIII, *Pst*I, *Hae*II KpnI and *Sst*II and the resulting fragments were analyzed by agarose gel electrophoresis. Fig. 4 shows a restriction enzyme map of the Rep fragment incorporating the results of these

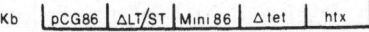

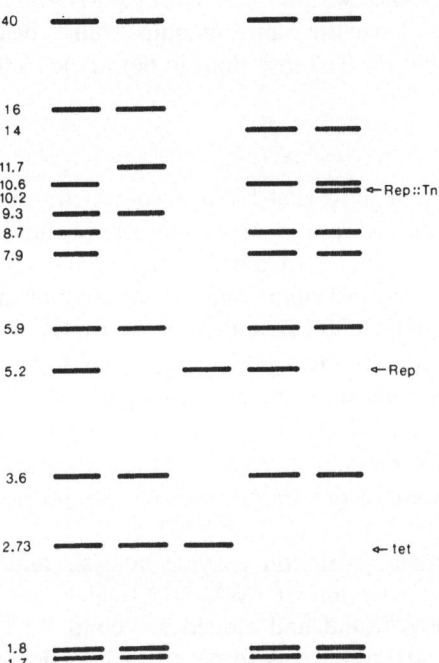

Fig. 3. Migration in a vertical 0.7% agarose gel of *Bgl*II cleared plasmids pCG86, pWM2982 (LT/ST), pWM5 (mini 86), pWM2981 (tet) and its Htx type 1 and type 2 mutants.

enzyme digests. It may be seen that the left arm of the map shows a striking similarity to the sequence of sites mapped in the incompatibility group FII miniplasmid pSM1, derived from the R plasmid R100. This miniplasmid has been studied extensively, including the determination of its DNA sequence[7]. The similarity between pWM5 and pSM1 may be traced as far as the second *Hae*II site at position 1740 b.p. However, the second *Pst*I site at 2470 b.p. in pSM1 is absent in pWM5 and the *Xho* 1 site at 2589 b.p. on pWM5 is absent in pSM1.

It seems likely that pCG86 was formed by recombination between a plasmid like Ent P307 and a group FII R plasmid like R100. This is indicated by the finding that pCG86 is incompatible with group FII R plasmids and with Ent-P307[8]. The same incompatibility behavior is found for pWM5. On the basis of the mapping data shown in Figs. 2 and 4 and the incompatibility properties of pWM5 we may suppose that one recombination event in the formation of pCG86 occurred between the *Hae*II site at 1740 b.p. and the *Pst*I site at 2470 b.p. of pSM1.

For further restriction enzyme analysis of pWM14 and pWM17, double digestions were carried out with *BglII* and each of the following enzymes: *BamHI*, *PvuI* and *RstI*. These 3 enzymes have cutting sites within Tn3. Analysis of the fragment seen in agarose gels leads to the conclusion that in pWM14 the Tn3 is inserted in position about 300 b.p. and in pWM17 in position about 230 b.p. (Fig. 4). In the corresponding region of pSMl there is a gene, *copB*, which controls copy number, but not incompatibility[9, 10]. Mutations in *copB* result in increased copy number. Since we find that both pWM14 and pWM17 show increased copy number, but have the same incompatibility behavior as pWM5, it is reasonable to expect that the Tn3 insertions in both type 1 and in type 2 are in *copB*.

Conclusions

The results presented show that LT hyperproduction by the Tn3 Htx mutants we studied is due to an increase in copy number, presumably resulting from the insertion of Tn3 into a gene controlling copy number. We find that the levels of plasmid-mediated drug resistance and LT production are raised 4 to 8 fold. The gene controlling copy number and affected by the Tn3 insertions (*copB*) is located in a hybrid "basic replicon" formed by recombination between a group FII R factor and an Ent plasmid similar to Ent P307. It is to be noted that among Tn3 insertions into Ent P307 we have not found any Htx mutants. This finding suggests that Tn3 is preferentially inserted into the *copB* gene of group FII plasmids.

It will be of interest to determine precisely the portions of the hybrid basic replicon in pWM5 contributed by Ent P307 and by the group FII R plasmid. This will involve further restriction enzyme analysis and DNA sequencing.

In regard to the replication of pWM2982, which lacks the *BglII* 5.1 kb Rep fragment, we have now found and cloned a second "basic replicon", which is also present in Ent P307 and seems to control its replication. In pCG86, the second replicon appears to be silent, as judged by incompatibility properties, but

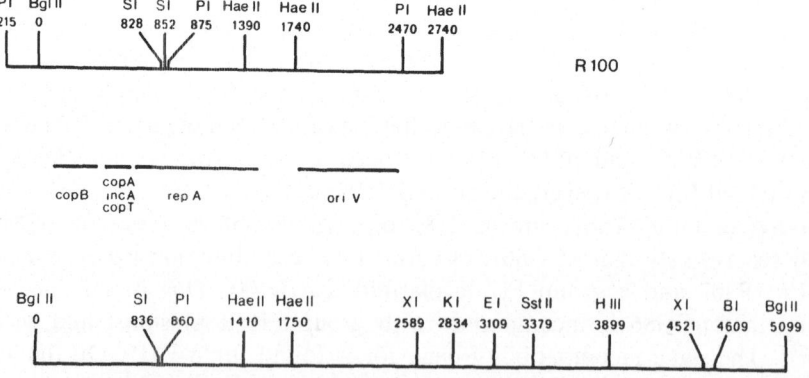

Fig. 4. Restriction enzyme map of the sequenced "Rep" portion from R100[7] and of the 5.1 kb "Rep" fragment from pCG86 drawn to the same scale. Numbers refer to base pair coordinates measured from the left terminal *BglII* site at 0 b.p. The positions of genes associated with replication functions are indicated. P1 = *Pst*I, S1 = *Sal*I, X1 = *Xho*I, K1 = *Kpn*I, E1 = *Eco*RI, H111 = *Hind*III, B1 = *Bam*HI.

when the first replicon is deleted, as in pWM2982, it is turned on and functions in the autonomous replication of the plasmid.

The work reported here was supported by grant PCM-7725134 from the National Science Foundation, grant 59-2369-0-2-109-0 from the U. S. Department of Agriculture and by grant GM06048 from the National Institutes of Health. W. K. M. is the holder of Public Health Service Research Career Award GM-15129 from the National Institute of General Medical Sciences.

REFERENCES

1. Gyles, C. K., S. Palchaudhuri, and W. K. Maas. 1977. Naturally occurring plasmid carrying genes for enterotoxin production and drug resistance. Science **198**: 198–199.
2. Silva, M. L., W. K. Maas, C. L. Gyles. 1978. Isolation and characterization of enterotoxin-deficient mutants of *Escherichia coli*. Proc. Natl. Acad. Sci. U.S.A. **75**: 2242–2246.
3. Mazaitis, A. J., R. Maas, and W. K. Maas. 1981. Structure of a naturally occurring plasmid with genes for enterotoxin production and drug resistance. J. Bact. **145**: 97–105.
4. Bramucci, M. G., and R. K. Holmes. 1978. Radial passive immune hemolysis assay for detection of heat-labile enterotoxin produced by individual colonies of *Escherichia coli* or *Vibrio cholerae*. J. Clin. Microbiol. **8**: 252–255.
5. Goebel, W., W. Lindernmaier, F. Pfeifer, H. Schremph, and B. Schelle. 1977. Transposition and Insertion of Intact, Deleted and Enlarged Ampicilli Transposon Tn3 from Mini-Rl (Rsc) Plasmids into Transfer Factors. Molec. Gen. Genet. **157**: 119.
6. Kretschmer, P. J., and S. N. Cohen. 1977. Selected Translocation of Plasmid Genes: Frequency and Regional Specificity of Translocation of the Tn3 Element. J. Bact. **130**: 888–899.
7. Rosen, J., T. Ryder, H. Inokuchi, H. Ohtsubo, and E. Ohtsubo. 1980. Genes and sites involved in replication and incompatibility of an R100 plasmid derivative based on nucleotide sequence analysis. Molec. Gen. Genet. **179**: 527–537.
8. McConnell, M. M., H. R. Smith, G. A. Willshaw, S. M. Scotland, and B. Rowe. 1980. Plasmids coding for Heat-Labile Enterotoxin production isolated from *Escherichia coli* 078: Comparison of Properties. J. Bacteriol. **143**: 158–167.
9. Molin, S., P. Stougaard, J. Light, M. Nordstrom, and K. Nordstrom. 1981. Isolation and characterization of New Copy Mutants of Plasmid Rl, and identification of a Polypeptide involved in copy number control. Molec. Gen. Genet. **181**: 123–130.
10. Danbara, H., G. Brady, J. K. Timmis, and K. N. Timmis. 1981. Regulation of DNA replication: "Target" Determinant of the replication control elements of Plasmid R6-5 Lies within a control element gene. Proc. Natl. Acad. Sci. U.S.A. **78**: 4699–4703.

Bacterial Diarrheal Diseases, eds., Y. Takeda, T. Miwatani, 209–218.
Copyright © 1985 by KTK Scientific Publishers, Tokyo.

EVALUATION OF THE BIKEN TEST FOR THE DETECTION OF LT-PRODUCING *ESCHERICHIA COLI**

R. G. A. Sutton[1], M. Merson[1], J. P. Craig[2], P. Echeverria[3], S. L. Moseley[4], B. Rowe[5], L. R. Trabulsi[6], T. Honda[7] and Y. Takeda[7]

Diarrhoeal Diseases Control Programme, World Health Organization, Geneva, Switzerland[1]; Downstate Medical Center, State University of New York, Brooklyn, N. Y., USA[2]; Armed Forces Institute of Medical Sciences, Bangkok, Thailand[3]; Stanford University, School of Medicine, Stanford, California, USA[4]; Central Public Health Laboratory, Colindale, London, England[5]; Escola Paulista de Medicina, Sao Paulo, Brazil[6]; and Research Institute for Microbial Diseases, Osaka University, Suita, Osaka, Japan[7].

A more detailed understanding of the role of enterotoxigenic *Escherichia coli* as a cause of diarrhoea, and of its epidemiology and mode of transmission within the community has been hampered by the lack of simple, reliable laboratory procedures for the detection of these organisms. Present methods rely on animal models (suckling mouse, rabbit loop, rabbit skin), tissue culture procedures (Yl adrenal cells, CHO cells) or, more recently, passive immune haemolysis (PIH), and DNA hybridization techniques. Although reliable in the hands of experienced workers, these techniques are, nevertheless, relatively expensive and often require materials that are not available in routine laboratories, particularly in the developing countries. The development of simpler, reliable and inexpensive techniques for the detection of both the heat-stable (ST) and heat-labile (LT) toxins of *E. coli* has therefore been given high priority by the Diarrhoeal Diseases Control Programme.

One such technique for the detection of LT that appears to satisfy these conditions is the modified Elek Test (Biken test) developed in 1981 by Honda, Taga, Takeda and Miwatani[1]. The principle of this technique is that of the Elek test whereby specific antitoxin reacts with toxin liberated by an actively growing culture of the test organism to produce a line of precipitation at the site of optimal toxin-antitoxin reaction.

In order to evaluate the accuracy and reproducibility of this technique, the Programme's Scientific Working Group on Bacterial Enteric Infections undertook an interlaboratory trial in which five investigators tested an identical set of "100" unknown strains of *E. coli*, using the Biken technique and one or more other techniques with which they were familiar.

---

* A collaborative study coordinated by the Scientific Working Group on Bacterial Enteric Infections of the Diarrhoeal Diseases Control (CDD) Programme, World Health Organization, Geneva.

MATERIALS AND METHODS

Organization of the evaluation trial

Five laboratories, each of which had considerable experience in the detection of LT by other methods, but no prior experience with the use of the Biken test, took part in the trial. Each received an identical set of 100 strains of *E. coli* prepared by a sixth laboratory not participating in the actual testing of the strains. On receipt, each culture was subcultured to ensure that it was not contaminated, although testing for heat-labile enterotoxin (LT) production was done directly from the original culture.

Each laboratory tested all 100 strains using the Biken test, and at least one other method (see Table 1 for methods used by the individual laboratories). The reagents and materials used in the Biken test, together with the protocol to be followed when performing the test, were common to all laboratories and were provided by Y. Takeda. The reagents, materials and methods used in other test systems (GM₁-ELISA, cell cultures, DNA-Probe, PIH or skin test) were those routinely used in the participating laboratory. As the objective of the trial was to evaluate the Biken (and other) test as a routine diagnostic procedure, all tests were carried out in a routine manner, and no special care or attention, above that normally given, was used.

Selection of test organisms

All strains of *E. coli* included in the study were isolated at Osaka Airport Quarantine station from patients with travellers' diarrhoea. The set of 100 cultures (50 LT positive, 50 LT negative) sent to each participating laboratory consisted of:
1. 82 different strains of *E. coli* (21 strains LT-ST, 20 strains LT only, 21 strains ST only and 20 non-toxigenic strains).
2. 9 replicate cultures of one of the LT only strains (536-2); all being prepared from one parent colony.
3. 9 replicate cultures of one of the non-toxigenic strains (8-669-1); all being prepared from one parent colony.

The LT positive and negative strains were randomly mixed throughout the

Table 1.   Collaborative results obtained by five participating laboratories for the identification of LT producing strains of *E. coli*.

LAB	Biken test	GM1 ELISA	YIA cells	CHO cell	Probe	PIH	PF
A	82 (100)	99	100		100		
B	100		100			100	
C	89 (100)				97 (100)		
D	92 (100)	77	100	100			
E	99						68

Results are expressed as percent correlation with "true" identity of test strain. Figures in brackets show results obtained after 'retesting' set, and sets of cultures sent to each laboratory were identical in that all five subcultures of each test organism (numbered 1-100) were prepared from one parent colony. The participating laboratories did not know the identity of the cultures, nor that the set of 100 organisms contained two organisms that were each included ten times.

Testing of E. coli strains

1. The "Biken" test
   The procedure* used by all laboratories was as follows:
   (i) Biken agar No. 2 (15 ml) was melted in a boiling water bath, cooled to 50 – 60°C and added to 0.5 ml of lincomycin solution, (2.7 mg/ml) previously warmed to 50°C, in a 85–90mm petri-dish. The agar was mixed well to obtain an even distribution of lincomycin, and allowed to solidify.
   (ii) The surface of dried plates was inoculated with the test organisms, using a prepared template provided to each laboratory. The spacing and size of the inoculum are shown in Fig. 1. Instructions were given to inoculate the plates so that the distance between the centre well (see below) and the edge of the colony, would be approximately 4 mm.
   (iii) The inoculated plates were incubated at 37°C for 48 hours.
   (iv) A polymyxin B containing disc was placed on the surface of each in-oculum (Fig.1).
   (v) Using a gel puncher and template provided, wells were punched in the agar, as shown in Fig. 1.
   (vi) The plates were reincubated at 37°C for a further 5-6 hours.
   (vii) Anti-LT antiserum (20 μl) was placed in each well.
   (viii) The plates were incubated at 37°C for a further 20 hours prior to being read.
   (ix) A positive result was indicated by a precipitin line between the colony and the well containing the antiserum. Reading was made easier by the use of a light box with a black background.
   (x) Results were confirmed after a further 15-20 hours incubation at 37°C.
2. *Other test procedures*
   As stated above, each laboratory tested the set of 100 cultures using at least one other method in addition to the Biken test. Other test systems used are briefly described below. It should be emphasized that although the procedures used in carrying out the Biken test were standardized and were common to all five laboratories, the procedures used for the other laboratory test methods were not standardized; the laboratories used the method with which they were most familiar.
   Chinese hamster ovary (CHO) cell assay: Bacterial strains were inoculated into 10 ml trypticase soy broth in 250 ml flasks and grown with shaking for 18 hours. Cultures were centrifuged and supernatants filtered. Trypsinized CHO cells were suspended in tissue culture medium, with 1% foetal calf serum. 0.2 ml CHO

---

* The materials, reagents and procedures used to carry out the Biken test were standardized for all laboratories and supplied in the form of a "Kit".

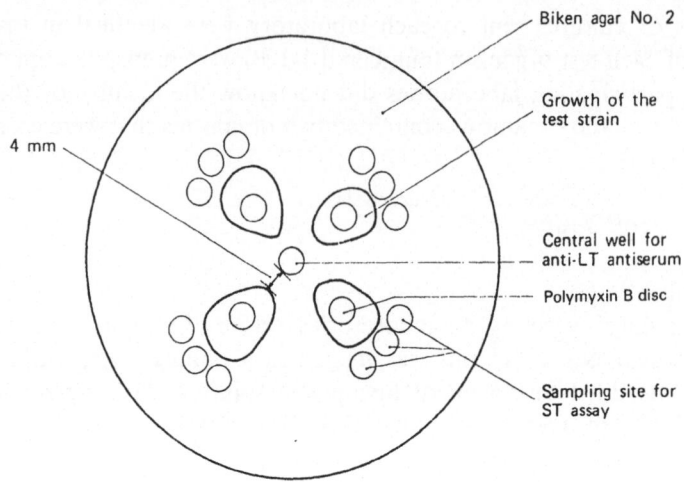

Fig. 1. Schematic presentation of the Biken test.

cell suspension was dispensed in each well of a microtitre plate. 0.025 ml filtrate was added to a well. After 24 hour incubation at 37°C, cells were fixed and observed for elongation.

Yl adrenal cell assay: This assay was performed essentially as described by Sack and Sack[2]. The following modifications were made by laboratory A.

(i) Colonies were inoculated into 2 ml of trypticase soy broth containing 0.6% yeast extract in 12 × 100 mm tubes with loose closures and incubated at 37°C for 48 hours before being tested.

(ii) 200 µl of whole bacterial culture were added to each well and only alternate wells were used.

(iii) The bacterial growth was exposed to the Y-1 adrenal cell monolayers for ten rather than five minutes.

Mini Yl assay: (laboratory D). Bacterial strains were grown 18 hours in 0.5 ml syncase-glucose medium in 'universal' bottles without shaking. Yl cells were grown three days in micro-titre plates to give a monolayer. On the day of test fresh medium was added to the monolayers, then 0.05 ml of whole, live bacterial culture was added to a well. After five minutes this was removed and the cells washed once with phosphate buffered saline. 0.2 ml tissue culture medium was replaced with medium containing penicillin, streptomycin and gentamicin. After 24 hours the cells were fixed, stained and observed for rounding.

ELISA test: 100 µl ganglioside GM_1 (2 µg/ml) were absorbed overnight at room temperature to micro ELISA plates (Dynatech Immulon). After washing 3 times with PBS Tween (0.05%), unoccupied binding sites were blocked with 1% bovine serum albumin (Sigma) for 30 minutes at 37°C. After washing, as above, 100 µl test filtrate prepared as for CHO test was added for 18 hours at room temperature. After washing, 100 µg anti-cholera toxin diluted 1/200 in PBS Tween was added for 2 hours at room temperature. After washing, 100 µl antirabbit IgG alkaline phosphatase conjugate (Sigma, 1/500) was added for 18 hours at room temperature. After washing, 200 μl p-nitrophenyl phosphate (1 mg/ml in carbonate buffer pH 9.8) was added. After 100 minutes the reaction was stopped with 25 μl NaOH (1M) and extinction read at 405 nm.

Minor modifications to this procedure were made by laboratory A.

LT "probe" assay: This was used by two laboratories and was essentially that described by Mosley et al.[3]

Passive immune hemolysis (PIH): This test was used by one laboratory and was carried out as described by Serafim et al.[4]

Rabbit skin vascular permeability factor (PF) assay: This test was used by one laboratory and was carried out as a modification of the method originally described by Kusama and Craig[5]. Organisms were grown in 5 ml casamino acid-yeast extract medium containing 0.2% glucose in resting 50 ml Erlenmeyer flasks for 24 hours at 37°C. Culture filtrates were mixed with an equal volume of borate-gelatin buffer pH 7.5 and a sample was heated at 70°C for 30 min. Blueing scores of heated and unheated samples and of appropriate dilutions of control cholera toxin were calculated by multiplying mean blueing diameter by mean blueing intensity of 4 lesions on two rabbits. Strains were considered positive if the unheated blueing score was greater than 12 and more than 3-fold greater than that of the heated material.

RESULTS

The general design and conduct of this study generated qualitative results, in which (a) the identity (LT positive or LT negative) of strains examined in the five participating laboratories was compared with the designated "true" identity of the strains, as determined by the reference laboratory supplying the strains and (b) the results obtained by different laboratory methods, within the one laboratory, could be compared. The overall objective was to assess the potential value of the Biken test as a routine diagnostic procedure for laboratories in both developed and developing countries.

Table 1 shows the results obtained by the five laboratories using the Biken test and at least one other procedure. In the case of laboratory A, some difficulty was initially experienced in reading the Biken test, although this was overcome with experience. This laboratory obtained excellent results with the GM_1-ELISA, Y1 adrenal cell and the DNA-probe tests. Laboratories A, C and D retested those strains which, on first testing, did not give uniform results with all methods. By so doing they were able to increase the number of "correct" results obtained with the Biken test.

Laboratory E achieved only 68% agreement between the rabbit skin PF assay and the designated Biken results. This was due entirely to false negative PF test results. No false-positive PF tests were found. A significant number of LT-producing *E. coli* did not produce enough toxin in culture filtrates under the conditions of growth which were used in this laboratory to yield a positive PF test. Further tests are being carried out with these strains under different growth conditions.

In general, the results obtained with other test systems were excellent; this was to be expected as the participating laboratories had all had considerable experience in the use of these test systems. The two exceptions were the results of the GM$_1$-ELISA assay in laboratory D and of the rabbit skin assay in laboratory E. Laboratory D was using GM$_1$-ELISA for the first time. Laboratory E has used the rabbit skin assay extensively for both cholera enterotoxin and LT assays and there is at present no ready explanation for the failure of many known LT-producing strains to give positive skin tests.

Table 2 shows the results obtained with the Biken test in the five laboratories. Using this data, the sensitivity, specificity and predictive accuracy of the Biken test were determined (Table 3). Specificity and protective accuracy were excellent. Sensitivity was only moderately good on initial testing, but improved greatly when retesting was carried out in three laboratories.

An attempt was made to more closely examine those strains on which an incorrect result was obtained by the Biken test. No one strain was incorrectly identified by all five laboratories, although one strain was incorrectly identified by 3 laboratories. Further analyses of incorrect results, according to the type of toxin produced by the test strain, are shown in Table 4. From these results it is clear that (a) with LT producing strains, an incorrect result is equally likely to occur with both LT-ST or LT only strains, (b) similarly with LT negative strains, an incorrect result in equally likely to occur with both ST producing and non-toxigenic strains. However, the results indicate that incorrect results are less likely

Table 2. Distribution of positive and negative results obtained with the Biken test within the five participating laboratories.

Laboratory	True positive	False positive	True negative	False negative
A	40 (50)	8 (0)	42 (50)	10 (0)
B	50	0	50	0
C	41 (50)	2 (1)	48 (49)	9 (0)
D	42 (50)	0	50 (50)	8 (0)
E	50	1	49	0

Test set is 50 positive and 50 negative strains. Figures in brackets give results after 'retesting'.

Table 3. Sensitivity, specificity and predictive accuracy of the 'Biken' test in each of the five participating laboratories.

Participating laboratory	Sensitivity (%)	Specificity (%)	Predictive accuracy (%)
A	80 (100)	84 (100)	83 (100)
B	100	100	100
C	82 (100)	96 (100)	95 (100)
D	84 (100)	100	100
E	100	98	98

Figures given in brackets show results obtained after 'retesting'.

to be reported with LT negative strains than with LT producing strains (X^2 = 7.29, p = <0.01). This of course correlates with data shown in Table 3 in which the specificity is shown to be higher than the sensitivity of the test.

In order to test the reproducibility of the Biken test, 10 replicate cultures of an LT producing strain, and 10 replicate cultures of an LT negative strain were included within the set of 100 test organisms. The results obtained with these organisms are given in Table 5. It is also interesting to note that despite the fact that laboratory D obtained 23 "incorrect" results using the GM_1-ELISA test, no incorrect results were obtained with this test using the two replicate strains. Reproducibility was 100% with the replicate strains for both the LT positive and LT negative cultures.

Claimed advantages of the Biken test are that it is relatively simple, requires no special or expensive equipment, and despite the fact that the elapsed time between setting up the test and reporting the final result is relatively long (at least 72 hours), the actual test "bench" time is relatively short. All participating laboratories were therefore asked to report their experience in this regard. The results are given in Tables 6 and 7.

Table 4. Distribution of "incorrect" results according to type of toxin produced by the test strains.

Toxins produced	Strains included in study	A	B	C	D	E	Total (all labs)
LT + ST	21	4	—	5	4	—	13/105
LT only	29	6	—	4	4	—	14/145
ST only	21	3	—	—	—	1	4/105
Non-toxigenic	29	5	—	2	—	—	7/145

X^2:	LT + ST vs LT only	0.0833	p = 0.76
	ST only vs non-toxigenic	0.147	p = 0.70
	All LT positive vs LT negative strains	7.29	p = <0.01

Results are based on initial finding and not those recorded on retesting.

Table 5. Reproducibility of initial test results obtained using the Biken test with 10 replicate strains of LT positive *E. coli* and 10 replicate strains of LT negative *E. coli*.

Laboratory	Percent reproducibility	
	LT positive strain	LT negative strain
A	100	100
B	100	100
C	90	80
D	100	100
E	100	100

Table 6. Timing of tests.

Test	Approximate total bench time (hours)	Time to test one strain*	Total time for result
Biken	2.5	15 Min	3–5 days
GM₁-ELISA	10	?	4 days
CHO	7.5	40 Min	3 days
Mini Y1	7.5	20 Min	3 days

Results for one laboratory only-chosen as representative of overall pattern observed by other laboratories.
*Time for one strain is very difficult to estimate.

Table 7. Ease of performance of Biken and other tests.

Test	Comments
Biken	Reading and test easy, special requirements (some difficulty to read test initially if light box not used) (+)
GM₁-ELISA	Reading easy, test laborious-many stages at interrupted intervals, special requirements (+ +)
PIH	Reading easy, test easy, special requirements (+ +)
CHO	Reading easy, test easy but slow, as many stages, special requirements (+ + +)
Mini Y1	Reading easy, test easy, special requirements (+ + +)
PF	Injection and reading relatively easy (some training desirable), no special equipment, reference rabbits and overnight housing needed

Discussion and Conclusions

There are two main conclusions to be drawn from the results of this interlaboratory trial; firstly, experienced laboratories, using their own methods, were, with one exception, able to correctly identify LT producing strains of *E. coli* with a high degree of accuracy. Secondly, bearing in mind that all laboratories were using the Biken test for the first time, the results indicate that this is a reliable and reproducible technique, and holds great potential for use as a routine diagnostic tool in developing countries.

The fact that most laboratories obtained best results using their "own" methods is not surprising. In a similarly conducted comparative study of laboratory media and methods used to isolate salmonella species, Edel and Kampelmacher[6] found that more samples were found positive with a laboratory's "own" method, than with a new, standardized technique with which they were less familiar. This is further illustrated in the present trial, by the results obtained by laboratory D, using GM₁-ELISA for the first time. This laboratory obtained only 77% correct results with the Yl adrenal cells and CHO cells (with which it was very familiar) and the Biken tests. On the other hand, laboratory E obtained excellent results with the Biken test, but only 68% correct results with the PF test with which it was familiar.

All laboratories reported that they were able to read the Biken test results more easily as they became familiar with the use of the technique. This is borne out by the fact that laboratories A, C and D all obtained 100% correct results when the test was repeated a second time (the true identity of the strains was still unknown to these investigators at this time).

Despite the most encouraging results obtained with the Biken test, one laboratory did obtain relatively unsatisfactory results on initial testing, and in general had difficulty reading the test. This was investigated further so that minor modifications could be made to the test protocol to make it even more suitable for use in developing countries. In reviewing specific comments made by the participating laboratories and from other laboratories (Y. Takeda, personal communication), the following points can be made regarding the actual performance (and reading) of the test.

(i) In general, the test is easy to perform and most of the materials required are readily available and inexpensive.

(ii) It is equally suitable for use with small numbers of cultures and with large batches of cultures. This is of great benefit to routine diagnostic laboratories.

(iii) Results are usually easier to read 36-48 hours after adding antiserum to the centre well - rather than within 20 hours as initially described.

(iv) A major disadvantage is that the test results are not knows until 3-5 days after initial inoculation.

(v) Precipitin lines (positive results) are easier to detect if a "light box" and optimum lighting conditions are used.

(vi) The test agar should be clear, and free of any background precipitate or cloudiness.

(vii) It is essential that the lincomycin is thoroughly mixed with the agar medium. In this regard prior warming (50 - 60°C) of the lincomycin solution is recommended. It is felt that this may have accounted for the initially poor results obtained by laboratory A.

(viii) The distance between the edge of the bacterial growth and the serum well is critical (about 4 mm).

(ix) Similarly the size of the inoculum itself is important. A final colony size (after 48 hours incubation) of 15 - 20 mm is optimum.

Although the results of the trial demonstrated the potential value of the Biken test to detect LT producing strains of *E. coli*, it must be remembered that most laboratories wish to test strains of *E. coli* for their ability to produce both LT and ST. Therefore, a technique for the detection of LT production, which could be adapted, without significant additional work, to detect ST production, would be of great value. Clearly, many of the advantages associated with the Biken test would be lost if it was also necessary to grow the organism in shaking cultures and prepare a toxin filtrate for use in testing for ST.

Unfortunately, it has not been possible to use the Biken test directly for the detection of ST (by precipitation). However Honda *et al.*[7] have developed a technique which basically involves removal of a small amount of agar from the Biken plate, elution of toxin with phosphate buffered saline, and use of this elute in the suckling mouse test. Such a procedure eliminates any need for additional shaking cultures (and expensive shaking water baths), and thus enhances the potential value of the Biken test as a diagnostic tool for use in developing countries. Because of this, the Scientific Working Group on Bacterial Enteric Infections plans to evaluate further this adaptation of the Biken plates (through a small interlaboratory trial) in the near future.

REFERENCES

1. Honda, T., S. Taga, Y. Takeda, and T. Miwatani. 1981. Modified Elek test for detection of heat-labile enterotoxin of enterotoxigenic *Escherichia coli*. J. Clin. Microbiol. **13**: 1–5.
2. Sack, D. A., and R. B. Sack. 1975. Test for enterotoxigenic *Escherichia coli* using Y1 adrenal cells in miniculture. Infect. Immun. **11**: 334–336.
3. Mosley, S. L., I. Huq, A. R. M. A. Alim, M. So, M. Samadpour-Motalebi, and S. Falkow. 1980. Detection of enterotoxigenic *Escherichia coli* by DNA Colony Hybridization. J. Infect. Dis. **142**: 892–898.
4. Serafim, M. B., A. F. Pestana de Costro, M. H. Lemos dos Reis, and L. R. Trabulsi. 1979. Passive immune hemolysis for detection of heat-labile enterotoxin produced by *Escherichia coli* isolated from different sources. Infect. Immun. **24**: 606–610.
5. Kusama, H., and J. P. Craig. 1970. Production of biologically active substance by two strains of *Vibrio cholerae* Infect. Immun. **1**: 80–87.
6. Edel, W., and E. H. Kampelmacher. 1968. Comparative studies on Salmonella-isolation in eight European laboratories. Bull. Wld Hlth Org. **39**, 487–491.
7. Honda, T., M. Arita, Y. Takeda, and T. Miwatani. 1982. Further evaluation of the Biken test (modified Elek test) for detection of enterotoxigenic *Escherichia coli* producing heat-labile enterotoxin and application of the test to sampling of heat-stable enterotoxin. J. Clin. Microbiol. **16**: 60–62.

Bacterial Diarrheal Diseases, eds., Y. Takeda, T. Miwatani, 219–228.
Copyright © 1985 by KTK Scientific Publishers, Tokyo.

THE USE OF GERM-FREE MICE ASSOCIATED WITH HUMAN FECAL FLORA AS AN ANIMAL MODEL TO STUDY ENTERIC BACTERIAL INTERACTIONS

A. Andremont[1], P. Raibaud[2], C. Tancréde[1], Y. Duval-Iflah[2], and R. Ducluzeau[2]

*Service de Microbiologie Médicale, Institut Gustave-Roussy, 94800 Villejuif[1],
Laboratoire d'Ecologie Microbienne, Centre National de Recherches Zootechniques,
Institut National de la Recherche Agronomique, 78350 Jouy-en-Josas[2], France*

In 1964 Dubos and Schaedler first assimilated the complex intestinal microflora and its relationship with its animal host to an ecosystem[12]. Composition and functions of the intestinal ecosystem have since been widely studied. The same workers[10] and Freter previously described *in vivo* antagonisms of intestinal bacteria against enteric pathogens[21, 22]. Through the work of Abrams and Bishop[1], Ducluzeau and Raibaud[15], and Van der Waij [49], the existence of microbiological barriers, which enhance resistance to colonization by exogenous bacteria and help to prevent infection, has progressively emerged. Interactions between bacterial species within the lumen of the gut may include reciprocal promotion of a strain by another[43], partial[13] or total[35] inhibition of such or such bacterial population, exchange of genetic information through in vivo DNA transfer[18, 19, 28, 39]. These kinds of interactions may be of primary importance in several instances such as : (i): the pathogenesis of local or general infections by organisms originating in the gut, (ii): the chemoprophylaxis of certain forms of infectious diarrhea and of nosocomial infections in surgical and immunocompromised hosts, (iii): the regulation of the spread among bacterial species of pathogenicity and/or resistance genetic determinants.

The heteroxenic man-mice model

Studies of the composition of the intestinal microflora of man are difficult to perform for obvious practical reasons[23]. Some ingenious devices have been used to study human digestive flora at various sites but they cannot be used on a wide scale[24, 25]. It is also difficult for ethical reasons to challenge human volunteers with pathogens or antibiotic drugs in a repeated manner. Major differences between the intestinal microflora of conventional laboratory animals[14] and of man prevent in this matter the use of rats, mice or rabbits as experimental models.

In order to obtain informations on the nature and on the functions of the microbial interactions within the intestinal flora of man, without performing human volunteers experiments, we [36, 46] and others[26] have developed an animal model (Fig. 1). Basically the model consists of germ-free (axenic) C_3H mice (Centre de Sélection des Animaux de Laboratoire, Orléans-La-Source, 45100 France) maintained in flexible plastic Trexler-type isolators[48]. Complex human microbial flora can then be associated to the mice in the following manner: a freshly passed fecal sample of the human donor is weighted and immediately introduced in an anaerobic glove box[4]. A 10^{-2} dilution is made with the aid of an electric high speed mixer (Ultra-Turrax Bioblock, Paris, France). Two butyl rubber-stooped tubes (to prevent any oxgen contact) are transferred to the germ-free mice isolators. The mice are inoculated intragastrically and intrarectally on two consecutive days with 1 ml from each tube. The animals are water-deprived 12 hours before and 12 hours after inoculation (to prevent inhibition of the inoculum by the pH 3 drinking water). This method has been used to associate germ-free mice with rat, chicken, calves, pigs and human microflora[7, 8, 36]. The resulting animals are termed *"heteroxenic mice"*.

To ease the handle of these gnotobiotic animals we have used several technological improvements recently developed in the "Laboratoire d'Ecologie Microbienne" (Jouy-en-Josas, France) [17]. Isolators are automatically sterilized with a commercially available equipment that vaporizes the right quantity of peracetic acid through the inlet filter and then pulses filtered air for rising (Sterivap commercialized by Aerovap, Paris, France). Various sizes of flexible plastic isolators including "mini isolators"[32] have been used. These isolators are equipped with a "rapid transfer double door system"[38] which allows considerable time sparing by avoiding a maximum waste of time inherent in the classical transfer system. Furthermore it avoids the use of peracetic acid in most of the transfers. This

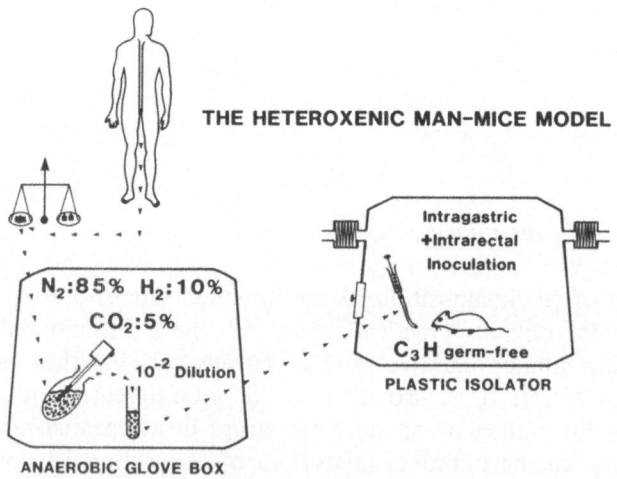

Fig. 1. The heteroxenic man-mice model (see text for explanation).

limits the potential hazards of this product for the personal, as well as the penetration of peracetic acid within the isolator as it happens with the standard lock chamber. An important gain of space is obtained by the use of mini isolators (Fig. 2A). They can be directly connected with a standard isolator (Fig. 2B). Material and axenic mice can be immediately introduced into it. Lastly the mice are fed with gamma irradiated (4 Mrad) sterile diet which allows the addition of such or such unsoluble additive to the diet.

Quantitative differential analysis of the microflora of the human donor and of the animal recipient have been performed in this system using the technics described by Raibaud et al.[34], and Aranki et al.[4]. Both quantitative and qualitative similarities can be observed in this model[36, 46, 26]. Total bacterial counts are identical around 5×10^{10} CFU/g of feces. This number is in agreement with those of literature when identical microbiological technics are used[20]. The equilibrium between the species of the dominant flora (over 10^8/g) (*Bacteroides,*

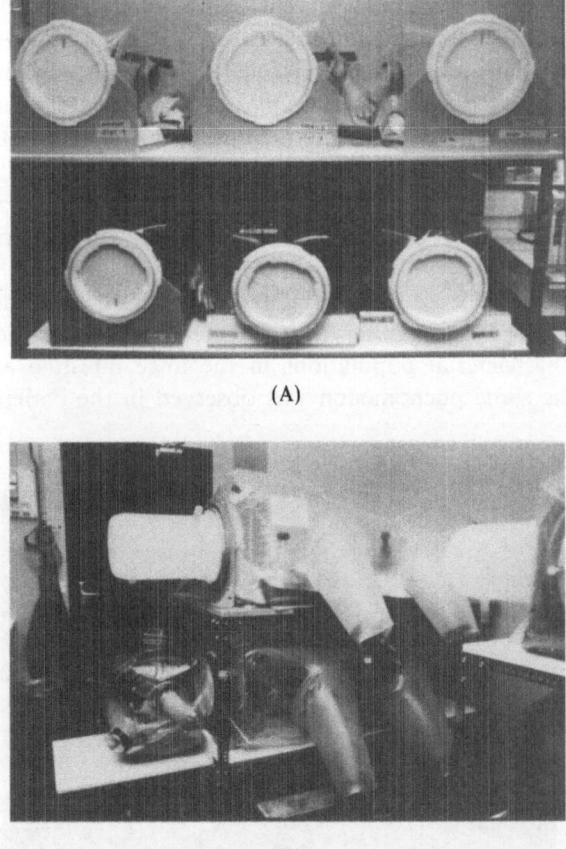

(A)

(B)

Fig. 2A.   Six "mini-isolators" can be stored on a 2 levels rank of 1.5 meter lenght.
Fig. 2B.   Mini-isolators and transfer cylinders can be instantaneously connected with standard isolators through a "setril transfer double door".

Eubacterium, Peptostreptococcus, Clostridium, and *Fusobacterium*) and of the subdominant flora (less than 10^8/g) (*Enterobacteriaceae, Streptococcus*) is reproduced in the mice intestine. An other criterion of the validity of the model can be obtained if one goes to its functional aspect. It is known that the concentration of the aerobic gram negative flora is rather constant in man between 5.10^6 and 5.10^7 CFU/g of feces[23]. This flora is maintained as subdominant flora by the barrier effect exerted by the anaerobic microbial species. Such an effect is called "a permissive barrier" (in contrast to "a drastic barrier" which allows the total elimination of the target strain). This permissive barrier effect is readily transferred to the recipient mice intestine with the same intensity as it was in the donor intestine[26, 36]. When longitudinal studies are performed (over 5 months) this effect persists all along (unpublished results).

The heteroxenic man-mice model to study intestinal decontamination of isolated immuno-compromised patients

We initially used this animal model to mimic the digestive microflora of leukemic patients during the post-chemotherapeutic period[46]. At that time they are severely neutropenic and most susceptible to both exogenous and gut-originated infections. We isolated them in flexible plastic large isolators initially sterile and maintained in positive pressure by sterile filtered air (Fig. 3). The mice are fed with the fecal flora of the patient at the time the patient enters the sterile environment with his endogenous microflora. We so obtain two comparable and stable ecosystems, one in the ward and one in the laboratory. Bacterial aerobic gram negative fecal populations and their qualitative and quantitative modifications are similar in man and in mice when identical antibiotics are used in the diet. Moreover, in some instances we have observed the emergence of previously undetected antibiotic-resistant bacterial populations in the mice intestine after several days of treatment. The same phenomenon was observed in the patient intestinal flora

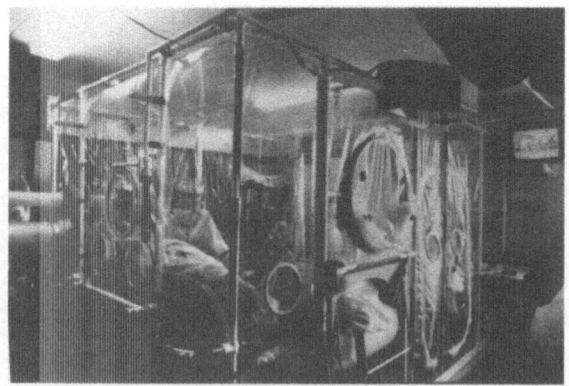

Fig. 3.   Large isolator fitted with the "steril transfer double door" system which allows strict microbial isolation and easy care of the patient.

(Fig. 4). Such information is important because these patients are at high risk of generalized septicemic infection by bacteria that reach high colonic population levels[44]. In the heteroxenic man-mice model we can thus:

- check concomitantly in separate mini isolators several procedures of antibiotic decontamination on a specific flora,

- select the most appropriate antibiotic regimen in the corresponding patient,

- appreciate the infectious risk that can be induced by the emergence of initially repressed bacterial species after the use of such antibiotics.

The heteroxenic man-mice and the chemoprophylaxis of traveller's diarrhea

We next used the heteroxenic man-mice when we approached the chemoprophylaxis of traveller's diarrhea. We had previously shown that oral

GF. C₃H MICE WERE FED INTRAGASTRICALLY WITH
DILUTION 10⁻² OF FECES ON DAY 0 .

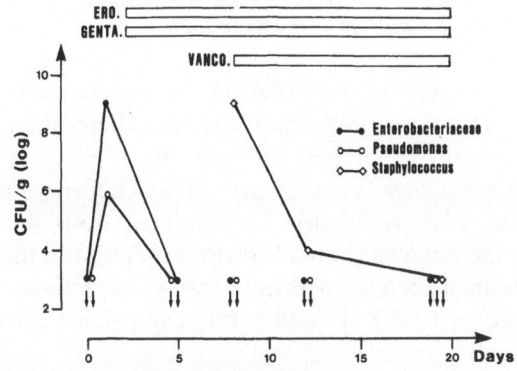

PATIENT IN ISOLATOR

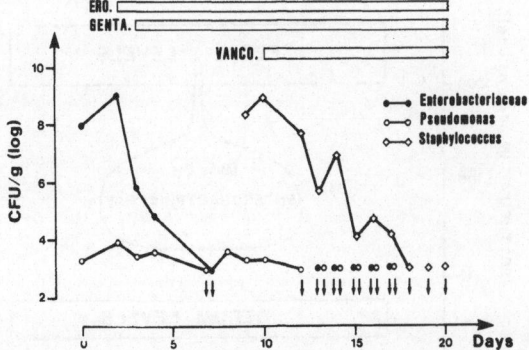

Fig. 4. Correspondance between the heteroxenic man-mice (up) and the donor microflora (down) under identical antibiotic decontamination and secondary emergence of previously undetected bacterial population (see text).

erythromycin (ero) could eliminate the aerobic gram negative bacterial flora from the digestive tract of man during prolonged period of time[45]. This paradoxical effect of ero is due to the high fecal concentrations of the drug when compared to the Minimum Inhibitory Concentrations on *Enterobacteriaceae*. The reproductibility of this effect and its persistance are due to the occurrence of exceptionally high level erythromycin resistant *Enterobacteriaceae* (Fig. 5). Bacterial species that cause traveller's diarrhea are also sensitive to concentrations of ero much lower than achieved in the lumen of the gut[2]. We have demonstrated that daily oral ero would prevent colonization by these bacterial species and so might be used for prophylaxis of traveller's diarrhea[2]. It is known however that during some oral antibiotic treatment the colonization resistance against potential pathogens is lowered[11, 21, 41]. This may lead to an increase incidence of "translocation" (i.e.: passage of viable bacteria from the GI tract to mesenteric lymph nodes) of intestinal bacteria[5]. However, after the end of the treatment with oral ero there is no overwhelming growth of the aerobic gram negative microflora[45], indicating that the barrier effect is still functional. The persistance of this barrier effect exerted by the remaining flora under erythromycin treatment has been further studied[3]: this barrier effect is effective against exogenous erythromycin-resistant strains (*P. aeruginosa, E. coli, C. albicans*).

In associating axenic mice with the fecal microflora of the human volunteer taking 3 g/day of ero base, we have obtained *Enterobacteriaceae*- free heteroxenic man-mice (Fig. 6). The interesting feature is that these animals are *not* treated with ero and can be orally challenged with ero-susceptible strains such as bacteria that cause traveller's diarrhea most often[2]. This challenge mimics what would happen to a traveller who would stop its treatment while being still exposed to contamination. We have shown (unpublished results) that in this situation the barrier effect of the intestinal flora is still drastic against *V. cholerae* 569B and, although slower, against *S. flexneri* DKR115 and permissive against enterotoxigenic *E. coli* H10407.

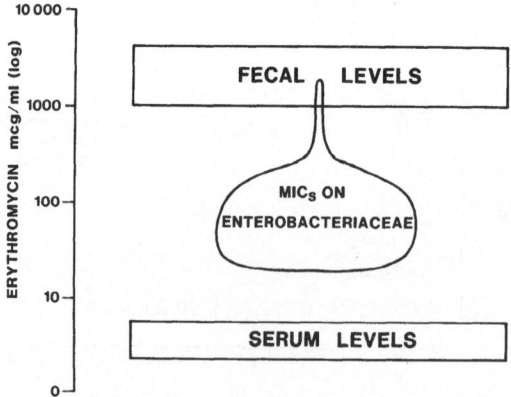

Fig. 5. Comparison between the MIC$_s$ of erythromycin against *Enterobacteriaceae* and serum and fecal levels obtained in man during a 1-3g/day treatment.

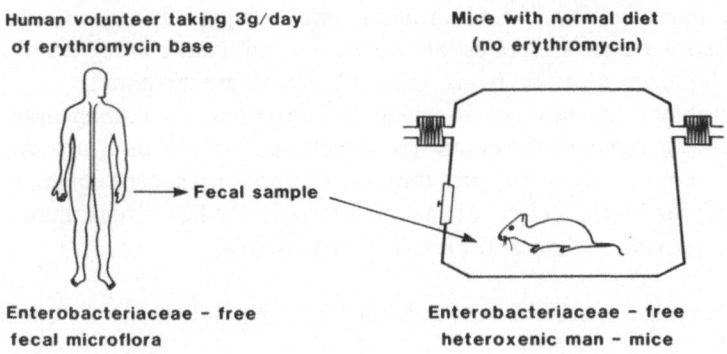

Fig. 6. *Enterobacteriaceae* - free heteroxenic man-mice which allows to test colonization resistance against erythromycin-sensitive aerobic gram negative species.

The heteroxenic man-mice model and the plasmid transfer in vivo

The heteroxenic man-mice model has also been used to study genetic transfer of R factors in vivo. The cotransfer of resistance to 14 antibiotics obserded *in vitro* between a strain of *Serratia liquefaciens* and *E. coli* occurred *in vivo*, in the digestive tract of axenic or heteroxenic mice. Mating occurred even when the donor strain was only transient in the digestive tract of the gnotobiotic animals. A dense population of *Bacteroides* did not hinder this mating. All matings occurred in the absence of any antibiotic selection pressure. However, during antibiotic administration to mice, and even after the end of the drug intake, the transconjugant became established in the dominant population and replaced the parental recipient strain[19].

DISCUSSION

Through these three examples of the use of the heteroxenic man-mice model we have tried to stress its multiple potential uses. The lack of disease of gnotobiotic adult rodents colonized with enteric pathogens of man (exept *Salmonella*) allows to prolong the period of observation and of experimentation[29, 37]. For instance the immunological conversion of *Vibrio cholerae* observed in gnotobiotic mice may lead to hypothesis on the mechanisms by which *V. cholerae* changes its serotype away from the immunological pressure of the population in endemic areas[30]. Human healthy carriers might play an important role in this phenomenon[30]. Descriptive and functional studies of the intestinal flora of such individuals are difficult[25] and could be more easily performed in the heteroxenic man-mice model.

Our model does not pretend to mimic a human disease. It is an ecological system in which bacterial interactions within the lumen of the gut are reproduced. It is known that synergism exists between ecologic and immunologic control mechanisms of intestinal flora[42]. Persistence of the strain in the colon is a major factor in oral immunogenicity even with pathogens that exert their pathogenicity in the jejunum like *V. cholerae*[6,40] and this persistence is controlled by the en-

226

dogenous microbial flora[27]. Gnotobiotic mice can provide a good model to study the competitive effects of intestinal microflora on *V. cholerae*[31] and thus be of primary importance when living vaccinal strains are prepared.

Gnotobiotic animals can also help to understand the pathogenesis of enteric infections that occur in the colon like shigellosis[16, 21, 47] or *Clostridium difficile* colitis[9, 33]. Control of the proliferation of these pathogens might be achieved in studying the barrier effects of the microflora in the heteroxenic man-mice model and thus provide a new approach for prophylaxis.

This work has been supported in part by the "Contrat de Recherche Clinique, Institut Gustave Roussy n = 80A5"

REFERENCES

1. Abrams, G. D., and J. E. Bishop. 1966. Effect of the normal microbial flora on the resistance of the small intestine to infection. J. Bact. **92**: 1604–1608.
2. Andremont, A., and C. Tancrède. 1981. Reduction of the aerobic gram negative bacterial flora of the gastro-intestinal tract and prevention of traveller's diarrhea using oral erythromycin. Ann. Microbiol. (Inst. Pasteur). **132 B**: 419–427.
3. Andremont, A., P. Raibaud, N. Guerlin, and C. Tancrède. 1981. Resistance to colonization by various pathogen organisms after selective decontamination of the gut with oral erythomycin. VII International Symposium on Gnotobiology pp 51 June 29 – July 3, Tokyo Japan.
4. Aranki, A., S. A. Syed, E. B. Kenney, and R. Freter. 1969. Isolation of anaerobic bacteria from human gingiva and mouse cecum by means of a simplified glove box procedure. Appl. Microbiol. **17**: 568–576.
5. Berg, R. D. 1981. Promotion of the translocation of enteric bacteria from the gastrointestinal tracts of mice by oral treatment with Penicillin, Clindamycin or Metronidazole. Infect. Immun. **33**: 854–861.
6. Bloom, L., and D. Rowley. 1979. Persistance in the mouse gut as an important factor in oral immunogenicity of strains of *V. cholerae*. Aus. J. Exp. Biol. Med. Sci. **57**: 325–333.
7. Corpet, D., and J. L. Nicolas. 1979. Antagonistic effect of intestinal bacteria from the microflora of holoxenic (conventional) piglets against *Clostridium perfringens* in the digestive tract of gnotobiotic mice and gnotobiotic piglets. pp. 169. *In*:Clinical and Experimental Gnotobiotics, T. Fliedner, H. Heit, D. Meithammer and H. pfigler(eds.) Zbl. Bakt. Suppl. 7, Stuttgart: Gustave Fisher.
8. Corpet, D. 1980. Influence de faibles doses de chlortétracycline sur la résistance à la chlortetracycline de *E. coli* dans le tube digestif de souris axéniques hébergeant des flores complexes d'enfant, de veau ou de porcelet. Ann. Microbiol. (Inst. Pasteur) **131 B**: 309–318.
9. Dabar, D., F. Dubos, L. Martinet, and R. Ducluzeau. 1979. Experimental reproduction of neotal diarrhea in young gnotobiotic hares simultaneously associated with *Clostridium difficile* and other *Clostridium* strains. Infec. Immun. **24**: 7–11.
10. Dubos, R. J., and R. W. Schaedler. 1960. The effect of the intestinal flora on the growth rate of mice, and their susceptibility to experimental infections. J. Exp. Med. **111**: 407–417.
11. Dubos, R., R. W. Schaedler, and M. Stevens. 1963. The effect of antibacterial drugs on the fecal flora of mice. J. Exp. Med. **117**: 131–243.
12. Dubos, R., and R. W. Schaedler. 1964. The digestive tract as an ecosystem. Am. J. Med. Sci. **248**: 49/267–53/271.
13. Ducluzeau, R., J. C., Salomon, and J. Huppert. 1967. Ensemencement d'une souche lysogène et d'une souche sensible d'*E. coli*K12 dans le tube digestif de souris axéniques. Etablissement d'un équilibre. Ann. Inst. Pasteur (Paris) **112**: 153–161.
14. Ducluzeau, R. 1969. Influence de l'espèce zoologique sur la microflore du tractus gastro-intestinal. Rev. Immunol. **33**: 345–384.
15. Ducluzeau, R., M. Bellier, and P. Raibaud. 1970. Transit digestif de divers inoculums bactériens

introduits per os chez des souris axéniques et "holoxéniques" (conventionnelles) : Effect antagoniste de la microflore du tractus gastrointestinal. Zbl. Bakt. Parasit. Infection. Kr. Hyg., 1 Orig., **213**: 533-548.

16. Ducluzeau, R., M. Ladire, C. Callut, P. Raibaud, and G. D. Abrams. 1977. Antagonist effect of extremely oxygen-sensitive *Clostridia* from the microflora of conventional mice and of *Escherichia coli* against *Shigella flexneri* in the digestive tract of gnotobiotic mice. Infec. Immun. **17**: 415-424.

17. R. Ducluzeau, C. Moreau, D. Corpet, C. Tancrède, D. Meyer, and M. Saint-martin. 1979. Improvement of techniques leading to time sparing in rearing gnotoxenic animals. pp.83-85 T. Fliedner, H. Heit, D. Meitheimmer and H. Pfigler(eds.), Zbl. Bakt. Suppl. 7, Stuttgart : Gustave Fisher.

18. Duval-Iflah, Y. 1972. Recombination in vivo et in vitro entre phages de *Staphylococcus pyogénes*. Cr. Acad. Sc. Paris **275** D 3035-3038.

19. Duval-Iflah, Y., P. Raibaud, C. Tancrède, and M. Rousseau. 1980. R-plasmid tranfer from *Serratia liquefaciens* to *Escherichia coli In Vitro* and *In Vivo* in the digestive tract of gnotobiotic mice associated with human fecal flora. Infect. Immun. **28**: 981-990.

20. Finegold, S. M., V. L. Sutter, P. T. Sugihaka, H. A. Elder, S. M. Lehman, and R. L. Phillips. 1977. Fecal microbial flora in seven day adventists population and control subjects. Am. J. Clin. Nutr. **30**: 1781-1792.

21. Freter, R. F. 1956. Experimental enteric *Shigella* and *Vibrio* infections in mice and in guinea pigs. J. Exp. Med. **104**: 411-418.

22. Freter, R. 1962. In vivo and in vitro antagonism of intestinal bacteria against *Shigella* flexneri. J. Infect. Dis. **110**: 38-46.

23. Gorbach, S. L., L. Nahas, P. I. Lerner, and L. Weinstein. 1976. Studies of intestinal microflora : I Effects of diet, age, and periodic sampling on numbers of fecal microorganisms in man. Gastroenterol. **53** 845-855.

24. Gorbach, S. L., A. G. Plaut, L. Nahas, L. Weinstein, G. Spaknebel, and R. Levitan. 1967. studies of intestinal microflora. II. Microorganisms of the small intestine and their relations to oral and fecal flora. Gastroenterol. **53**: 856-867.

25. Gorbach, S. L., J. G. Banwell, N. F. Pierce, B. D. Chatterjee, and R. C. Mitra. 1970. Intestinal microflora in a chronic carrier of *Vibrio cholerae*. J. Infec. Dis. **121**: 383-390.

26. Hazenberg, M. P., M. Bakker, and A. Verschoor-Burggraaf. 1981. Effects of the human intestinal flora on germ-free mice. J. Appl. Bacteriol. **50**: 95-106.

27. Horsfall, D. J., and D. Rowley. 1978. Modifications of the local immune response to *Vibrio cholerae* attributed to the intestinal microbial flora of the mouse. Aus. J. Exp. Biol. Med. Sci. **56**: 579-586.

28. Kasuya, M. 1964. Transfer of drug resistance between enteric bacteria induced in the mouse intestine. J. Bacteriol. **88**: 322-328.

29. Klipstein, F. A., C. A. Goetsch, R. F. Engert, H. B. Short, and E. A. Schenk. 1978. Effect of monocontamination of germ-free rats by enterotoxigenic bacteria. Gastroenterol. **76**: 341-347.

30. Miller, C. E., K. H. Wong, J. C. Feeley, and M. E. Forlines. 1972. Immunological conversion of *Vibrio cholerae* in gnotobiotic mice. Infect. Immun. **6**: 739-742.

31. Miller, C. E., J. C. Feeley. 1975. Competitive effects of intestinal microflora on *Vibrio cholerae* in gnotobiotic mice. Lab. Anim. Sci. **25**: 454-458.

32. Moreau, M. C., R. Ducluzeau, and D. Meyer. 1978. Utilisation d'isolateurs miniaturisés pour l'expérimentation sur animaux "gnotoxéniques". Sci. Tech. Anim. Lab. **3**: 117-120.

33. Onderdonk, A. B., R. L. Cisneros, and J. G. Bartlett. 1980. *Clostridium difficile* in gnotobiotic mice. Infec. Immun. **28**: 277-282.

34. Raibaud, P., A. B. Dickinson, E. Sacquet, H. Charlier, and G. Mocquot. 1966. La microflore du tube digestif du rat. I. Techniques d'étude et milieux de culture proposés. Ann. Inst. Pasteur (Paris;) **110**: 568-590.

35. Raibaud, P., R. Ducluzeau, and C. Tancrède. 1977. L'effect de barrière microbien dans le tube digestif : moyen de défense de l'hôte contre les bactéries exogènes. Med. et Mal. Infect. **1**: 130-134.

36. Raibaud, P., R. Ducluzeau, F. Dubos, S. Hudault, H. Bewa, and M. C. Muller. 1980. Implantation of bacteria from the digestive tract of man and various animals into gnotobiotic mice. Am. J. Clin. Nutr. **33**: 2440–2447.

37. Sack, R. B., and C. E. Miller. 1969. Progressive changes of *Vibrio* serotypes in germ-free mice infected with *Vibrio cholerae*. J. Bact. **99**: 688–695.

38. Saint-Martin, B., R. Ducluzeau, J. C. Ghnassia, C. Griscelli, and B. Lauvergeon. 1975. Amélioration de la technologie des enceintes stériles permettant leur application à la médecine et à la chirurgie. Rev. Franc. Gynec. **70**: 585–593.

39. Sansonetti, P., J. P. Lafont, A. Jaffe-brachet, J. F. Guillot, and E. Shaslus-Dancla. 1980. Parameters controlling interbacterial plasmid spreading in a gnotoxenic chicken gut system : influence of plasmid and bacterial mutations. Antimicrob. Agents Chemother. **17**: 327–333.

40. Sasaki, S., N. Ohnishi, R. Suzuki, K. Adachi, M. Miyashita, T. Shimamura, and S. Tazume, *et al*. 1970. The relation between the persistence of *El tor Vibrio* in the intestines of germ-free mice and the so-called coproantibody. J. Infect. Dis. **121**: 5124–5131.

41. Savage, D. C., and R. Dubos. 1968. Alterations in the mouse cecum and its flora produced by antibacterial drugs. **128**: 97–110.

42. Shedlofsky, S., R. Freter. 1974. Synergism between ecologic and immunologic control mechanisms of intestinal flora. J. Infec. Dis. **129**: 296–303.

43. Syed, S. A., G. D. Abrams, and R. F. Freter. 1970. Efficienty of various intestinal bacteria in assuming normal functions of enteric flora after association with germ-free mice. Infect. Immun. **2**: 376–386.

44. Tancrède, C., P. Azzizi, P. Raibaud, and R. Ducluzeau. 1977. Conséquences de la destruction des barrières écologiques de la flore du tube digestif par les antibiotiques : perturbation des relations entre l'hôte et les bactéries potentiellement pathogènes. Med. et Mal. Infect. **7**: 145–149.

45. Tancrède, C., A. Andremont, and N. Guerlin. 1980. Effect de l'Erythromycine sur les populations d'Entérobactéries du tube digestif chez l'homme. Nouv. Presse Med. (Paris) **9**: 2742–2743.

46. Tancrède, C., A. Andremont, and A. M. Kherbiche. 1981. Germ-free mice associated with human flora as a means of bacteriological surveillance of neutropenic patients in sterile environment. VII International symposium on Gnotobiology p-72 June 29–July 3 - Tokyo, Japan.

47. Tazumes, S., K. Mashimoto, and S. Sasaki. 1979. Intestinal flora and bile acids metabolism. Influence of bile acids on rejection of *Shigella flexneri* 2a from the intestine. Jap. J. Bacteriol. **34**: 745–754.

48. Trexler, P. C., and L. I. Reynolds. 1957. Flexible film apparatus for the rearing and use of germ-free animals. Appl. Microbiol. **5**: 406–412.

49. van der Waaij, D., J. M. Berghuis-de-Vriies, and van der Weesje, Lekkerkerk. 1971. Colonization resistance of the digestive tract in conventional and antibiotic treated mice. J. Hyg. (Lond) **69**: 405–407.

Bacterial Diarrheal Diseases, eds., Y. Takeda, T. Miwatani, 229–232.
Copyright © 1985 by KTK Scientific Publishers, Tokyo.

EXPERIMENTAL CHOLERA IN PIGLET MODELS

N. Ohtomo, T. Muraoka, E. Tokunaga, K. Kudo, and S. Akiyama

The Chemo-Sero-Therapeutic Research Institute, Kumamoto 860, Japan

Many kinds of animal models have been developed for studies on cholera[1]. Although these models have been useful, problems are often encountered in interpretation of results, because the models do not resemble cholera in humans. Moreover, because, with many models, inoculation of *Vibrio cholerae* or cholera toxin must be done by surgical manipulation, the pathogenicity rarely represents severe diarrhea but rather localized fluid accumulation. Dogs are known to show the cholera syndrome after ingestion of *V. cholerae* or cholera toxin, but this requires a large inoculum and is poorly reproducible[2,3]. Since swine like humans, are natural host for enterotoxigenic *E. coli*, LT of which is etiologically closely related to *V. cholerae*, we studied the sensitivity of piglets to oral challenge with *V. cholerae* and/or cholera toxin[4,5].

We used three kinds of piglets: (1) those purchased conventional, (2) hysterectomy-produced, colostrum-deprived (HPCD) and germ-free piglets and[3] HPCD-gnotobiotic piglets. The latter two kind were kept in sterile isolators from birth. Piglets of 2 to 5 weeks old (usually 2 weeks old), were given various strains of *V. cholerae* or cholera toxin through a silicon rubber tube. Samples were given in 30 ml of 6% bicarbonate solution. Then the health, stools, excretion of vibrios, etc. were examined at interval until the end of the experiment.

Experiments on conventional piglets

Piglets of 2 weeks old, were inoculated orogastrically with *V. cholerae* strain 569B of doses of 10^6 to 10^{10} cfu. Diarrheal of varied severity appeared in only some individuals, irrespective of the dose. Mild diarrhea was also noticed in control animals. Other piglets, inoculated with 5 to 100 μg of cholera toxin, also showed varied responsed, some developing severe diarrhea and others transient diarrhea or none. Control animals also demonstrated transient symptoms. The sensitivity of this kind of piglet to cholera toxin, and probably also to *V. cholerae* seemed to vary in different fallows (Table 1).

Experiments in HPCD-germ-free piglets

HPCD piglets being fed on sterile SPF milk in isolators, were challenged

Table 1. Diarrhea in conventional piglets after orogastric challenge with *V. cholerae* or cholera toxin

Piglet fallow	*V. cholerae* strain or Cholera toxin	Challenge dose	No. responding with			No. death/ No. tested
			soft stool	diarrhea	watery diarrhea	
C1	569B classic. Inaba	10^6 cfu	0	1	1	0/2
		10^8	1	0	1	0/2
		10^{10}	1	0	0	0/1
	Control	0	0	2	0	0/2
C2	Cholera toxin	20 μg	0	0	1	0/1
		70	0	0	1	0/1
C3	Cholera toxin	5 μg	0	1	0	0/2
		10	2	0	0	0/2
		20	2	0	0	0/2
		40	1	1	0	0/2
	Control	0	0	2	0	0/2
C4	Cholera toxin	10 μg	0	2	0	0/2
		50	0	0	1	0/2
		100	0	2	0	0/2
	Control	0	1	0	0	0/1

Conventional piglets, aged 2 weeks, were challenged orogastrically with *V. cholerae* or cholera toxin in 6% bicarbonate, and were observed periodically for approximately 2 days until piglets were sacrificed.

with *V. cholerae*. The strains used were 569B classical Inaba, NIH 41 classical Ogawa, P6973 Eltor Inaba and T348 Eltor Inaba and doses were from 10^6 to 10^9 cfu., (mainly 10^8 cfu). Clear results were obtained: All animals showed a severe cholera-like syndrome, with diarrhea starting 6 to 18 hr after challenge, which was soon followed by watery diarrhea. Another group of piglets was challenged with cholera toxin at doses of 10 to 100 μg. Animals that received 10 μg of toxin developed diarrhea but not watery flow, but those receiving 25 μg or more toxin developed severe cholera-like diarrhea after a short incubation of 3 hr. In both challenge experiments on germ-free piglets, a few animals died during the period of severe diarrhea but most recovered gradually within a few days (Table 2).

Germ-free piglets challenged with *V. cholerae* continued to excrete vibrios in their stools even when they became convalescent. Measurement of the number of vibrios in diarrheal stool showed that when diarrhea started, the number of vibrios reached 10^{10} to 10^{11} cfu/ml of stool, and then gradually decreased to about 10^8 cfu/ml.

Histological studies were also carried out on intestinal specimens obtained from a piglet during severe diarrhea. Major changes were observed in the ileum, such as oedema in the lamina propria and submucosal tissue, dilatation of the lymphatics and vacuoles in epithelial cells of villi.

Experiments in HPCD-gnotobiotic piglets

HPCD piglets were given *Enterobacter cloacae* and *Staphylococcus epider-*

231

Table 2. Diarrhea in HPCD piglets after orogastric challenge with *V. cholerae* or cholera toxin

V. cholerae strain or Cholera toxin	Challenge dose	No. responding with			Excretion of *V. cholerae*	No. death/ No. tested
		soft stool	diarrhea	watery diarrhea		
HPCD-germ-free piglets						
569B classic. Inaba	10^6 cfu	0	0	3	3	0/3
	10^7	0	0	1	1	0/1
	10^8	0	0	3	3	0/3
	10^9	0	0	1	1	1/1
NIH 41 classic. Ogawa	10^8	0	0	2	2	0/2
P6973 Eltor Inaba	10^7	0	0	2	2	1/2
T348 Eltor Inaba	10^8	0	1	1	2	0/2
Cholera toxin	10 μg	0	2	0		0/2
	25	0	0	1		1/1
	50	0	0	1		0/1
	100	0	0	1		1/1
Control	0	0	0	0		0/8
HPCD-gnotobiotic piglets						
569B classic. Inaba	10^8 cfu	0	0	4	4	0/4
Cholera toxin	50 μg	0	0			0/2
Control	0	0	0	0		0/2

Hysterectomy-produced colostrum-deprived (HPCD) piglets, aged 2 weeks predominantly, were challenged orogastically with *V. Cholerae* or cholera toxin in 6% bicarbonate, and were observed periodically for approximately 7 days until piglets were sacrificed. All the challenge strains were recovered by swab test during the test period.

midis concomitantly before experiment and were challenged with either 50 μg of cholera toxin or 10^8 cfu of *V. cholerae* strain 569B. Like germ-free piglets, all of them developed cholera-like diarrhea. Other gnotobiotic piglets, with a species of gram-positive anaerobes, were also challenged with *V. cholerae*. They also clearly responded to the challenge developing cholera-like diarrhea (Table 2).

The chronological change in the number of vibrios excreted in the stools of the latter gnotobiotic piglets was also measured. Contrary to results in germ-free piglets the curve appeared to have an upward convex form coinciding with the severity of diarrhea.

CONCLUSION

From the present work we conclude that not only HPCD-germ-free piglets, but also various HPCD-gnotobiotic piglets are sensitive to oral challenge with either *V. cholerae* or cholera toxin. Since they respond to the challenge very clearly, showing a typical cholera syndrome, they seem to be useful as animal models, especially in studies on choleragenicity.

REFERENCE

1. Burrows, W. and R. B. Sack. 1974. Animal models of Cholera. pp. 189–205. *In* Barua, D. and Burrows, W. (ed.). Cholera. Saunders Company, Philadelphia, London and Toronto.
2. Sack, R. B. and C. C. J. Carpenter. 1969. Experimental canine cholera. I. Development of the model. J. Infect. Dis., **119**: 138–149.
3. Sack, R. B. and C. C. J. Carpenter. 1969. Experimental canine cholera. II. Production by cell-free culture filtrates of *Vibrio cholerae*. J. Infect. Dis., **119**: 150–157.
4. Ohtomo, N., T. Muraoka, E. Tokunaga, S. Akiyama, K. Kudo, and H. Taneno. 1980. Experimental cholera in hysterectomy-produced colostrum-deprived (HPCD) piglets. *In* Proceedings of 16th US-Japan Joint Cholera Conference, Gifu, 266–275.
5. Tokunaga, E., T. Muraoka, S. Akiyama, K. Kudo, and N. Ohtomo. 1983. Experimental cholera in germ-free and gnotobiotic piglets. pp. 127–134. *In* Kuwahara, S. and Pierce, N. F. (ed.). Advances in Research on cholera and Related Diarrheas. Martinus Nijhoff Publishers, Boston.

Bacterial Diarrheal Diseases, eds., Y. Takeda, T. Miwatani, 233–239.
Copyright © 1985 by KTK Scientific Publishers, Tokyo.

CAMPYLOBACTER ENTERITIS

J. P. Butzler

*Infectious Disease Unit and WHO Collaborating Center for Campylobacter jejuni,
St Pierre Hospital 322, Rue Haute, 1000 Brussels, Belgium*

In the last few years *Campylobacter jejuni* has been recognized as one of the commonest causes of bacterial diarrhea. In many industrialised countries as Belgium[1], Great Britain[2], the Netherlands[3], Spain[4], Finland[5], France[6], Australia[8], Canada[9] and the United States[10], workers have reported its isolation from 5–14% of diarrhea cases and from less than 1% of asymptomatic persons. The prevalence of *C. jejuni* in developing countries a Zaire[11], Rwanda[12], Brazil[13], Peru[14], South Africa[15], Indonesia[16] and Bangladesh[17] is far greater than that in industrialized countries and seems directly related to socioeconomic factors. Although the global magnitude of the problem of *C. jejuni* enteric infection in the world has still to be determined it seems that this infection is as-if not more common than salmonellosis.

Clinical features

Firstly not all *Campylobacter* infections produce symptoms. Symptomless excreters occur among the close contacts of infected patients, although their incidence in industrialized countries is less than 1%. In some developing countries 40 per cent of children, nine to 24 months of age, are asymptomatic excreters[17]. For symptomatic patients the average incubation period is about 5 days but ranges 2 to 11 days. The patient may experience malaise, headache, backache, aching limbs and fever 2 to 3 days before the onset of bowel symptoms (Table 1). This prodromal state is followed by nausea and abdominal cramps, which are typically peri-umbilical. These are rapidly followed by diarrhea, which may be profuse, watery or slimy and foul smelling. In 30 to 50% of cases dysenteric stools characterized by blood and mucus may appear and most diarrheal stool samples that have been examined microscopically contain an inflammatory exsudate with leucocytes. In some severely affected patients, dehydration and electrolyte imbalance necessitate hospital admission. However the most frequent reason for hospital admission has probably been abdominal pain, which can be severe enough to mimic an acute abdomen and is usually seen in young adults and teenagers. Some undergo emergency surgery and occasionally they do indeed have peritonitis from an acute appendicitis, but most of these that undergo laparotomy have inflammation of some part of the ileum and jejunum coupled with mesenteric adenitis (Table 2).

Another potential surgical complication may arise in young infants with *Campylobacter* infection. They sometimes pass blood in their stools and have little diarrhea[18]. This has led in some cases to a mistaken diagnosis of intussusception, resulting in an unnecessary laparotomy. The sites of tissue injury include the jejunum, ileum and colon. The illness may be localized to the upper gastrointestinal tract: *C. jejuni* could be cultured from ileal aspirates in children with *Campylobacter* enteritis[19] and post mortem examinations of patients who died of *C. jejuni* enteritis showed hemorrhagic lesions of the jejunum and ileum[28]. However many patients have erythrocytes and leucocytes in their stools which suggests colonic involvement cause infectious proctitis in homosexual men [23]. A variety of other clinical syndromes have been associated with the isolation of *C. jejuni* : meningism[24], meningitis[25], cholecystitis[26], Reiter's syndrome[27] and reactive arthritis in men with and without HLA-B$_{27}$ histocompatibility antigen[5]. Septicemia appears to be uncommon but this may reflect a failure to take blood cultures early enough in the disease[28, 29].

Laboratory Diagnosis Direct Microscopy

The direct examination of stools by dark-field or phase contrast microscopy is a specific and sensitive method for diagnosis provided the samples are not more than a few hours old[9]. The test is particularly useful in the acute phase of the illness. Campylobacters can be recognized by their characteristic morphology and rapid darting and oscillating motility. Microscopy is also useful for the detection of pus cells and red blood cells which are commonly found in *Campylobacter*

Table 1. *Main Symptoms of Campylobacter enteritis*

Prodromal phase:	a few hours to a few days-not always present-general feeling of weakness, headache, malaise, myalgia, arthralgia, fever.
Diarrheal phase:	2 to 5 days (10 days) abdominal cramps, diarrhea (profuse, watery of slimy) stools show inflammatory exsudate with leucocytes and fresh blood.
Recovery phase:	2 days to 3 weeks abdominal pain may persist, sometimes dehydration.

Table 2. *Camplications of C. jejuni enteritis*

	severe abdominal pain	
	appendicitis	
	cholecystitis	
	peritonitis	
	emergency surgery	
exceptional		*in general*
cholecystitis		inflammation of
peritonitis		ileum or
		jejunum with
		mesenteric
		adenitis

enteritis.

Stoolculture

The introduction of selective culture media has made the diagnosis of *Campylobacter* enteritis a simple procedure for a clinical laboratory. Three types of media are in common use:[10, 11] Campy-BAP[10] which consists of brucella agar base, 10% sheep erythrocytes and Blaser's formulation of antimicrobials per liter : vancomycin, 10 mg; trimethoprim, 5 mg; polymyxin B, 2500 IU; amphotericin B, 2 mg; and cephalotin, 15 mg. b) Butzler's medium virion[30]: columbia agar with 7% sheep blood with the following concentrations per liter : cefoperazone, 15 mg; rifampicin, 10 mg; colistin, 10,000 units and amphotericin B, 2 mg. c) Skirrow's medium[2]: Oxoid Base no. 2 with 7% lysed horse blood with following antibiotics per liter: vancomycin, 10 mg; trimethoprim, 5 mg; and polymyxin B sulfate, 2,500 IU. Blaser's and Butzler's are preferable to Skirrow's medium for use in developing countries because they are more selective, they can be used at 37°C and they do not require horse blood (often difficult to obtain). Either fresh stool or rectal swabs can be used for culture. If swabs must be transported and stored, Cary Blair semisolid transport medium should be used, which will maintain the viability of *C. jejuni* for up to 72 hours[17]. Swabs or liquid stools should be applied directly to 1/4 of a selective agar plate and streaked for separation with a loop. If solid stool is being cultured, it should first be emulsified with saline before it is applied to the agar. With all media, plates must be incubated under conditions of reduced oxygen tension, preferable with added carbondioxide. *C. jejuni* grows best at 42°C in an atmosphere of 5% O_2, 10% CO_2 and 85% N_2 or H_2[18]. Various methods for creation of this atmosphere are available to clinical microbiological laboratories. They must be adapted in respect of cost and workflow to each laboratory. In well equiped laboratories which handle a large amount of specimens we recommend the evacuation replacement system where in an incubator 2/3 of the air are replaced by a mixture of 95% N_2 on 5% CO_2. In developing countries we recommend the use of the inexpensive candle jar, where the oxygen level is reduced to approximately 17%. A candle jar is usually satisfactory for isolation but has the disadvantage that at a temperature of 37°C the total incubation time should be extended to 72 hours in order to detect *C. jejuni* whick grows slower at 37°C than at 42°C. Therefore incubation in a candle jar at 42°C is recommended. Plates containing 1.5% agar or less and incubated at 42°C should be examined at 24 and, 48 hours for gray, flatty glossy and effuse colonies, which have a tendency to spread along the tracks left by the inoculating wire. When well spaced they resemble droplets of fluid that have been spattered on the agar. The moisture content of the medium produced a profound effect on the colony morphology of *C. jejuni*. If the medium is fresh and excessively moist it produced flat, spreading colonies with a watery appearance. Any suspicious colonies should be smeared and stained with a strong stain such as crystal violet or carbol fuchsin, as campylobacters do not take up stain readily. *C. jejuni* can be seen as slender, gram-negative, spiral or S-shaped organisms with tapering ends. Occasionally the spiral morphology is not obvious and in some cases spindle-shaped bacilli predominate. A highly characteristic feature of *C. jejuni* is that they degenerate into coccoid forms after a few days of culture, especially when grown on solid media. Generally those coccoid forms have lost their motility and fail to subculture. In general the spiral morphology and the rapid darting and oscillating motility are sufficiently characteristic to allow isolation and identification of *C. jejuni* from stools. When the microscopy looks like a *Campylobacter* simple oxidase and catalase tests are performed and if found positive, the organism can be presumptively identified as *Campylobacter jejuni*. This information is frequently available within 24 hours of plating and can provide very useful information to the physician for patient management.

Serological response

The great majority of patients infected with *C. jejuni* acquire specific antibodies, which appear during the first few days of illness. The antibody response has been measured by a number of assays including tube agglutination[18], complement fixation tests[18], bactericidal assays[10] and indirect immunofluorescence[10]. In the near future diffusion-in gel-Enzyme Linked Immunosorbent assyas[31] and complement fixation tests[32] both using a common antigen from *C. jejuni* will probably allow serological survey. It is not known whether specific serum antibody protects against reinfection by homologous or heterologous organisms.

Antibiotic sensitivites

The minimum inhibitoty (MIC) and minimum bactericidal concentrations have been described by different investigators[32-36]. Aminoglycosides, furazolidone, erythromycin, doxycycline, minocycline and chloramphenicol are the most active compounds. *Campylobacter jejuni* is weakly to not susceptible to metronidazole and trimethoprim-sulphamethoxazole. 30% of *C. jejuni* strains are resistant to ampicillin. Almost all strains are resistant to penicillin, most of the cephalosphorins, rifampin, vancomycin, trimethoprim and polymyxin B[34]. Some strains produce a betalactamase[3]. In a recent study Vanhoof and coll[38] have compared the antibiotic sensitivities of human *C. jejuni* strains to those of animal *C. jejuni* strains. In general the distribution for human and animal strains were very similar, confirming the previous hypothesis that *C. jejuni* infection should be considered as a zoonosis. Furazolidone, gentamicin and chloramphenicol have the lowest MIC's. The MIC distibutions for tetracycline and erythromycin are very comparable for the human and animal strains. The tetracycline resistance in the animal population is exclusively due to the chicken strains. In the human population 4.2% of the strains are resistant to erythromycin. In the animal population the proportion of erythromycin resistant strains is comparable with that of the human population, i.e. 4.3%. There too the erythromycin resistance is mainly attributed to chickenstrains[38].

Prognosis and treatment

In general *Campylobacter* enteritis has a very good prognosis and the isolation of *C. jejuni* form stools does not necessary warrant chemotherapy. Indeed by the time a bacteriological diagnosis is made, it is common to find that the patient is already recovering. *Campylobacter* enteritis can be treated successfully by diet but if the abdominal pain is severe or there is the possibility of a complication, it is preferable to administer antibiotics. Erythromycin seems the drug of choice on the basis of the high susceptibility of the organism, the ease of administration, the high tissue levels and the lack of serious toxicity. Because of the risk of cholestatic hepatitis due to erythromycin estolate, ethylsuccinate or stearate is preferred. Erythromycin stearate 500 mg. b.i.d. for adults or erythromycin ethylsuccimate 40 mg/kg/day given for 7 days are treatment regimens that have been used successfully. It is preferably to carry out sensitivity tests because cases of erythromycin and tetracycline resistance have been described[37, 38]. In Campylobacter septicemia gentamicin is the drug of choice but tetracyclines, erythromycin and chloramphenicol are good altervatives. It should be noted that penicillins and the first and second generations of cephalosorins are totally ineffective[33]. The prognosis in septicemic cases is difficult to evaluate because most patients recover after a few days of treatment and because self limited or asymptomatic bacteremia due to *C. jejuni* has been observed. An unfavourable course is likely to be due to the presence of an underlying disease[18]. Chloramphenicol should be considered in patients with meningitis, since it is difficult to attain an adequate concentration of aminoglycosides in the cerebrospinal fluid.

Pathogenesis

The mechanisms by which *C. jejuni* causes disease still need further research. Until now some evidence of heat-labile or heat stabile toxin has been found. Tests for invasiveness in guinea pig conjunctivae (Sereney test) were negative, but tests for invasiveness using chicken embryo cells and Hela cells were positive in all strains tested[18]. After intragastric inoculation of 8 day-old chicks Campylobacter jejuni could be isolated from the blood in 50% of the animals[18]. In many documented cases, *Campylobacter* has been isolated from both the blood and the feces of patients with enteritis without underlying pathology[18]. These patients develop high sepcific antibody titers towards their infecting organism[18]. Two human volunteers suffered a typical attack of *Campylobacter* enteritis within 3 to 4 days after swallowing a glass milk with a living culture of *C. jejuni* that had recently been isolated from a patient with the disease. Several investigators have shown that *Campylobacter jejuni* can like *Shigella, Salmonella* and Yersinia enterocolitica, cause acute inflammation of the colonic mucosa[18, 41]. All these findings suggest that *Campylobacter jejuni* produces a predominantly invasive type of infection.

Evidence for the enteropathogenic character of C. jejuni

There are a number of arguments suggesting that *C. jejuni* is an etiologic

238

agent of diarrheal disease in men.

1. In industrialized countries *C. jejuni* has been isolated from the stools of 5-14% of patients with diarrhea and in less than 1% from normal stools of healthy persons.

2. *C. jejuni* has been isolated form both the feces and the blood in patients with gastroenteritis.

3. Most of patients with *Campylobacter* enteritis have had a specific serum antibody response to the infecting *Campylobacter* strain.

4. Many outbreaks of Campylobacter enteritis were reported.

REFERENCES

1. Butzler, J. P., P. Dekeyser, M. Detrain, and F. Dehaen. 1973. Related vibrio in Stools. J. Pediat., **82**: 493-495.
2. Skirrow, M. B. 1977. *Campylobacter* enteritis: a new "disease". Brit. Med. J., **2**: 9-11.
3. Severin, W. P. 1978. *Campylobacter* en enteritis. Ned. Tijdsch. Geneeskd., **122**: 499-504.
4. Lopez Brea M., D. Molina and Baquero, M. 1979. *Campylobacter* enteritis in Spain. Trans. Roy. Soc. Trop. Med. Hyg., **73**: 474.
5. Kosunen, T. U., O. Kauranen, and J. Martio. 1980. Reactive arthritis after *Campoylobacter jejuni* enteritis in patients with HLA-B27. Lancet, **1**: 1312-1313.
6. Delorme, L., T. Lambert, C. Branger, and J. F. Acar. 1979. Enterites a *Campylobacter jejuni* dans la region parisienne. Med. Mal. Infect., **9**: 675-681.
7. Megraud, F., and J. Latrille. 1981. L'enterite a *Campylobacter* Bilan d'une recherche systematique en milieu pediatrique. Sem. Hop. Paris. in press.
8. Steele, T. W., and S. McDermott. 1978. *Campylobacter* enteritis in South Australia. Med. J. Austr., **2**: 404-406.
9. Karmali, M. A., and P. C. Fleming. 1979. *Campylobacter* enteritis in children. J. Pediat., **94**: 527-534.
10. Blaser, M. J., I. D. Berkowitz, F. M. La Force, J. L. B. Reller, and W. L. Wang. 1979. *Campylobacter* enteritis: clinical and epidemiologie features. Ann. Int. Med., **91**: 179-185.
11. Butzler, J. P. 1973. Related vibrios in Africa Lancet, **2**: 858.
12. Demol, P., and E. Bosmans. 1978. *Campylobacter* enteritis in Centra Africa. Lancet, **1**: 604.
13. Ricciardi, I. D., M. C. Ferreira, S. S. Otto, N. Oliveira, A. Sabra, and C. F. Fontes. 1979. Thermophilic *Campylobacter* associated diarrhea in Rio de Janeiro. Rev. Bras. Pesq. Med. Biol., **12**: 189-191.
14. Grados, O., N. Bravo, E. Salazar, T. Serano, S. Lauwers, and J. P. Butzler. 1982. *Campylobacter* enteritis in Peru Proceedings of Annual Meeting of the American Society for Microbiology, Atlanta, 7-12th March.
15. Bokkenheuser, V., N. J. Richardson, J. P. Bryner, and *et al.* 1979. Detection of enteric Campylobacteriosis in children. J. Clin. Microbiol. **9**: 227-232.
16. Ringertz, S., R. C. Rockhill, O. Ringertz, and A. Sutomo. 1980. *Campylobacter* fetus subsp. jejuni as a cause of gastroenteritis in Jakarta, Indonesia. J. Clin. Microbiol. **12**: 538-540.
17. Blaser, M. J., R. I. Glass, M. I. Huq, B. Stoll, G. M. Kibriya, and A. Alim. 1980. Isolation of *Campylobacter* fetus ssp. jejuni from Bangladeshi children. J. Clin. Microbiol., **12**: 744-747.
18. Butzler, J. P., and M. B. Skirrow. 1979. *Campylobacter* enteritis. Clin. Gastroent., **8**: 737-765.
19. Cadranel, S., P. Rodesch, J. P. Butzler, and P. Dekeyser. 1973. Enteritis due to related vibrio in children. Amer. J. Dis. Child., **126**: 152-155.
20. Lambert, M. E., P. F. Scholfield, A. G. Ironside, and B. K. Mandal. 1979. *Campylobacter* colitis. Brit. Med. J., **1**: 857-859.
21. Willoughby, C. P., J. Piris, and S. C. Truelove. 1979. *Campylobacter* colitis. J. Clin. Path. **32**: 986-989.
22. Price, A. B., J. Jewkes, and P. J. Sanderson. 1979. Acute diarrhea: *Campylobacter* colitis and the role of rectal biopsy J. Clin. Path. **32**: 990-997.

23. Quinn, T. C., I. Corey, R. G. Chaffee, M. D. Schuffler, and K. K. Holmes. 1980. *Campylobacter* proctitis in a homosexual man. Ann Intern Med., **93**: 458–459.

24. Weight, C. P. 1979. Meningism associated with Campylobacter jejuni enteritis. Lancet, **1**: 1092.

25. Norrby, R., R. V. McCloskey, G. Zackrisson, and E. Falsen. 1980. Meningitis caused by *Campylobacter* fetus ssp. *jejuni*. Brit. Med. J., **1**: 1164.

26. Mertens, A. De Smet M. 1979. *Campylobacter* chlecystitis. Lancet., **1**: 1092–1093.

27. Leung, F. Y. 1980. Reiter's syndrome after *Campylobacter jejuni* enteritis. Althr. and Rheum., **83**: 948.

28. King, E. O. 1957. Human infections with vibrio fetus and a closely ralated vibrio. J. Infect. Dis., **101**: 119–128.

29. Dekeyser, P., M. Gossuin-detrain, J. P. Butzler, and J. Sternon. 1972. Acute enteritis due to a related vibrio first positiv stool cultures. J. Infect. Dis., **125**: 390–392.

30. Butzler, J. P., De Boeck, M., and Goossens, M. 1983. New selective medium for the isolation of campylobacter jejuni from fecal specimens. Lancet, **1**: 818.

31. Kayser, B. 1982. 82nd Annual Meeting of the American Society for Microbiology Atlanta, 7-12th March, personal communication.

32. Lauwers, S. 1982. 82nd annual Meeting of the American Society for Microbiology Atlanta, 7-12th March, Personal communication.

33. Butzler, J. P., P. Dekeyser, and Lafontaine, T. 1974. Susceptibility of related vibirios and vibrio fetus to twelve antibiotics. Antimicrob. Agent Chemother., **5**: 86–89.

34. Vanhoof, R., M. P. Vanderlinden, R. Dierickx, S. Lauwers, E. Yourassowsky and J. P. Butzler. 1978. Susceptibility of *Campylobacter* fetus subsp *jejuni* to twenty nine antimicrobial agents. Antimicrob. Agents Chemother., **14**: 553–556.

35. Vanhoof, R., B. Gordrs, R. Dierickx, H. Coignau, and J. P. Butzler. 1980. Bacteriostatc and bactericidal activities of 24 antimicrobial agents against *Campylobacter* fetus subsp *jejuni*. Antimicrob. Agents. Chemother., **18**: 118–121.

36. Walder, M. 1979. Susceptibility of Campylobacter fetus subsp jejuni to twenty antimicrobial agents. Antimicrob. Agents Chemother., **16**: 37.

37. Chow, A. W., V. Patten, and D. Bednorz. 1978. Susceptibility of Campylobacter fetus to twenty two antimicrobial agents. Antimicrob. Agent. Chemother., **13**: 416–418.

38. Vanhoof, R., H. Goosens, H. Coignau, G. Stas, and J. P. Butzler, J. P. 1982. Susceptibility pattern of *Campylobacter jejuni* from human and animal origin. Antimicro. Agent. Chemother., in press.

39. Karmali, M. A., R. M. Bannatyne, W. Leers, and K. Biers. 1980. Erythromycin-resistant *Campylobacter jejuni*. Canad. Med. Ass. J., **123**: 263–264.

40. Duffy, M. C., J. B. Benson, and S. J. Rubin. 1980. Mucosal invasion in *Campylobacter* enteritis. Amer. J. Clin. Path. **73**: 706–708.

Bacterial Diarrheal Diseases, eds., Y. Takeda, T. Miwatani, 241–251.
Copyright © 1985 by KTK Scientific Publishers, Tokyo.

BIOCHEMICAL AND SEROLOGICAL CHARACTERISTICS AND FATTY ACID COMPOSITION OF THERMOPHILIC *CAMPYLOBACTER*

M. Ohashi, S. Sakai, T. Itoh, K. Saito, A. Kai, and Y. Yanagawa

Department of Microbiology, Tokyo Metropolitan Research Laboratory of Public Health, 24-1, Hyakunin-cho 3-chome, Shinjuku-ku, Tokyo 160, Japan

Development of microbiological methods for selective isolation of thermophilic *Campylobacter* has now become a serious problem, since clinical and public health laboratories in various countries are reporting a significant number of cases of acute enteritis caused by this organism.

An outline in occurrence of the disease due to this organism in Tokyo and some bacteriological findings on isolates of human and animal origin, obtained in early stages of our investigation, were reported by Itoh *et al.* at the International Workshop on *Campylobacter* Infections in Reading in 1981[1]. A serological typing scheme, which was developed by us in an attempt to understand the epidemiology of enteritis caused by this organism, was also presented on the same occation[2].

The present paper describes the current status of *Campylobacter* enteritis in Tokyo. On the basis of biochemical and serological charactzization, and cellular fatty acids analysis of isolates, the relatedness between *C. jejuni* and *C. coli*, members of the thermophilic *Campylobacter*, is also discussed.

Incidence of Campylobacter enteritis in Tokyo

In January 1979, a routine test for *Campylobacter* was introduced in our laboratory, and immediately after this the organism was found to be responsible for having induced an outbreaks of enteritis in a nursery school in the outskirts of Tokyo[3]. This was the first outbreak recognized in Japan. From this time until December 1981, there have been 15 outbreaks attributed to this organism in Tokyo. As summarized in Table 1, 331 outbreaks of bacterial food poisoning, involving 8,910 cases, have occurred in Tokyo during the past three years. Thermophilic *Campylobacter* was responsible for 4.5% of these outbreaks, affecting 9.2% of the patients involved. This organism has 4th place after *Staphylococcus aureus, Vibrio parahaemolyticus*, and *Salmonella*.

As shown in Table 2, thermophilic *Campylobacter* was detected in 3.7% of

Table 1. Outbreaks of bacterial food poisonings in Tokyo (1979–1981)

Causative agents	Number of outbreaks (%)	Number of patients involved (%)
S. aureus	120 (36.3)	2,168 (24.3)
V. parahaemolyticus	118 (35.6)	2,488 (27.9)
Salmonella	48 (14.5)	705 (7.9)
C. jejuni	15 (4.5)	858 (9.2)
E. coli	13 (3.9)	1,123 (12.6)
C. perfringens	11 (3.3)	1,540 (17.3)
B. cereus	6 (1.8)	28 (0.3)
Total	331 (100)	8,910 (100)

the recent cases of diarrhea in travellers from overseas. Most of these cases were assumed to have been infected in Southeast Asian countries, such as Thailand, the Philippines, Indonesia, and the Indian Subcontinent, though some may have been infected in Korea, Taiwan or Mainland China, suggesting an extensive distribution of the organism throughout Asia.

Biochemical characterization of thermophilic Campylobacter isolated from human and animal sources

A total of 1,389 isolates of thermophilic *Campylobacter* were submitted to biochemical characterization. They include 1,005 human strains isolated from cases of diarrhea and 384 animal strains obtained from cattle, dogs, pigs and poultry.

Table 2. Detection of thermophilic *Campylobacter* and other enteropathogens from overseas travellers' diarrheal cases in Tokyo (1979–1981)

Number of cases examined[a]	1,002
Number of pathogen positives	596 (59.5%)
Number of positives for:	
Enterotoxigenic *E. coli*	342 (34.1%)
Salmonella	119 (11.9)
V. parahaemolyticus	100 (10.0)
Shigella	62 (6.2)
C. jejuni/coli	37 (3.7)
V. cholerae, non O-1	18 (1.8)
V. cholerae, O-1	4
Enteropathogenic *E. coli*, serotypes	18 (1.8)
Enteroinvasive *E. coli*	7
V. fluvialis	6
Y. enterocolitica	1

[a] cases in an acute phase.

For isolation of *Campylobacter*, Skirrow's method was employed with slight modifications[3], and isolates were identified by the method of Véron and Chatelain[4]. Their biochemical characteristics were further studied by the methods described by Skirrow and Benjamin[5].

Results are summarized in Table 3. In all, 964 of 1,005 (96%) of the human isolates were hippurate hydrolysis-positive (*C. jejuni*), the remaining 41 being negative (*C. coli*). Most of the former isolates were H_2S-negative in iron medium, and therefore, were identified as biotype 1 described by Skirrow and Benjamin, but 14 strains were H_2S-positive, or biotype 2. Most human isolates were sensitive to nalidixic acid when examined by 30 μg discs, but 9 (5 hippurate-positives and 4 hippurate-negatives) from cases of travellers' diarrhea or sporadic domestic cases were not sensitive to nalidixic acid.

Table 4 outlines the biological characteristics of the isolates derived from animals. All 34 isolates from cattle and 34 isolates from dogs were classified as *C. jejuni*, and most of them met the criteria of biotype 1. All 105 strains from

Table 3. Biochemical characteristics of thermophilic *Campylobacter*[a] isolates of human origin

Characteristics		Number of strains from:			
Hippurate hydrolysis	H_2S production in iron medium	Outbreaks cases	Sporadic cases	Travellers' diarrhea cases	Total
+	−	319	563 (5)[b]	68	950 (5)
+	+	3	11	—	14
−	−	—	16 (1)	25 (3)	41 (4)
−	+	—	−	−	−
Total		322	159 (6)	93 (3)	1,005 (9)

[a] Catalase-positive *Campylobacter* which grew at 43°C but not at 25°C.
[b] Figures in parentheses indicate number of nalidixic acid-resistant strains.

Table 4. Biochemical characteristics of thermophilic *Campylobacter*[a] isolates of animal origin

Characteristics		Number of strains from:				
Hippurate hydrolysis	H_2S production in iron medium	Cattle	Dogs	Pigs	Poultry	Total
+	−	33	33	13 (2)[b]	105 (6)	184 (8)
+	+	1	1	—	—	2
−	−	—	—	197 (4)	—	197 (4)
−	+	—	—	1	—	1
Total		34	34	211 (6)	105 (6)	384 (12)

[a] Catalase-positive *Campylobacter* which grew at 43°C but not at 25°C.
[b] Figures in parentheses indicate number of nalidixic acid-resistant strains.

porltry were identified as *C. jejuni* biotype 1, but 6 of them were found to be nalidixic acid-resistant.

On the contrary, 198 of 211 (94%) of the isolates from pigs were identified as *C. coli*, and only 13 strains (6%) were *C. jejuni*. Four of the former and two of the latter were nalidixic acid-resistant.

The nalidixic acid-resistant thermophilic *Campylobacter* described by Skirrow and Benjamin[5] was hippurate hydrolysis-negative and H_2S-positive, but some of our resistant strains were hippurate-positive and H_2S-negative.

We found that the test for tolerance to brilliant green proposed by Véron and Chatelain[4] for differentiation between *C. jejuni* and *C. coli* was of little value since it was not capable of differentiating *C. jejuni* from more sensitive strains of *C. coli*, which were clearly distinguishable by the hippurate hydrolysis test.

Table 5. Cross agglutination reaction of reference strains of each serotype of thermophilic *Campylobacter*

Reference strains		Source	Hip[a]	Serotype (TCK)	1	2	3	4	5	6	7	8	9
CF	1	Human	+	1	1,280	—[c]	—	—	—	—	—	—	—
CF	57	Human	+	2	—	640	—	—	—	—	—	—	—
CF	60	Human	+	3	—	—	1,280	—	—	—	—	—	—
CF	88	Human	+	4	—	—	—	1,280	—	—	—	—	—
CF	129	Human	+	5	—	—	—	—	640	—	—	—	20
CF	229	Human	+	6	—	—	—	—	—	640	—	—	—
CF	256	Human	+	7	—	—	—	—	—	—	1,280	—	—
CF	41	Human	+	8	—	20	—	—	—	—	—	320	—
CF	17	Human	+	9	—	—	—	—	40	—	—	—	1,280
CF	54	Human	+	10	—	—	—	—	—	—	—	—	20
CF	77	Human	+	11	—	—	—	—	—	—	—	—	—
CF	181	Human	+	12	—	—	—	—	—	—	—	—	—
CF	97	Cattle	+	13	—	—	—	—	—	—	—	—	—
CF	227	Human	+	14	—	—	—	—	—	—	—	—	—
CF	68	Human	+	15	—	—	—	—	80	—	—	—	—
CF	356	Human	+	16	—	—	—	—	—	—	—	—	—
CF	314	Poultry	+	17	—	—	—	—	—	—	—	—	—
CF	30	Human	+	18	—	—	20	—	—	—	—	—	—
CF	571	Human	+	19	—	—	—	—	—	—	—	—	—
CF	598	Human	+	20	—	—	—	—	—	—	—	—	.
CF	601	Human	+	21	—	—	—	—	—	—	—	—	—
CF	618	Human	+	22	—	—	—	—	—	—	80	—	—
CF	627	Human	+	23	—	—	—	—	—	—	—	—	—
HP	5	Human	+	24	—	—	—	—	—	80	—	—	—
HP	18	Human	+	25	—	—	—	—	160	80	—	—	20
HP	118	Human	+	26	—	—	—	—	—	80	—	—	—

[a] Hippurate hydrolysis.
[b] Rattbit antisera against formalin-treated cells (unabsorbed)
[c] Agglutinin titer lower than 20×.

Serological typing of thermophilic Campylobacter

Serological typing systems have recently been reported by many workers[6, 7, 8, 9]. We also established a system, based on a rapid slide agglutination technique, using formalin-treated cells and absorbed antisera for detection of heat-labile antigenic factors. A preliminary scheme with 18 type-specific antisera was reported previously[2] and has since been extended to cover 8 newly defined antigenic types.

Table 5 shows the results of quantitative cross-agglutination tests on the reference strains for these 26 types selected mainly from human isolates and their corresponding antisera obtained by immunizing rabbits with formalin-treated whole cell suspensions. Each of these antisera showed the highest agglutination titer with its corresponding antigen, and cross reaction with heterologous antigen was rare and weak, if any. For routine use, antisera were absorbed for elimination of

Titer of typing antiserum[b]

10	11	12	13	14	15	16	17	18	19	20	21	22	23	24	25	26
—	—	—	—	—	—	—	—	—	—	—	—	—	—	—	—	—
—	—	—	—	—	—	—	—	—	—	—	—	—	—	—	—	—
—	—	—	—	—	—	—	—	160	—	—	—	40	—	—	—	—
—	—	—	—	—	—	—	—	—	—	—	—	—	—	—	—	—
—	—	—	—	—	—	—	—	—	—	—	—	—	—	—	—	—
—	—	—	—	—	—	—	—	—	—	—	—	—	—	—	—	—
—	—	—	—	—	—	—	—	—	—	—	—	—	—	—	—	—
—	—	—	—	—	—	—	—	—	—	—	—	—	—	—	—	—
—	—	40	—	—	—	—	—	—	—	—	—	—	—	—	—	—
5,120	—	—	—	—	—	—	—	—	40	—	—	—	—	—	—	—
—	2,560	20	—	—	—	—	—	—	—	—	—	—	—	—	—	—
—	—	1,280	—	—	—	—	—	—	—	—	—	—	—	—	40	—
—	—	—	1,280	—	—	—	—	—	—	—	—	—	—	—	—	—
—	—	—	—	640	—	—	—	—	—	—	—	—	—	—	—	—
—	—	—	—	—	2,560	—	—	80	—	—	—	—	—	—	—	—
—	—	—	—	—	—	2,560	—	—	—	—	—	—	—	—	—	—
—	—	—	—	—	—	—	640	—	—	—	—	—	—	—	—	—
—	—	—	—	—	80	—	—	320	—	—	—	—	—	—	80	—
80	—	40	—	—	—	—	40	—	640	—	—	—	—	—	—	—
—	—	—	—	—	80	—	—	—	—	320	—	—	—	—	—	—
—	—	—	—	—	—	—	—	—	—	—	640	—	—	—	—	—
—	—	—	—	—	—	—	—	—	—	—	—	320	—	—	—	—
—	—	—	—	—	—	—	—	—	—	—	—	—	320	—	—	—
—	—	—	—	—	—	—	—	—	80	—	—	—	—	1,280	—	—
—	160	80	—	—	—	—	—	—	—	—	—	—	—	—	1,280	80
—	—	—	—	—	—	—	—	—	—	—	—	—	—	—	160	640

antibodies to homologous heat-stable somatic antigens and heterologous cross-reactive antigens.

With this system, 1,030 isolates of thermophilic *Campylobacter*, 692 from human cases of enteritis and 338 from animals were serotyped, and results are summarized in Table 6 and 7, respectively. About 70% of the human strains could be typed with these 26 antisera, and the common types were TCK 1, 4, 9, 14, 18, 21 and 23. One strain from each of the outbreaks was included in the figures

Table 6. Serotypes of thermophilic *Campylobacter* isolates of human origin

Serotypes (TCK)	Number of strains:					
	Hip +[a]		Hip −		Total	
1	50**[b]		—		50	
2	18*		6		24	
3	13**		—		13	
4	28** (1)[c]		1		29 (1)	
5	7*		—		7	
6	4*		—		4	
7	24*		—		24	
8	23*		1		24	
9	29		—		29	
10	13		—		13	
11	5		—		5	
12	18		2		20	
13	14		1		15	
14	29**		2		31	
15	5 (1)		—		5 (1)	
16	16		1		17	
17	1		—		1	
18	56***		4		60	
19	2		—		2	
20	19		—		19	
21	34		1		35	
22	1		—		1	
23	30		—		30	
24	14		1		15	
25	3		—		3	
26	6		—		6	
Total, typable	462 (2)	71.0%	20	48.8%	482 (2)	69.7%
Routh	11		—		11	
Untypable	179 (3)		21 (4)		199 (7)	
Total	651 (5)	100%	41 (4)	100%	692 (9)	100%

[a] Hippurate hydrolysis.

[b] The number of asterisks indicates the number of outbreaks included in these figures represented by one strain per outbreak.

[c] Figures in parentheses indicate the number of nalidixic acid-resistant strains involved.

in Table 6. It is of interest that about 49% of the hippurate hydrolysis-negaitve, or *C. coli*, strains were found to share heat-labile antigens with hippurate hydrolysis-positive, or *C. jejuni*, strains. It is also of interest that some strains of biotype 1 of *C. jejuni* shared type specificities with strains of biotype 2. For example, 8 strains obtained in one outbreak, including those of both biotype 1 (5 strains) and biotype 2 (3 strains) were all found to have the specificity of serotype TCK 8.

On the other hand, about 45% of the non-human strains were typable into 22 serotypes. Among the serotypes encountered, types 9 and 18 also appeared

Table 7. Serotypes of thermophilic *Campylobacter* isolates of animal origin

Serotypes (TCK)	Number of strains:					
	Hip +[a]		Hip −		Total	
1	2		2		4	
2	6		5		11	
3	1		2		3	
4	3		3		6	
5	5 (1)[b]		—		5 (1)	
6	6		1		7	
7	7		3		10	
8	1		9		10	
9	9		1		10	
10	5 (2)		—		5 (2)	
11	—		—		—	
12	1		7		8	
13	3		—		3	
14	5		4		9	
15	2		—		2	
16	3		9		12	
17	4 (1)		6		10 (1)	
18	13 (1)		5		18 (1)	
19	3		—		3	
20	3		1 (1)		4 (1)	
21	6		—		6	
22	—		—		—	
23	1		—		1	
24	1		3		4	
25	—		—		—	
26	—		—		—	
Total, typable	90 (5)	48.9%	61 (1)	39.6%	151 (6)[c]	44.7%
Rough	2		1		3	
Untypable	92 (3)		92 (2)		184 (5)	
Total	184 (8)	100%	154 (3)	100%	338 (11)	100%

[a] Hippurate hydrolysis.
[b] Figures in parentheses indicate number of nalidixic acid-resistant strains involved.
[c] Typable strains involve 14 strains from cattle, 22 from dogs, 51 from poultry and 64 from pigs.

frequently in human strains. About 40% of the strains of *C. coli* derived from pigs also shared type specificities with *C. jejuni* of human origin. These results support the view that these animals play important roles as reservoirs for the human disease.

Cellular fatty acid compositions of thermophilic Campylobacter

To obtain a better understanding of the difference between *Campylobacter* species, especially *C. jejuni* and *C. coli*, we studied the cellular fatty acid compositions of a total of 55 *Campylobacter* strains from various sources, including the reference strains of each species.

Cellular fatty acids were analyzed by the procedure of Moss[10] with slight modifications. Samples of 10 - 20 mg of bacterial cells cultured on brain heart infusion agar at 37°C for 48 hrs in an atmosphere of 10% CO_2, 5% oxygen, and 85% nitrogen were harvested and suspended in 0.5 ml of sterile distilled water in a screw-capped Pyrex test tube. The suspension was mixed with 3.0 ml of 5% NaOH in 50% aqueous methanol and heated in a boiling water bath for 30 min. The saponified material was cooled to room temperature and adjusted to pH 2 with 6 N HCl. Then 3.0 ml of 10% boron trichloride-methanol reagent was added, and the mixture was heated for 5 min. in a water bath maintained at 80 - 85°C. The mixture was cooled to room temperature, 1.0 ml of saturated NaCl was added and the fatty acid methyl esters were extracted twice with 10 ml of a 1:1 mixture of ethyl ether and hexane. The combined ether-hexane phase was evaporated under a gentle flow of nitrogen gas. Residual moisture was removed by adding a small amount of Na_2SO_4 and the final volume of the sample was reduced to approximately 0.2 ml.

The fatty acid methyl esters were analysed in a Hitachi gas chromatograph instrument, type 163, equipped with a flame ionization detector and a computing integrator recorder, Shimadzu R1A. A glass column (3 mm × 2 m) was packed with 2% Silicone OV-101 on 80 - 100 mesh Chromosorb W · AW-DMCS. In the analysis, the column temperature was increased from 140°C to 200°C at a rate of 2°C/min. The flow rate of carrier N_2 gas was adjusted to 30 ml/min. The fatty acid methyl esters were identified by comparing their retention times with those of purified methyl ester standards (Gasukuro Kogyo), and by mass spectrometry.

Gas chromatograms of esterified fatty acids of *C. jejuni* strain CF 1(top), *C. coli* strain NCTC 11366 (middle), and *C. fetus* strain ATCC 27374 (bottom) are shown in Fig. 1. Tirty three strains of *C. jejuni*, 28 H_2S-negatives in iron medium, or biotype 1 of Skirrow and Benjamin, and 5 H_2S-positives, or biotype 2, including 26 different serotypes, profiled chromatograms essentially identical to each others, and are exemplified by that of strain CF 1 in the figure.

As shown quantitatively in Table 8, their profiles were characterized by the presence of a relatively large amount of hexadecanoic (16:0) acid, moderate amounts of octadecenoic (18:1), 19-cyclopropane (19 cyc) and tetradecanoic (14:0) acids, and a small amount of hexadecenoic (16:1) acid. The fatty acid composition of H_2S-negative strains was similar to that of H_2S-positive strains, although the former

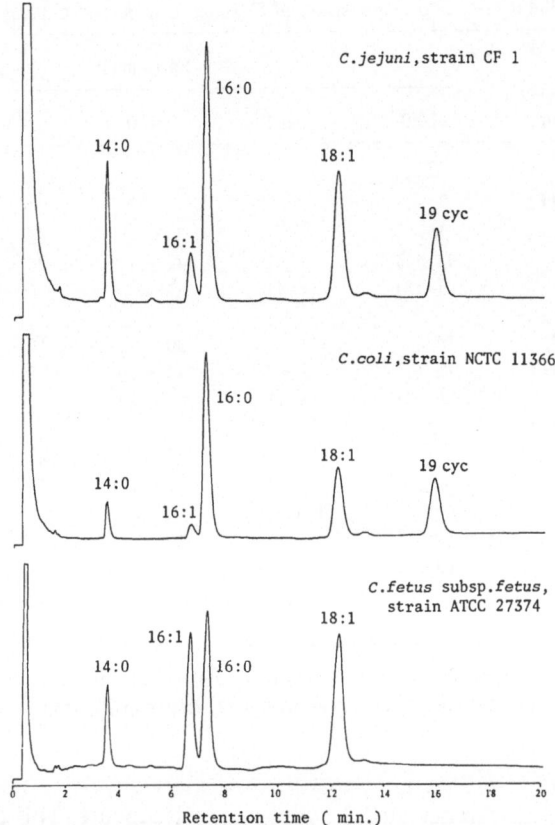

Fig. 1. Gas chromatograms of esterified fatty acids of representative strains of *C. jejuni* (top), *C. coli* (middle), and *C. fetus* (bottom). Column: Glass column (3mm × 2m) packed with 2% OV-101-coated Chromosorb W·AW-DMCS (80–100 mesh). Column temperature: 140-200°C (increased at a rate of 2°C/min). Carrier gas: N₂ (30 ml/min). Detector: Flame ionization detector. Instrument: Hitachi GC-163.

contained a relatively larger amount of octadecenoic acid and less 19-cyclopropane acid. Our collection of hippurate hydrolysis-positive strains included one nalidixic acid-resistant strain, but its profile was similar to those of other sensitive strains.

The fatty acid profiles of 17 hippurate hydrolysis-negative strains of thermophilic *Campylobacter*, or *C. coli*, of defferent serotypes were essentially identical and are represented by that of the type strain of *C. coli*, NCTC 11366 in Fig. 1. The fatty acid compositions of these strains were similar to those of the hypputate-positive strains described above (Table 8).

These fatty acids profiles of thermophilic *Campylobacter* differed from that of *C. fetus*. As shown in Fig. 1 and Table 8, the fatty acid analysis of 5 strains of *C. fetus* revealed that they contained undetectable amount of 19-cyclopropane acid and relatively larger amount of hexadecenoic acid in comparison with strains of the *jejuni/coli* group.

The fatty acid profiles of the *jejuni/coli* group were essentially identical to those reported by Leaper and Owen[11], but different from those reported by Blaser,

Table 8. The cellular fatty acid composition of *C. jejuni*, *C. coli*, and *C. fetus*

Species and strains	Fatty acid[a]				
	14:0	16:1	16:0	18:1	19cyc
C. jejuni					
(Skirrow's biotype 1)					
Strain CF 1	8	4	34	26	15
27 isolates	11 ± 3	6 ± 2	42 ± 7	28 ± 8	13 ± 6
	(6–18)	(4–11)	(34–67)	(6–43)	(4–29)
C. jejuni					
(Skirrow's biotype 2)	14	8	30	12	28
Strain NCTC 11392	12 ± 3	5 ± 1	44 ± 14	13 ± 5	23 ± 6
4 isolates	(7–14)	(3–7)	(33–68)	(5–19)	(14–29)
C. coli					
Strain NCTC 11366[b]	5	4	48	23	21
16 isolates	7 ± 3	4 ± 1	49 ± 16	23 ± 12	13 ± 9
	(2–12)	(Trace-6)	(33–81)	(4–44)	(2–30)
C. fetus					
Strain ATCC 27374[b]	10	25	32	33	—
4 isolates	10 ± 1	26 ± 4	35 ± 4	29 ± 2	—
	(8–11)	(19–29)	(32–41)	(26–31)	—

[a] Mean value of the fatty acid concentration as a percentage of the total with standard deviation. Figures in parentheses indicate range among strains. Peaks with areas less than 2% are not recorded.
[b] Type strain.

Moss and Weaver[12], who detected 3-hydroxytetradecanoate. This discrepancy may have resulted from differences in experimental conditions and strains. However, we are in complete agreement with these two groups as far as significant differences in fatty acid compositions between the *jejuni/coli* group and *C. fetus* are concerned.

Comparison of *C. jejuni* and *C. coli* showed that, in spite of differing in being hippurate hydrolysis-positive and negative, the two species had indistinguushable fatty acid profiles and shared common heat-labile antigenic factors.

The findings obtained in the present investigations provide useful information on the ecology of thermophilic *Campylobacter* and the epidemiology of enteritis due to this organism.

REFERENCES

1. Itoh, T., K. Saito, Y. Yanagawa, S. Sakai, and M. Ohashi. 1982. *Campylobacter* enteritis in Tokyo, pp.5-12. *In* D. G. Newell (ed.), Campylobacter; Epidemiology, Pathogenesis, and Biochemistry. MTP Press Co., Lancaster.
2. Itoh, T., K. Saito, Y. Yanagawa, S. Sakai, and M. Ohashi. 1982. Serological typing of thermophilc campylobacters isolated in Tokyo, pp. 106-110. *In* D. G. Newell (ed.), Campylobacter; Epidemiology, Pathogenesis, and Biochemistry. MTP Press Co., Lancaster.
3. Itoh, T., K. Saito, T. Maruyama, S. Sakai, M. Ohashi, and A. Oka. 1980. An outbreak of acute enteritis due to *Campylobacter fetus* subspecies *jejuni* at a nursery school in Tokyo. Microbiol. Immunol. **24**: 371-379.

4. Véron, M., and R. Chatelain. 1973. Taxonomic study of the genus *Campylobacter* Sebald and Véron and designation of the neotype strain for the type species, *Campylobacter fetus* (Smith and Taylor) Sebald and Véron. Int. J. Syst. Bacteriol. **23**: 122–134.

5. Skirrow, M. B., and J. Benjamin. 1980. Differentiation of enteropathogenic campylobacter. J. Clin. Pathol **33**: 1122.

6. Butzler, J. P., and M. B. Skirrow. 1979. *Campylobacter* enteritis, pp. 737–765. *In* Ian A. D. Bouchier *et al.* (ed.), Clinics in Gastroenterology. W. B. Saunders Co., London.

7. Abbott, J. D., B. Dale, J. Eldridge, D. M. Jones, and E. M. Sutcliffe. 1980. Serotyping of *Campylobacter jejuni/coli*. J. Clin. Pathol. **33**: 762–766.

8. Penner, J. L, and J. N. Hennessy. 1980. Passive hemagglutination technique for serotyping *Campylobacter fetus* subsp. *jejuni* on the basis of soluble heat-stable antigens. J. Clin. Microbiol. **12**: 732–737.

9. Lior, H., D. L. Woodward, J. A. Edgar, and L. J. Laroche. 1981. Serotyping by slide agglutination of *Campylobacter jejuni* and epidemiology. Lancet, **ii**: 1103–1104.

10. Moss, C. W. 1979. Analysis of cellular fatty acids of bacteria by gas-liquid chromatography, pp. 118-122. *In* G. L. Jones, and G. Ann Hébert(ed.), "Legionnaires" the disease, the bacterium and methodology. Center for Disease Control, Atlanta.

11. Leaper, S., and R. J. Owen. 1981. Identification of catalase-producing *Campylobacter* species based on biochemical characteristics and on cellular fatty acid composition. Current Microbiol. **6**: 31–35.

12. Blaser, M. J., C. W. Moss, and R. E. Weaver. 1980. Cellular fatty acid composition of *Campylobacter fetus*. J. Clin. Microbiol. **11**: 448–451.

Bacterial Diarrheal Diseases, eds., Y. Takeda, T. Miwatani, 253-256.
Copyright © 1985 by KTK Scientific Publishers, Tokyo.

CAMPYLOBACTER JEJUNI/COLI SERPTYPING IN DEVELOPED AND DEVELOPING COUNTRIES

S. Lauwers

Infectious Diseases Unit, Free University of Brussels

Since *C. jejuni/coli* became established as an important etiologic agent in enteritis[1-6] there was an obvious need for further differentiation of isolates in order to elucidate the epidemiology of campylobacter disease. Lior described a serotyping scheme for *C. jejuni* based on a rapid slide agglutination technique, using live bacteria and absorbed antisera for the detection of heat-labile antigenic factors[7]. We developed a serotyping system based on heat-stable antigens, using the passive haemagglutination technique in microtiterplates[8, 9], similar to the technique described by Penner[10].

Antisera are prepared in rabbits by subcutaneous injections of a Mac Farland nr. 9 suspension of live cells mixed with complete Freund's adjuvant, followed one week later by 3 intravenous injections (without adjuvant) with a few days interval each. Homologous titers of at least 1/12,800 are obtained. 47 different rabbit antisera are now included in our scheme : 37 were prepared against Belgian reference strains from our collection of strains (22 *C. jejuni* and 15 *C. coli*) and 10 against reference strains of J. L. Penner (7 *C. jejuni* and 3 *C. coli*) that were untypable in our system. 23 antisera do not react with any heterologous type strain and are thus monospecific. The exact nature of interstrain relations in crossreacting serotypes remains to be established. For each *C. jejuni/ coli* strain to be typed a suspension is heated at 100°C for 2 hours and adsorbed on human O-Rhesus negative erythrocytes. Antigens are first screened with pooled antisera. Up to 15 undiluted antisera are mixed in equal amount to constitute one pool. Following the results of crosstitrations 5 different pools were establised, in such a way that an isolate would agglutinate in only one pool. In a second step the antigens are tested with the specific antisera contained in the pool that gave a positive haemagglutination reaction. The isolates are assigned to the serotype correspondig to the antiserum or antisera in which they agglutinated.

From January 1980 until December 1981, 778 *C. jejuni/coli* strains isolated from 559 patients at the St. Pierre hospital in Brussels were assayed in our serotyping system. All patients – mostly children – suffered from enteritis.

From 61 patients two strains were available, isolated with an interval of 0 to 23 days. In 82% of these patients the same serotype was recovered for the 2 isolates. From 42 patients 3 or more strains were isolated which all belonged to the same serotype in 78% of cases. These results suggest that over 20% of patients could have been infected by two different serotypes during one infectious episode. Both serotypes were probably present in the two or more faecal samples, but since routinely only one colony is chosen from the primary culture plate, only one type can be detected in one sample. Serotyping subcultures of several colonies from the primary culture, as mentioned by Karmali *et al.*[11], is indicated in such cases. About 18% of all our patients harbored an untypable strain.

In two cases of neonatal *C. jejuni/coli* infection, the same serotype was recovered from the baby and the mother. From the first neonate *C. jejuni* serotype 6 was isolated from 5 samples : 3 stools, 1 rectal biopsy and 1 colon biopsy, as well as from a faecal specimen of the mother. In the second case, *C. jejuni* serotype 1 was present in the faeces of both mother and neonate.

In 3 patients with *C. jejuni/coli* bacteremia, faecal and blood isolates belonged to the same serotype : one case was serotype 1, the second serotype 39, the third serotype PEN 15 (corresponding to Penner's type 15).

38 different serotypes were encountered in the 778 stools from the St. Pierre hospital. The two most common serotypes : 1 and 2 occured in 14 and 11% of all the strains examined.

The 12 most common serotypes cover about 60% of the strains (Table 1). Strains isolated in other areas in Belgium show the same distribution of serotypes.

Also in other European countries (the U.K., Sweden, Germany, The Netherlands) as well as in the U.S.A. and Canada, common Belgian serotypes seem to occur frequently. For example, more than 40% of 57 Swedish and 22 German *C. jejuni/coli* strains belonged to our 12 most common belgian serotypes (Table 2). A recent food-borne outbreak of *C. jejuni* diarrhea in Sweden was caused by our most common serotype 1 : all 17 *C. jejuni* isolated about 10 days

Table 1. The 12 most common serotypes in Brussels

Serotype	nr. (%) of patients			
	1980 (231 patients)		1981 (328 patients)	
2	30	(13,0)	31	(9,4)
1	27	(11,7)	51	(15,5)
5,8	15	(6,5)	14	(4,3)
52	14	(6,1)	10	(3,0)
3	13	(5,6)	25	(7,6)
45	11	(4,8)	3	(1)
4	9	(3,9)	13	(4,0)
25	8	(3,5)	26	(7,9)
PEN 17	8	(3,5)	4	(1,2)
6	7	(3,0)	11	(3,3)
7	6	(2,6)	2	(1)
11	5	(2,2)	4	(1,2)
		66,4		57,4

Table 2. Occurence of the 12 most common Brussels serotypes in other European countries

Serotype	57 Swedish C. jejuni	22 German C. jejuni
2	4	1
1	1	1
5,8	1	2
52	—	
3	8	2
45	1	—
4	1	1
25	7	1
PEN17	—	—
6	—	—
7	1	—
11	1	—
	25 (44%)	9 (41%)

after onset of illness were serotype 1. Among 60 strains isolated from blood cultures in the U.S.A. and in the U.K., 17 different serotypes were recognized. The U.S.A. strains were isolated over a period of more than ten years, the U.K. strains were recent isolates.

60% and 70% of U.S.A. and U.K. blood isolates respectively, belonged to the 12 most common Belgian serotypes (found in faecal isolates). Although it is difficult to compare the serotype distibution of faecal and blood C. jejuni strains isolated from different populations at different time-intervals, these results suggest that there should be no relationship between serotype and invasiveness or virulence of strains.

To assess the role of several animal species in human campylobacter infections, 146 strains from cows, pigs, chickens, turkeys, dogs and a few gulls were examined. 70% of these strains were typable, and 20 different serotypes were identified. The 3 most common human serotypes (1; 2 and 5,8) were frequently seen in cows and chickens, supporting the view that these animals constitute important sources of human infections (12,13), at least in developed countries.

The distibution of human serotypes in strains isolated in Thailand, Bangladesh[14], South Africa[15,16] and Peru[17] seems to be different from that in Europe and in North America. Up to 50% of the 133 strains examined remained untypable in our system. Several of our common serotypes were identified, but they represented only a minority of the typable strains.

CONCLUSION

Although more than 40 different serotypes were identified with our serotyping scheme based on heat-stable antigens, a set of only 12 serotypes are more common than others, covering about 60% of our Belgian isolates, and being also frequently encountered in other European countries and in North America.

A different distibution of serotypes seems to exist in other continents, perhaps reflecting different epidemiological situations, but more strains need to be examined.

C. jejuni/coli serotyping, based on both heat-stable and heat-labile antigens has already a proven value in the epidemiological study of campylobacter infections, and can be of great help in the future for the solution of remaining problems related to pathogenicity and epidemiology.

We thank P. Echeverria, R. I. Glass, O. Grados, M. Kist, J. Oosterom, N. J. Richardson, M. B. Skirrow, Å. Svedhem and R. I. Weaver for the C. jejuni/coli strains that they provided.

REFERENCES

1. Butzler, J. P., P. Dekeyser, M. Detrain, and F. Dehaen. 1973. Related Vibrio in stools. J. Pediatrics **82**: 318–321.
2. Skirrow, M. B. 1977. *Campylobacter* enteritis : a "new" disease. Br. Med. J. **ii**: 9–11.
3. Lauwers, S., M. De Boeck, and J. P. Butzler. 1978. *Campylobacter* enteritis in Brussels. Lancet **i**: 604–605.
4. Butzler, J. P., and M. B. Skirrow. 1979. *Campylobacter* enteritis Clin. Gastoenterol. **8**: 737–765.
5. Svedhem, Å., and B. Kaijser. 1980. *Camplobacter* fetus subspecies jejuni : a common cause of diarrhea in Sweden. J. Infect. Dis. **142**: 353–359.
6. Blaser, M. J., and L. Barth Reller. 1981. *Campylobacter* enteritis. N. Engl. J. Med. **24**: 1444–1451.
7. Lior, H., D. L. Woodward, J. A. Edgar, and L. J. LaRoche. 1981. Serotyping by slide agglutination of *Campylobacter jejuni* and epidemiology. Lancet **ii**: 1103–1104.
8. Lauwers, S., L. Vlaes, and J. P. Butzler. 1981. *Campylobacter* serotyping and epidemiology. Lancet **i**: 158–159.
9. Lauwers, S. Serotyping of *C. jejuni*: a useful tool in the epidemiology of campylobacter diarrhoea. *In* : Newell D. (ed.), 1982. *Campylobacter*. Epidemiology, Pathogenesis and Biochemistry.
10. Penner, J. L., and J. N. Hennessy. 1980. Passive haemagglutination technique for serotyping *Campylobacter* fetus subspecies jejuni on the basis of soluble heat-stable antigens. J. Clin. Microbiol. **12**: 732–737.
11. Karmali, M. A., M. Kosoy, A. Newman, M. Tischler, and J. L. Penner. 1981. Reinfection with *Campylobacter jejuni*. Lancet **ii**: 1104.
12. Brouwer, R., M. J. A. Mertens, T. H. Siem, and J. Katchaki. 1979. An explosive outbreak of *Campylobacter* enteritis in soldiers. Antonie van Leeuwenhoek **45**: 517–519.
13. Robinson, D. A., W. J. Edgar, G. L. Gibson, A. A. Matchett, and L. Robertson. 1979. *Campylobacter* enteritis associated with consumption of unpasteurised milk. Br. Med. J. **1**: 1171–1173.
14. Blaser, M. D., R. I. Glass, M. Imdadul Huq, B. Stool, G. M. Kibriya, and A. R. M. A. Alim. 1980. Isolation of *Campylobacter* fetus subspecies *jejuni* from Bangladeshi children. J. Clin. Microbiol. **12**: 744–747.
15. Bokkenheuser, V. D., N. J. Richardson, J. H. Bryner, D. J. Roux, A. B. Schutte, H. J. Koornhof, I. Freimand, and E. Hartman. 1979. Detection of enteric campylobacteriosis in children. J. Clin. Microbiol. **9**: 227–232.
16. Richardson, N. J., H. J. Koornhof, and V. D. Bokkenheuser. 1981. Long-term infections with Campylobacter fetus subspecies jejuni. J. Clin. Microbiol. **13**: 846–849.
17. Grados, O., N. Bravo, E. Salazar, T. Serano, S. Lauwers, and J. P. Butzler. 1982. *Campylobacter* enteritis in Peru. Abstracts of the annual meeting, American Society of Microbiology.

Bacterial Diarrheal Diseases, eds., Y. Takeda, T. Miwatani, 257–265.
Copyright © 1985 by KTK Scientific Publishers, Tokyo.

DRUG RESISTANCE OF *SHIGELLA* AND EXPERIMENTAL CHEMOTHERAPY OF SHIGELLOSIS

R. Nakaya[1], N. Okamura[1], M. Ogawa[1], N. Goto[1], A. Nakamura[2], H. Yoshikura[2]*, and H. Ogawa[2]**

Department of Microbiology, Tokyo Medical and Dental University School of Medicine, Yushima, Bunkyo-ku, Tokyo 113, Japan[1], National Institute of Health, Kamiosaki, Shinagawa-ku, Tokyo 141, Japan[2]

This paper reports the epidemiological trend of emergence of antibiotic resistant isolates of *Shigella* in Japan over a period of recent 25 years, and a method for in vivo evaluation of chemotherapeutic agents against shigellosis by infection of tissue culture monolayers of virulent *Shigella*.

Drug resistance and conjugative R plasmids in isolates of Shigella in Japan

We found that 90% of the isolates from patients with bacillary dysentery in 1950 in Tokyo were resistant to sulfa drugs(Su)[6]. In 1952, 110,000 cases of dysentery were reported in Japan, the incidence being the highest since 2nd world War. In 1956, antibiotic resistant *Shigella* were isolated at a discernible frequency after wide use of tetracyclines (Tc) and chloramphenicol (Cm) in chemotherapy since 1950. The incidence of drug-resistant isolates increased yearly until 1966, when about 80% of the isolates were resistant to Cm, Tc, streptomycin(Sm), or Su or more than one of these drugs[4, 6]. Most isolates in this period were resistant to four drugs, and some were resistant to Tc or Cm, Sm, and Su[6]. Since the late 1960, resistance to kanamycin(Km) or ampicillin(Ap) has increased, resulting in the emergence of more complex resistance patterns. We demonstrated that 47 of 67 resistant strains (70%) harbored R plasmids[6]. This incidence has remained unchanged up to now, though the resistance patterns mediated by some R plasmids have become more complicated. Table 1 shows the latest data on the incidence of resistance of isolates in Japan. It is noteworthy Ap and Km resistances have reached 35 and 4.1%, respectively. We think that the increased clinical use of

* Present address: Department of Bacteriology, Faculty of Medicine, University of Tokyo, Hongo, Bunkyo-ku, Tokyo 113, Japan.
** Present address: Research Institute, Daiichi Seiyaku Co., Ltd., Kitakasai, Edogawa-ku, Tokyo 134, Japan.

258

Table 1. Incidence of drug resistant isolates of *Shigella* in Japan (1979–1981)[a]

Drug	% Resistant[b]
Ampicillin	35
Cephalexin	0.4
Cefoperazone	0.4
Chloramphenicol	40
Tetracycline	47
Gentamicin	0
Kanamycin	4.1
Streptomycin	67
Nalidixic acid	1.1
Pipemidic acid	0
Rifampicin	0

[a] A total of 266 isolates from patients in 12 main Isolation Hospitals isolated between 1979 and 1981 were tested. (M. Ogawa et al., to be published)

[b] Percent of resistant isolates, whose growth were not inhibited at 100 µg per ml, except gentamicin. All isolates were susceptible to gentamicin at 6.25 µg/ml.

a variety of β-lactam antibiotics in recent years has caused this increase in Ap-resistant organisms.

Experimental chemotherapy of shigellosis using tissue culture cell infection by Shigella

It has been established that virulent *Shigella* organisms are intracellular pathogens[3, 5, 7, 8]. This demands that the drugs used in chemotherapy of shigellosis should have potent antibacterial activity against intracellular organisms at low concentration. Various animal models of experimental shigellosis have been developed[3, 7], and the Serény test of keratoconjunctivitis in guinea pigs has been shown to be suitable for evaluating the efficacy of drugs[2, 10, 14, 15]. We established a more sensitive assay system for assessing the in vivo effectiveness of drugs by the infection of tissue culture cells with virulent *Shigella* (A. Nakamura, R. Nakaya, H. Yoshikura and H. Ogawa, Abstr. 21st Gen. Meet. Kanto Branch Jpn. Soc. Bactriol. 1966. A-5, p.11). Results with this system correlate well with experience in clinical treatment of patients with dysentery.

METHODS

L, Mlg, and HeLa cell monolayers were used in cell culture assay by the cover slip technique as described previously[5, 9] (see legends to Figs. 1 and 4 for details). The assay was based on inhibition of intracellular multiplication of *Shigella* bacilli after entry of drugs into the cells. The number of infected cells containing one or more bacteria was counted in Giemsa stained preparations by microscopy, and equations (1) and (2) were used to estimate the cell infection rate and the relative cell infection rate, respectively:
Cell infection rate (%)

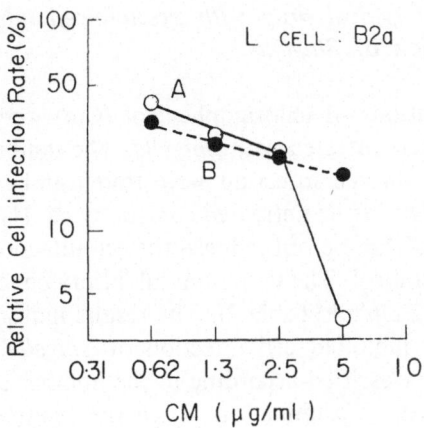

Fig. 1.   Effect of chloramphenicol on relative cell infection rate. (A, ○); *Shigella flexneri* 2a 5503 (B2a) was grown on L agar plates. L cell monolayers (3×10^5 cells) grown on cover slips in Leighton tubes were infected with 10^8 bacteria and incubated at 37°C. At 2 h after infection, various concentrations of chloramphenicol were added to the medium. At 7 h after infection, the monolayers were washed with phosphate-buffered saline, fixed, and stainded with Giemsa solution. (B, ●); The cells were infected with bacilli in the presence of chloramphenicol for 2 h, then washed and incubated for 5 h without the drug. The cell infection rate was calculated from the number of infected cells containing 1 or more organisms among 2,000 or more cells counted. See text for definition of relative cell infection rate.

$$\alpha = \frac{\text{No. of infected cells}}{\text{total no. of cells counted}} \times 100 \tag{1}$$

Relative cell infection rate (%)

$$\alpha_K = \frac{\alpha_t}{\alpha_c} \times 100 \tag{2}$$

where α_c is the cell infection rate of controls (without drug) and α_t is that of specimens treated with drug.

Equations (3) and (4) were also used:
Relative number of infected cells

$$N_K = \alpha_k \frac{C_b}{100} \tag{3}$$

where C_b is the percent of infected cells containing a given number of intracellular bacilli, b, and equals 2^i (i = 0, 1, 2, $\cdots$, n).
Relative number of intracellular bacilli

$$B = \sum_{i=0}^{n} b \cdot N_b \tag{4}$$

Chloramphenicol as a typical drug with pronounced inhibitoty activity on intracellular multiplication of Shigella

Various concentrations of chloramphenicol (Cm) were added to tubes containing L cell monolayers infected with *Shigella*. The inhibitory effects of various concentrations of Cm on cell infection were tested and rates of infection were calculated relative to that of the untreated control by eq. (1) (Fig. 1). For example, treatment with 2.5 μg of Cm per ml reduced the cell infection rate to approximately 20% of that of the control. The minimum inhibitory concentration (MIC) determined in vitro was 3.12 μg/ml (Table 2). The results indicate that reasonably low concentrations of Cm inhibited cell infection of *Shigella*.

Infected cells were classified according to the number of intracellular bacteria determined by microscopic examination. Then the relative numbers of infected cells in each class were determine by eqs. (2) and (3). Figure 2 shows that relation between the concentration of Cm and the distributions of relative numbers of infected cells. For example, at a concentraion of 0.63 μg of Cm per ml, most of the infected cells contained 3 to 5 organisms, whereas those harboring either fewer or more bacilli were lower. As the concentration of Cm increased, the peak shifted to the left and at 5 μg of Cm per ml, the number of infected cells decreased greatly, and there were only 1 or 2 intracellular bacteria per cell. The data shown in Fig. 2 were employed to calculate the relative number of intracellular bacilli by eq. (4). Figure 3 illustrates the relation of the drug concentration to the relative number of intracellular bacteria. It is clear that the higher the concentration, the fewer the bacteria per cell. These results indicate that Cm at sufficiently low concentration inhibited the multiplication of organisms that had penetrated the cell.

Microscopic observation showed certain morphological changes of intracellular *Shigella* (data not shown). We also confirmed that Tc had similar inhibitory effects to Cm on the cell infection rate and the intracellular multiplication of dysenery bacilli (data not shown).

Table 2. Minimum inhibitory concentrations (MICs) and median inhibitory doses (ID$_{50}$) of antibiotics for HeLa cell infection with *Shigella flexneri* 5503–01 [15]

Antibiotic	MIC[a] (μg/ml)	ID$_{50}$[b] (μg/ml)
Chloramphenicol	3.12	0.32
Tetracycline	25	4.7
Ampicillin	6.25	0.70
Piperacillin	0.19	0.06
Cephaloridine	3.12	0.50
Cefroxadine	6.25	1.0

[a] Determined by the agar dilution method using Penassay broth agar (Difco).
[b] Calculated by Probit analysis.

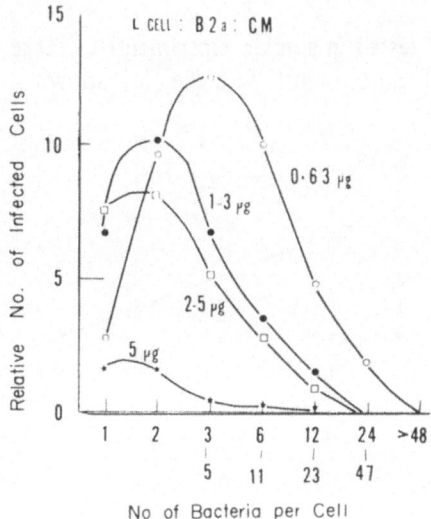

Fig. 2. Effect of concentrations of chloramphenicol on distribution of numbers of infected L cells containing given numbers of organisms of *Shigella flexneri* 2a 5503 (B2a). See text for definition of the relative number of infected cells and the number of bacteria per cell. See footnote to Fig. 1 for details of experimental procedures.

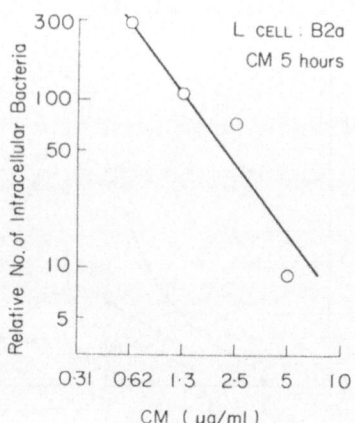

Fig. 3. Inhibition by chloramphenicol of intracellular multiplication of *Shigella flexneri* 2a 5503 (B2a) within L cells. See text for definition of relative number of intracellular bacteria. See footnote to Fig. 1 for details of experimental procedures.

Kanamycin as a typical drug with weak activity on intracellular multiplication of Shigella

Km and Sm were tested in similar experiments to those on Cm and Tc described above. The results of experiments with Km are shown in Figs. 4, 5, and 6, and

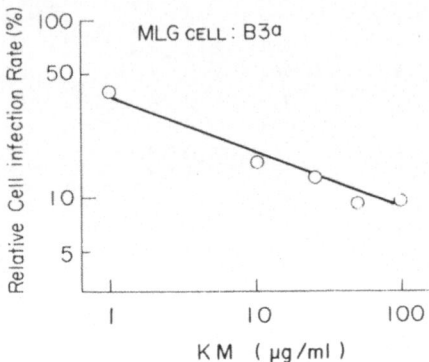

Fig. 4. Effect of kanamycin on relative cell infection rate. *Shigella flexneri* 3a 638–66 (B3a) was grown on L agar plates. Mlg cell monolayers (3 × 10⁵ cells) grown on cover slips in Leighton tubes were infected with 10⁸ bacteria and incubated at 37°C. At 2 h after infection, various concentrations of kanamycin were added to the medium. At 7 h after infection, the monolayer was washed with phosphate-buffered saline, fixed, and stained with Giemsa solution. See text for definition of relative cell infection rate.

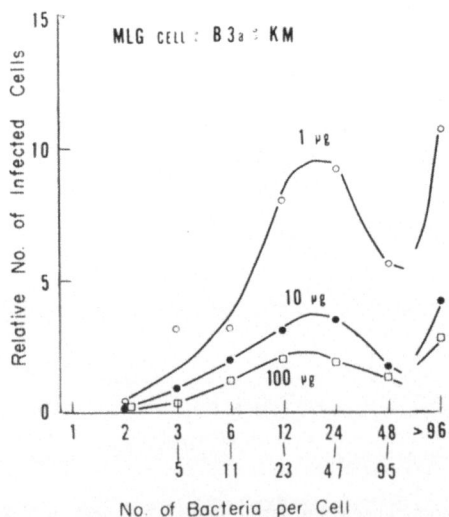

Fig. 5. Effect of concentrations of kanamycin on distribution of numbers of infected cells containing given numbers of organisms of *Shigella flexneri* 3a 638–66 (B3a). See text for definition of relative number of infected cells and the number of bacteria per cell. See footnote to Fig. 4 for details of experimental procedures.

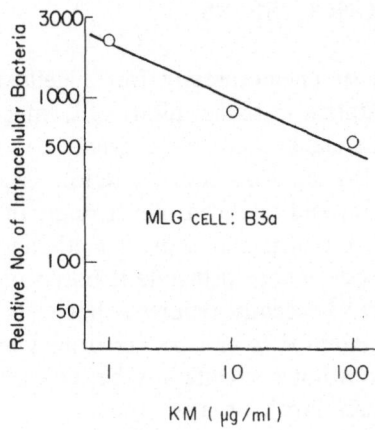

Fig. 6. Inhibition by kanamycin of intracellular multiplication of *Shigella flexneri* 3a 638–66 (B3a) within Mlg cells. See text for definition of relative number of intracellular bacteria. See footnote to Fig. 4 for details of experimental procedures.

can be summarized as follows: Km inhibited cell infection at relatively higher concentrations, but it did not significantly suppress intracellular multiplication of bacteria even at 100 μg per ml. The former finding may be explained by the inhibitory effect of Km on extracellular bacilli released from infected cells that otherwise would penetrate uninfected cells.

Some changes in morphology of intracellular bacilli were noticed in experiment with Km (data not shown). We also carried out similar experiments with Sm to those with Km, and obtained much the same results (data not shown).

Sensitivity of the assay and its application to β-lactam *antibiotics*

Although the Serény test can be used for in vivo evaluation of the effects of drugs on shigellosis, this test is rather qualitative, and cannot be used for testing penicillins, because of their lethal toxicity to guinea pigs and rabbits[2, 10, 14, 15]. In contrast, the cell infection assay system seems to be useful for quantitative determination of the effectiveness of antimicrobial agents and for evaluation of the in vivo effects of penicillins and cephalosporins[11, 12]. To explore these possibilities, we carried out experiments with a variety of β-lactam antibiotics, including recently developed ones such as piperacillin(Pipc) and cefroxadine(Cxd)[15]. We used a cell infection system consisting of a combination of HeLa cell monolayers and *S. flexneri* 5503-01[9]. This strain is a rough mutant of *S. flexneri* 2a 5503 that still retains the ability to penetrate tissue culture cells and shows a higher infection rate than its parent[9]. Table 2 summarizes results on in vivo and in vitro susceptibilities. The median inhibitory doses (ID_{50}) for cell infection of the drugs tested were found to be 3-10 times lower than the MICs determined by the standard agar dilution method. These results indicate the cell infection assay system provides a sensitive, quantitative method for measurement of the in vivo antibacterial activity of drugs. It was also shown that this assay is applicable to β-lactams.

DISCUSSION AND CONCLUSIONS

The in vivo model of chemotherapy for shigellosis described in this communication, namely, treatment of tissue culture cells infected with *Shigella*, is useful for in vivo evaluation of chemotherapeutic agents (A. Nakamura, *et al.*, Abstr. 21st Gen. Meet. Kanto Branch Jpn. Soc. Bacteriol. 1966. A-5, p. 11; 11). It was shown that Tc, refampicin, and erythromycin strongly inhibited cell to cell transfer of intracellular *Shigella*, but Km and colistin methanesulfonate did not[12], in a similar cell infection model, whose principle is based on the studies of Schneider *et al.*[13]. Bacheson *et al.*[1] recently reported that tests on antimicrobial susceptibility to *Legionella pneumophila* can be performed in a tissue culture system, although this method does not correlate any better with in vivo observations for gentamicin efficiency than broth or agar systems.

Among the β-lactam antibiotics tested, Pipc, a newly developed semi-synthetic penicillin, and Cxd, a new oral cephalosporin, seem potentially useful for clinical treatment of bacillary dysentery, judging by results of cell infection assay on these drugs. It may also be worthwhile to evaluate some recently developed cephalosporins and monobactams that are resistant to β-lactamases encoded by R plasmids as chemotherapeutics for shigellosis with this assay system.

This paper reports changes in drug resistance and conjugative R plasmids of isolates of *Shigella* in Japan. It is important to select a suitable drug for chemotherapy of shigellosis in relation to changes in resistance. The method for testing antimicrobial susceptibility of *Shigella* in an intracellular environment described may be useful in determining whether drugs are effective in inhibiting intracellular multiplication of organisms that have penetrated into the cells.

We thank Sankichi Horiuchi and Harumi Shibaoka for technical assistance, and Kiyomi Hashimoto for aid in preparation of the manuscript.

REFERENCES

1. Bacheson, M. A., H. M. Friedman, and C. E. Benson. 1981. Antimicrobial susceptibility of intracellular *Legionella pneumophila*. Antimicrob. Agents Chemother. **20**: 691–692.
2. Cross, W. R., and M. Nakamura. 1970. Chemoprophylaxis of *Shigella flexneri* keratoconjunctivitis in rabbits. Appl. Microbiol. **20**: 505–507.
3. Formal, S. B., H. L. DuPont, R. B. Hornick, M. J. Snyder, J. P. Libonati, and E. H. LaBrec. 1971. Experimental models in the investigation of the virulence of dysentery bacilli and *Escherichia coli*. Ann. N. Y. Acad. Sci. **176**: 190–196.
4. Imagawa, Y. 1982. Present status of clinical dysentery in Japan. Bacterial. Diarrheal Diseases. KTK Scientific Publishers, Tokyo.
5. LaBrec, E. H., H. Schneider, T. J. Magnani, and S. B. Formal. 1964. Epithelial cell penetration as an essential step in pathogenesis of bacillary dysentery. J. Bacteriol. **88**: 1503–1518.
6. Nakaya, R. 1976. Drug Resistance. Kodansha, Tokyo.
7. Nakaya, R., N. Okamura, H. Ogawa, and Y. Osada. 1977. Cell penetration by dysentery bacilli. Jpn. J. Bactriol. **32**: 785–804.
8. Ogawa, H., A. Nakamura, R. Nakaya, K. Mise, S. Honjo, M. Takasaka, T. Fujiwara, and K. Imaizumi. 1967. Virulence and epithelial cell invasiveness of dysentery bacilli. Jpn. J. Med. Sci. Biol. **20**: 315–328.
9. Okamura, N., and R. Nakaya. 1977. Rough mutant of *Shigella flexneri* 2a that penetrates tissue

culture cells but does not evoke keratoconjunctivitis in guinea pigs. Infect. Immun. **17**: 4–8.

10. Osada, Y., M. Nakajo, and H. Ogawa. 1972. Application of experimental keratoconjunctivitis shigellosa in chemotherapeutic evaluation of rifampicin to bacillary dysentery. Jpn. J. Microbiol. **16**: 329–332.
11. Osada, Y., M. Nakajo, T. Une, H. Ogawa, and Y. Oshima. 1972. Application of cell culture in studying antibacterial activity of refampicin to *Shigella* and enteropathogenic *Escherichia coli*. Jpn. J. Microbiol. **16**: 525–533.
12. Osada, Y., T. Une, and H. Ogawa. 1973. Inhibition of cell to cell transfer of *Shigella* by treatment with some antibiotics. Jpn. J. Mcrobiol. **17**: 233–235.
13. Schneider, H., H. Ogawa, A. Nakamura, and R. Nakaya. 1967. intercellular transfer of infection in HeLa cell cultures challenged with virulent *Shigella flexneri*. Jpn. J. Bacteriol. **22**: 398.
14. Serény, B. 1958. Aetiotropic treatment of experimental shigellosis. Acta Microbiol. Hung. **5**: 179–191.
15. Tomita, M. 1980. Studies on experimental chemotherapy of bacillary dysentery. Ochanomizu Med. J. **28**: 171–182.

Bacterial Diarrheal Diseases, eds., Y. Takeda, T. Miwatani, 267–271.

THE PATHOGENESIS OF BACILLARY DYSENTERY

S. B. Formal, P. Sansonetti, T. L. Hale, L. S. Baron, and D. J. Kopecko

Walter Reed Army Institute of Research Walter Reed Army Medical Center Washington, DC 20012 U.S.A.

Shigellosis is a disease which is endemic throughout the world but is of special concern in tropical regions and in developing countries. Not only does the organism cause point source outbreaks of dysentery, but, because of its low infectious dose (the ID_{50} is approximately 200 cells), can be spread by person-to-person contact. The severity of disease may range from a mild diarrhea to a severe dysentery (multiple stools of small volume which contain blood mucous and inflammatory cells). Other signs of illness include fever, cramps, tenesmus, and, in severe cases hypotensive shock. In cases which include both diarrhea and dysentery, the diarrheal phase usually occurs early, and is followed by dysentery. Disease is observed only in man and in sub-human primates.

One of the first steps in the pathogenesis of bacillary dysentery is the penetration of the intestinal epithelial cell by the pathogen[1, 2]. Mutant shigella strains which do not possess this ability do not cause disease when fed either to experimental animals or to man. Several laboratory models are available to test for an organism's ability to invade epithelial cells. These include a) the Sereny test[3] which detects an organism's ability to produce keratoconjunctivitis in rabbits or guinea pigs and which in turn is a reflection of the penetration of the corneal epithelial cell by the pathogen[4]; b) a test employing cultured mammalian cells which determines an organism's capacity to penetrate into the cytoplasm[1, 5]; and c) the histologic or electronmicroscopic examination of the intestines of experimentally infected animals for the presence of organisms in their intestinal epithelial cells[1, 6, 7].

Little is known about the process of epithelial cell invasion or the properties which a bacterial cell must have to complete this event. In order to reach the intestinal epithelial cell, the dysentery bacillus must traverse both the mucous and the glycocalyx layers which coat the epithelium. How this step is achieved is not known and is only now being addressed[8]. A general pattern of the events of invasion following contact of the pathogen with the epithelial cells has been revealed from electron microscopic studies[6, 7, 9]. The first observed alteration is a localized destruction of the brush border of the intestinal epithelial cell. The pathogen is then engulfed by an invagination of the cell membrane and is subsequently found in a vacuole (consisting of the host cell membrane) within the epithelial cell. The integrity of the cell membrane and the brush border is apparently restored following invasion. The bacterium is then observed free in the cell cytoplasm. In the case of a dysentery infection, the organism invades an adjacent cell, and through this repeated process causes death of the epithelium resulting in the formation of an ulcerative lesion. Dysentery bacilli which reach the lamina propria evoke an intense inflammatory reaction and the bacteria are efficiently killed; they rarely reach the submucosa.

Genetic studies have indicated that several factors are most likely involved in the pentration process. If the *pur*E region of the virulent *S. flexerni* is replaced by that of *E. coli* K-12, the resulting *S. flexneri* hybrids are uniformly unable to produce keratoconjunctivitis[10]. This loss of ability to produce a positive Sereny test is a reflection of this particular test system, since these hybrids retain the ability to invade epithelial cells in other models. In other experiments the virulence was restored to avirulent mutants of *S. flexneri* in one case by transferring the *glp* K region from a virulent donor[11] and in another case the *mal* B region from and *E. coli* K-12 donor strain[12]. The particular property which was transferred to restore the virulence of these two mutant strains is not known. Other studies have identified the *his* chromosomal region with the expression of the group antigen of *S. flexneri* and the *pro* region with the synthesis of the type-specific antigen[13]. Expression of the group antigen is necessary for virulence because rough strains lacking this, although able to invade cultured mammalian cells, are highly susceptible to the normal defense mechanisms of the intact host[14].

Recently interest has focused on the role of plasmids in the virulence of shigellae. The previously described colonial variation which occurs in *S. flexneri* and results in the loss of ability to penetrate epithelial cells is not accompanied in an alteration of the plasmid profile of the mutant strain[15]. However, all *S. flexneri* thus far examined (and these represent all serotypes) contained at least one plasmid of approximately 140 Mdal in size. Strains in which the large plasmid had been eliminated were still smooth in colonial morphology but were always avirulent and unable to penetrate epithelial cells. When this plasmid was transferred to avirulent *S. flexneri* strains lacking the large plasmid, the transconjugants regained virulence[16]. Although plasmid genes are clearly responsible for the invasive property, the products that they encode or regulate are not yet identified. Since penetration requires surface interaction between the bacterium and the host cell, plasmid-coded outer membrane proteins may be important in this process.

A large 120 Mdal plasmid is also involved in the virulence of *S. sonnei*. Virulent *S. sonnei*, termed form I, dissociate at a high frequency to yield rough avirulent varients termed form II. The form I to form II variation is irreversible and it is accompanied by the loss of the form I somatic antigen, and by the loss of the large plasmid[17, 18]. Transfer of this plasmid from a form I strain to an avirulent form II strain results in the restoration of form I antigen expression and virulence[19]. It is not known whether restoration of just the ability to express the form I antigen is sufficient to confer virulence on the form II cells or if additional virulence encoding genes on the plasmid are also involved. Cloning the genes responsible for form I antigen expression may resolve this question.

After penetration and multiplication, a complex series of events occurs which may result in mucosal inflammation and ulceration, fluid loss, cramps, tenesmus, fever and shock. Ulceration, due to death of epithelial cells, is characteristic of shigella infections, and may be due to the fact that shigellae rapidly inhibit protein synthesis within a cell. This ability to inhibit protein synthesis may be due in large part to a cytotoxin (Shiga toxin) which is elaborated by shigellae[20, 21, 22]. This toxin has been demonstrated to inhibit protein synthesis in intact cells[23] and, in high dilution, to kill HeLa cells[20].

Intestinal perfusion studies in monkeys infected with shigellae demonstrate that the most consistent transport and morphological abnormalities occur in the colon. The magnitude of the colonic transport defect roughly correlates with the severity of the invasive process. Interestingly, in shigella-infected monkeys, abnormalities of small intestinal salt and water transport were also seen. In these animals, a correlation between the site of transport abnormalities and the type and magnitude of dysentery or diarrhea was apparent. In those animals with classical dysentery (i.e., multiple stools of small volume with blood, pus, and mucus), abnormal transport occurred only in the colon. However, in animals that manifested watery diarrhea, either alone or in combination with dysentery, jejunal water secretion was regularly observed[25]. We believe that dysentery is strictly a colonic process and that diarrhea is the result of jejunal secretion superimposed on absorption abnormalities occurring in the colon. Diarrhea results because the colon is unable to absorb fluid entering it from the small intestine.

The classical "Shiga toxin" of S. dysenteriae 1 is, as noted above, cytotoxic, and it has also been shown to be enterotoxic[26]. Strains of S. flexneri and S. sonnei also elaborate a similar toxin[21, 22], albeit in much smaller amounts, and it is likely that this material is responsible for the fluid loss in shigellosis. But again, the evidence is not yet clear, for non-penetrating but toxin-producing S. dysenteriae 1 mutants fail to cause disease when fed to monkeys[27] or volunteers[28]. Only invasive organisms cause disease, and invasion of the jejunum, the site of fluid secretion in shigella diarrhea, has not been observed. Nevertheless, shigella must pass through the small intestine in order to elicit a watery diarrhea. Monkeys challenged intracecally develop only classical dysentery (stools of small volume containing blood, mucus, and inflammatory cells), but the small volume of fluid is secreted only from the cecum, not form the jejunum[29]. Since shigella cause jejunal fluid secretion only if transmitted through the small intestine, an enterotoxic substance such as Shiga toxin probably mediates this secretion. From our experience with cholera and enterotoxigenic E. coli, the secretion of enterotoxins by shigellae is highly suggestive of a role in pathogenesis and work should be supported to define their function.

Other signs of disease which result from penetration and multiplication in the bowel wall are fever, shock, cramps and tenesmus. Research in the former two areas has been pursued for many years. However, little work has been addressed to the basic causes of cramps or tenesmus which may well result from an alteration in normal patterns of bowel motility. Techniques which measure electrical activity in the bowel wall are now available, and studies have commenced to approach the problem of hypermotility in the infected bowel. Since intestinal cramps are among the most debilitating symptoms of dysentery, this area should

270

be studied intensively in the future.

REFERENCES

1. LaBrec, E. H., H. Schneider, T. J. Magnani, and S. B. Formal. 1964. Epithelial cell penetration as an essential step in the pathogenesis of bacillary dysentery. J. Bacteriol., **88**: 1503–1518.
2. Voino-Yasenetsky, M. V., and T. N. Khaokin. 1964. A study of intraepithelial localization of dysentery causative agents with the aid of fluorescent antibodies. J. Microbiol. **12**: 98–100.
3. Sereny, B. 1957. Experimental keratoconjunctivitis is *Shigellosa*, Acta Microbiol. Hung. **4**: 367–376.
4. Piechaud, M.,, S. Szturn-Rubinstein, and D. Piechaud. 1958. Evolution histologique de la keratoconjunctivite a bacille dysenterique du cobaye. Ann. Inst. Pasteur. **94**: 298–309.
5. Ogawa, H., A. Nakamura, R. Nakaya, K. Mise, S. Honko, M. Takeuchi, T. Fujiwara, and K. Imaizumi. 1967. Virulence and epithelial cell invasiveness of dysentery bacilli. Jap. J. Med. Sci. biol. **20**: 315–318.
6. Polotsky, Yu., E. Snigireskay, and E. S. Dragunskaya. 1974. Electron microscopic data on the mode of penetration of *Shigella* in the intestinal epithelial cells. Bull. Exp. Biol. Med. (Moscow) **77**: 110–114.
7. Takeuchi, A., H. Sprinz, E. H. LaBrec, and S. B. Formal. 1965. Experimental bacillary dysentery: an electron microscopic study of the response of the mucosa to bacterial invasion. Am. J. Pathol. **47**: 1011–1044.
8. Prizont, R., and W. P. Reed. 1980. Possible role of colonic content in the mucosal association of pathogenic shigella. Infect. Immun. **29**: 1197.
9. Takeuchi, A. 1967. Electron microscope studies of experimental *Salmonella* infection. I. Penetration into the intestinal epithelium of *Salmonella typhimurium*. Am. J. Pathol. **50**: 109–136.
10. Formal, S. B., P. Gemski, Jr., L. S. Baron, and E. H. LaBrec. 1971. A chromosomal locus which controls the ability of *Shigella flexneri* to evoke keratoconjunctivitis. Infect. Immun. **3**: 73–79.
11. Kim, R., and DL. M. Corwin. 1974. Mutation in *Shigella flexneri* resulting in loss of ability to penetrate HeLa cells and loss of glycerol kinase activity. Infect. Immun. **9**: 916–923.
12. Formal, S. B., E. H. LaBrec, H. Scheneider, and S. Falkow. 1965. Restoration of virulence to a strain of *S. flexneri* by mating with *Escherichia coli*. J. Bacteriol. **89**: 835–838.
13. Formal, S. B., P. Gemski, Jr., L. S. Baron, and E. H. LaBrec. 1970. Genetic transfer of *Shigella flexneri* 2a antigens to *Escherichia coli* K-12. Infect. Immun. **1**: 279–287.
14. Okamura, N., and R. Nakaya. 1977. Rough mutant of *Shigella flexneri* 2a that penetrates tissue culture cells but does not evoke keratoconjunctivitis in guinea pigs. Infect. Immun. **17**: 4–8.
15. Kopecko, D. J., J. Holcombe, and S. B. Formal. 1979. Molecular characterization of plasmids from virulent and spontaneously occurring avirulent colonial mutants of *Shigella flexneri*. Infect. Immun. **24**: 580–582.
16. Sansonetti, P. J., D. J. Kopecko, O. Washington, and S. B. Formal. Evidence that a large plasmid participates in the virulence of *Shigella flexneri*. In press.
17. Kopecko, D. J., O. Washington, and S. B. Formal. 1980. Genetic and physical evidence for plasmid control of *Shigella sonnei* form I cell surface antigen. Infect. Immun., **29**: 207–214.
18. Sansonetti, P., M. David, and M. Toucas. 1980. Correlation entre la perte d' ADN plasmidique et le passage de la phase I virulents a'la phase II avirulente chez *Shigella sonnei* C.R.Acad. Sc. Paris 290(d): 879–882.
19. Sansonetti, P., D. J. Kopecko, and S. B. Formal. 1980. *Shigella sonnei* plasmids: Evidence that a large plasmid is necessary for virulence. Infect. Immun. **34**: 75–83.
20. Vicari, G., A. L. Olitski, and Z. Olitski. 1960. The action of the thermolabile toxin of *Shigella dysenteriae* on cells cultivated *in vitro*. Br. J. Exp. Pathol. **41**: 179–189.
21. Keusch, G. T., and M. Jaceqicz. 1977. The pathogenesis of shigella diarrhea VI. Toxin and antitoxin in *Shigella flexneri* and *Shigella sonnei* infections in humans. J. Infect. Diseases. **135**: 552–556.
22. O'Brien, A. D., M. R. Thompson, P. Gemski, B. P. Doctor, and s. B. Formal. 1977. Biological

properties of *Shigella flexneri* 2a toxin and its serological relationship to *Shigella dysenteriae* 1 toxin. Infect. immun. **15**: 796–798.

23. Brown, J. E., S. W. Rothman, and B. P. Doctor. 1980. Inhibition of protein synthesis in intact HeLa cells by *Shigella dysenteriae* 1 toxin. Infect. Immun. **29**: 98–107.

24. Keusch, G. T., P. R. Papenhausen, M. Jacewitz, and K. Hirschorn. 1976. Comparison of *Shigella* and cholera toxin effects using lymphocytes as target cells. Clin. Res., **24**: 287A.

25. Rout, W. R., S. B. Formal, R. A. Giannella, and G. J. Dammin. 1975. Pathophysiology of shigella diarrhea in the rhesus ;monkey: intestinal transport, morphological, and bacteriological studies. Gastroenterology **68**: 270–278.

26. Keusch, G. T., G. F. Grady, L. J. Mata, and J. McIver. 1972. Pathogenesis of *shigella* diarrhea. I. Enterotoxin production by *Shigella dysenteriae* 1. J. Clin. Invest. **51**: 1212–1218.

27. Gemski, P. Jr., A. Takeuchi, O. Washington, and S. B. Formal. 1972. Shigellosis due to *Shigella dysenteriae* 1: relative importance of mucosal invasion versus toxin production in pathogenesis. J. Infect. Dis. **5**: 523–530.

28. Levine, M. M., H. L. DuPont, S. B. Formal, R. B. Hornick, A. Takeuchi, E. J. Gangarosa, M. J. Snyder, and J. P. Libonati. 1973. Pathogenesis of *Shigella dysenteriae* 1 (Shiga) dysentery. J. Infect. Dis. **127**: 261–270.

29. Kinsey, M. D., S. B. Formal, G. J. Dammin, and R. Giannella. 1976. Fluid and electrolyte transport in rhesus monkeys challenged intracecally with *Shigella flexneri* 2a. Infect. Immun. **14**: 368–371.

Bacterial Diarrheal Diseases, eds., Y. Takeda, T. Miwatani, 273–295.
Copyright © 1985 by KTK Scientific Publishers, Tokyo.

ECOLOGY OF *VIBRIO CHOLERAE, VIBRIO PARAHAEMOLYTICUS* AND RELATED VIBRIOS IN THE NATURAL ENVIRONMENT

R. R. Colwell, F. L. Singleton[1], A. Huq, H. -S. Xu and N. Roberts[2]

Department of Microbiology, University of Maryland, College Park, Maryland 20742 USA, Department of Biological Sciences, Old Dominion University, Norfolk, Virginia 23508 USA[1], Lake Charles Regional Laboratories, P.O.Box 1322, Lake Charles, Louisiana 70601 USA[2]

Since the discovery of the ubiquitous distribution of *Vibrio parahaemolyticus* in estuarine and coastal waters, several new species of the genus *Vibrio* have been identified as human pathogens during the past few years, including *Vibrio vulnificus, Vibrio fluvialis, Vibrio hollisae, Vibrio damsela*, and *Vibrio mimicus*. Brackish and estuarine waters have been identified as a common habitat for many of these and related *Vibrio* spp. *Vibrio cholerae*, the causative agent of epidemic cholera, has been isolated from a variety of clinical and environmental samples. The majority of *V. cholerae* from environmental sources have been non-01 serovars, although isolation of 01 serovars has been reported in areas where limited outbreaks of cholera have occurred[1]. Evidence has been accumulating rapidly indicating that the pathogenic *Vibrio* spp., including *Vibrio cholerae*, are naturally occurring members of the aquatic ecosystem[1-6]. Ecological studies reported to date have described the spatial and temporal distribution of *Vibrio parahaemolyicus* and related pathogenic vibrios in the water column of the aquatic environment[4, 7, 8].

All pathogenic *Vibrio* species elaborate an extracellular chitinase and, to date, only one study has fully investigated the significance of the association between pathogenic vibrios and chitin-containing zooplankton in the water column. In the study of Kaneko and Colwell[8], *Vibrio parahaemolyticus* was shown to adsorb onto copepods, with the efficiency of this effect being dependent on pH and salinity. Furthermore, both pH and salinity were concluded to be major factors influencing the distibution of *V. parahaemolyticus* in estuarine ecosystems, such as Chesapeake Bay[7].

The patchy distribution of serovars of *V. cholerae* in coastal and estuarine waters has been found to be unrelated to sewage contamination or to the presence of wastes which can serve as a potential vehicle of entry into the environment[4]. To account for the apparent sporadic distribution of *V. cholerae* in the aquatic environment, as well as the repeated occurrence of the 01 serovar in regions with no reported outbreaks of cholera, Colwell *et al.*[9] hypothesized that *V. cholerae* is a member of the autochthonous microbial flora of brackish water and estuaries.

Many of the results reported concerning the occurrence of *V. cholerae* in aquatic environments, as well as sporadic outbreaks of cholera in localities without an apparent source of the organism, can, in fact, be explained by the autochthonous nature of *V. cholerae* in brackish water and estuarine environments.

Interaction with abiotic environmental parameters

Although it is known to occur in diverse aquatic systems, the influence of environmental parameters on growth of *V. cholerae*, until recently, has not been examined under controlled conditions. Salinity and nutrient concentrations have been reported to influence the growth and viability of *V. cholerae* and results of such studies may, in part, explain the apparent selective distribution of *V. cholerae* in estuarine systems[4, 10].

Evaluating the influence of selected environmental parameters on a bacterial population is difficult because of the spatial and temporal heterogeneity of such populations *in situ* and the constantly changing conditions of the environment, especially in tidal estuaries. Application of laboratory microecosystems, i.e., microcosms, valuable in ecological studies since they allow for replication of experimental units, have proven useful in defining physical, chemical, and biological parameters of a given environment and controlling those parameters during experimentation[11]. Microcosms were used by Singleton *et al.*[5, 6] to elucidate the effect of temperature, salinity, and nutrient concentrations on *V. cholerae*. Details of the experiments are published elsewhere[5, 6, 12]. Samples for viable, i.e., "culturable", counts were enumerated by spread plating onto tryptic soy agar. Samples for enumeration were diluted in sea-salts solution prepared to the same salinity as the microcosms being sampled. A statistically designed sampling regime was established, based on a principal component of variance analysis[11], to estimate accurately the mean number of culturable bacteria. Total cell numbers were also determined by acridine orange direct counts (AODC)[13, 14, 15]. Heterotrophic activity of *V. cholerae* populations in the microcosms was measured by the ^{14}C-labeled amino acid uptake method described by Hobbie and Crawford[16].

The influence of different concentrations of NaCl on growth and viability of *V. cholerae* was measured, employing microcosms prepared with a salt solution consisting of (g/l) $MgSO_4.7H_2O$, 2.86; KBr, 0.07; H_3BO_3, 0.019; $MgCl_2.6H_2O$, 7.74; $CaCl_2$, 0.82; $SrCl_2$, 0.017; K_2CO_3, 0.05; amended with selected concentrations of NaCl. In order to minimize changes in total salinity, Cl^- and monovalent cation concentrations were conserved by substitution of molar equivalents of KCl or LiCl for NaCl, as the latter was decreased. The microcosms, as prepared, allowed determination of the extent to which the Na^+ requirement could be spared by K^+ or Li^+ [17-20].

Microcosms, for which salinity was adjusted to 25 ‰ and nutrient concentration adjusted to 500 µg/l tryptone (Difco), were incubated at 25°C and served as controls[6]. Growth and/or survival of ten strains *V. cholerae* isolated from diverse sources were compared in these control microcosms (Table 1). All isolates, including clinical and environmental 01 serovars, grew to approximately the same final cell concentration under the conditions employed. Cell numbers, determined

Table 1.   Population sizes of *Vibrio cholerae* strains in microcosms adjusted to a salinity of 25‰ and tryptone concentration of 500 µg/l[a]

Strain	Source	Mean Log$_{10}$ Colony count/ml	Mean Log$_{10}$ Total Cell Count
V-69[b]	Environmental	5.788 ± 0.055[c]	5.806 ± 0.054
N-19	Environmental	5.780 ± 0.029	5.908 ± 0.016
N-17	Environmental	5.730 ± 0.018	5.763 ± 0.055
N-1400	Environmental	5.845 ± 0.022	5.857 ± 0.130
N-1403	Environmental	5.769 ± 0.048	5.869 ± 0.063
N-33	Environmental	5.571 ± 0.060	5.716 ± 0.080
N-999	Environmental	5.685 ± 0.025	5.732 ± 0.110
SGN-7677[b]	Environmental	5.768 ± 0.034	5.748 ± 0.175
LA-4808[b]	Clinical	5.840 ± 0.010	5.954 ± 0.044
CA-401[b]	Clinical	5.746 ± 0.035	5.792 ± 0.051

[a] No significant difference between the mean colony counts, obtained by plating on a nutrient medium, for the different strains was detected using Duncan's multiple comparison (21).
[b] 01 serovar.
[c] Mean ± standard error.

by AODC, ranged from 5.2×10^5 to 9.0×10^5/ml, whereas viable counts, i.e., culturable counts, ranged from 3.7×10^5 to 7.0×10^5/ml.

Bacterial counts, obtained by spread plating, were analyzed statistically. The experimental design provided sufficient replication of experimental units to permit application of analysis of variance to the microcosm data[11]. A comparison of log$_{10}$ transformed mean culturable counts for the 10 strains of *V. cholerae*, using Duncan's multiple comparison[21], demonstrated that the counts were not significantly different ($p < 0.05$) (Table 1). Since all strains tested developed to approximately the same population size in the microcosms and corroborative data had been obtained for strain LA 4808 in previous studies[6], LA 4808 was selected as a representative strain. It should be noted, however, that similar results were obtained for other strains examined.

a) *Salinity and nutrient effects.* Studies on growth of *V. cholerae* LA 4808, a toxigenic 01 strain isolated from a patient in Louisiana who became ill following ingestion of improperly prepared seafood, showed that population sizes of *V. cholerae* in microcosms of salinities from 5 ‰ to 45 ‰ were influenced by organic nutrient, i.e., tryptone concentration (Fig. 1). Regardless of tryptone concentration, at 25°C, optimum growth of *V. cholerae*, indicated by maximum population size, as measured by both culturable and total count, occurred in the presence of an intermediate salinity of 25 ‰. However, at lower tryptone concentrations, i.e., less than 500 µg/1, a pronounced salinity effect was evident. Not only were there differences in population sizes at given tryptone concentrations, but also lack of recoverability of cells at the extremes of high or low salinity, coupled with low tryptone concentration. Above 500 µg/1 tryptone, however, the salinity effect was masked if larger concentrations of tryptone were present, indicating that the salinity requirement was spared by a high organic nutrient concentration.

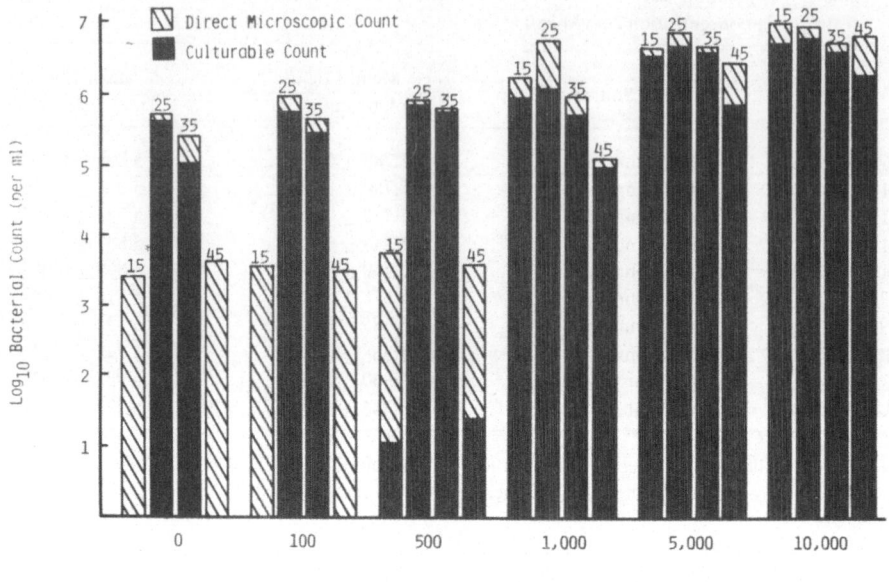

Fig. 1. Comparison of direct microscopic and culturable plate counts of *Vibrio cholerae* LA 4808 in a medium containing various concentrations of tryptone. (From Ref. 6.)

b) *Temperature and salinity effects.* From the conclusions of the previous study, the nutrient level in microcosms was fixed at 500 μg/1 tryptone.

Microcosms were prepared with salinities of 5, 15, 25 and 35 ‰ and incubated at 10, 15, 20 and 25°C. When inoculated with 4×10^2 cells/ml and incubated at 10°C, culturable colony counts declined for all salinities tested (Fig. 2). Changes in total direct cell counts could not be determined, since the number of cells comprising the inoculum was below the practical limit required in the AODC technique, which employs a microscope for direct counting of cells. However, in all microcosms examined, culturable *V. cholerae* were present throughout the 8-day test period, indicating extended survival at 10°C.

An incubation temperature of 15°C yielded similar results, except for microcosms for which the salinity was adjusted to 15 ‰, in which case both culturable and total cell counts increased (Fig. 3). At salinities of 5 and 35 ‰, the counts were lower. However, in the presence of 25 ‰, after the second day of incubation, the culturable counts gradually increased throughout the experiment. In microcosms adjusted to 15 ‰ salinity and incubated at 15°C, the total cell counts paralleled the culturable counts after the fourth day of incubation, when the cell concentration became sufficiently high to be monitored accurately by direct counting (Fig. 3).

The influence of salinity on cells of *V. cholerae* LA 4808 at 20°C is illustrated in Figure 4. Two days after inoculation, culturable colony counts for microcosms in which the salinity was adjusted to 5, 25 and 35 ‰, deviated very little from

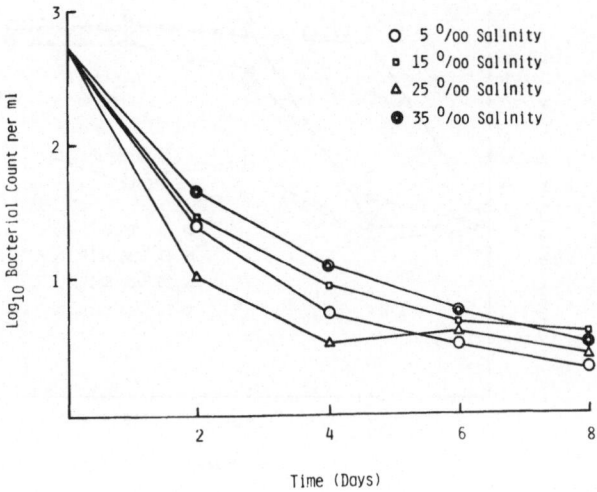

Fig. 2. Survival of *Vibrio cholerae* LA 4804 at 10°C, measured by plate count. (From Ref. 6.)

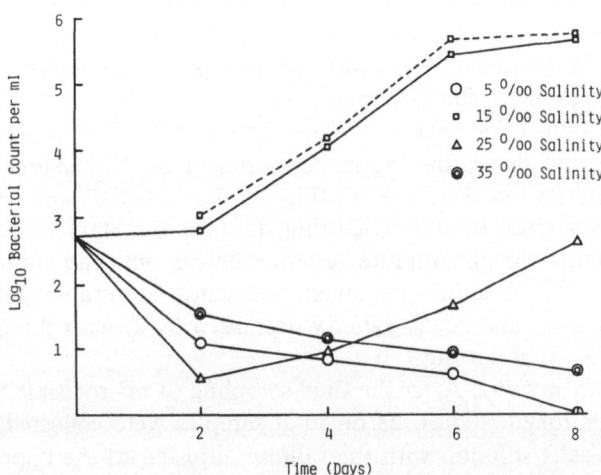

Fig. 3. Total cell count (- - -) and plate count (——) of *Vibrio cholerae* LA 4808 grown at 15°C. (From Ref. 6.)

the inoculation size. However, *V. cholerae* in microcosms adjusted to 15 ‰ salinity increased by approximately 2.5 $\log_{10}$ cycles. By the fourth day, populations of *V. cholerae* for all salinities demonstrated a significant increase ($p \le 0.05$) above the original inoculum size[21]. Maximum culturable populations were detected in 25 ‰ salinity microcosms, although these were not consistently significantly greater ($p \le 0.05$) than populations in 15 ‰ salinity microcosms. The smallest numbers of culturable *V. cholerae* were present in 5 ‰ salinity microcosms. Total cell populations (AODC) developed according to the same pattern as that of the

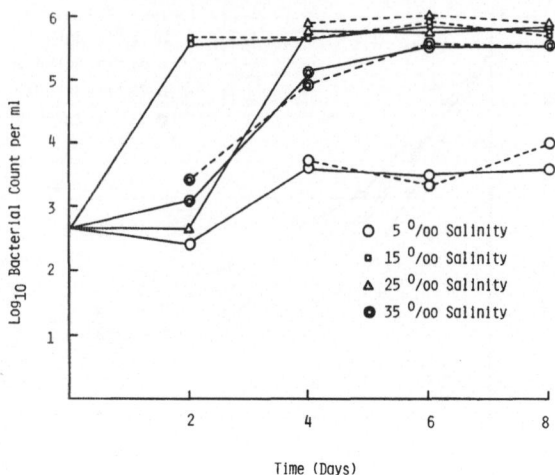

Fig. 4. Total cell count (- - -) and plate count (——) of *Vibrio cholerae* LA 4808 grown at 20°C. (From Ref. 6.)

culturable populations. Not only was development of the total and culturable populations parallel in the presence of different salinities, but also in population size, with 25 ‰ salinity microcosms containing the maximum populations and those of 5 ‰ salinity, the minimum.

Results obtained for microcosms incubated at 25°C were similar to those at 20°C, although no detectable lag in development of *V. cholerae* populations at any of the salinities tested was noted (Fig. 5). Both AODC and culturable counts increased to maximum by day 4. During the last four days of testing, total cell counts were stable for all salinities tested, whereas only the culturable counts at 15 ‰ and 25 ‰ salinities remained constant. Culturable colony counts in microcosms of 5 ‰ and 35 ‰ salinity decreased by at least 0.5 log cycle during the last four days of testing.

C) *Heterotrophic activity.* After the final sampling of microcosms for enumeration in the aforementioned studies, 25 or 50 μl samples were collected and inoculated into 25 ml sea-salts solution with the salinity adjusted to the appropriate concentration as the microcosms. Heterotrophic activity with ^{14}C-labeled amino acid mixture (Amersham Co., IL) was assayed[5]. Since the microcosms contained different numbers of bacteria, it was not unexpected that the largest uptake values were obtained from systems which received inocula from microcosms with the largest *V. cholerae* populations (Table 2). At 25°C and 20°C, populations of *V. cholerae* from microcosms for which the salinity was adjusted to 25 ‰ utilized more amino acids than populations at the other salinities tested. Also, at 25°C and 20°C, the lowest rates of uptake were obtained for populations in microcosms of 5 ‰ salinity.

In order to obtain a representation of the influence of salinity and temperature on heterotrophic activity, uptake of the ^{14}C-amino acid mixture on a per cell basis was calculated. When the total uptake of amino acids by *V. cholerae* in the microcosms was compared to total and culturable population sizes, with uptake per cell calculated, it was observed that both temperature and salinity influenced

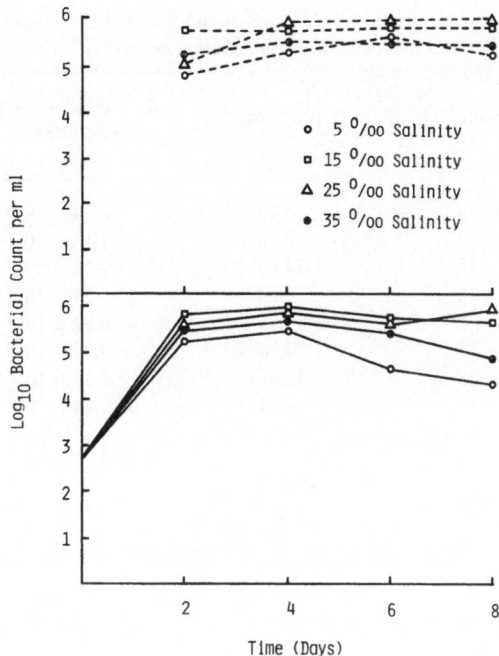

Fig. 5. Total cell count (- - -) and plate count (——) of *Vibrio cholerae* LA 4808 grown at 25°C. (From Ref. 6.)

activity (Table 2). In microcosms incubated at 25°C, for the total population, the largest uptake per cell was obtained for microcosms of 25 ‰. Up-take of cells of all other salinities were approximately equivalent and at a level approximately 50% less than that of the 25 ‰ microcosms. This was not true, however, when uptake per culturable cell was compared. Greater uptake per cell was obtained for 5 ‰ and 35 ‰ microcosms.

When microcosms were incubated at 20°C and the activity of the *V. cholerae* populations compared (Table 2), a higher rate of uptake was obtained for populations of 25 ‰ salinity. Although uptake per total cell number at 15, 25, and 35 ‰ was between 1.13×10^{-7} and 1.17×10^{-7} μg/1/hr, the 5 ‰ salinity microcosms yielded an uptake approximately 25 times larger, which was also the case for uptake per culturable cell.

d) *Ionic requirements.* Previous studies had indicated that *V. cholerae* LA 4808 remained culturable up to 42 days in 25 ‰ salinity at 10°C, but failed to survive longer than 8 days at 10°C in 5 ‰ salinity[5].

To determine whether the effect of salinity on stability and survival of *V. cholerae* was due, in part, to a requirement for specific ion(s), a series of microcosms were prepared, employing selected concentrations of NaCl or $MgCl_2$, the major salts in seawater. Growth of *V. cholerae* at different concentrations of NaCl and $MgCl_2$ were measured after incubation for 4 days at 25°C. When the concentration of $MgCl_2$ in the microcosms was varied, little or no effect was observed on total or culturable cell counts. However, an effect was evident when the NaCl concentration was altered. Both total and culturable cell counts followed the same

Table 2. Heterotrophic uptake of ^{14}C-labeled amino acid by *Vibrio cholerae* in basal-salts solution of varying salinities and incubated at selected temperatures[a]

Temperature (°C)	Salinity (‰)	Uptake rate[b] ($\mu g/l/hr \times 10^{-2}$)	Uptake rate/ culturable cell ($\mu g/l/hr$)	Uptake/total cell number ($\mu g/l/hr$)
25	5	2.43	6.93×10^{-7}	1.08×10^{-7}
	15	4.78	1.16×10^{-7}	8.68×10^{-8}
	25	14.40	1.75×10^{-7}	1.81×10^{-7}
	35	2.74	3.38×10^{-7}	8.64×10^{-8}
20	5	2.95	6.82×10^{-6}	3.58×10^{-6}
	15	7.36	9.97×10^{-8}	1.13×10^{-7}
	25	12.9	1.33×10^{-7}	1.66×10^{-7}
	35	4.94	1.14×10^{-7}	1.71×10^{-7}
15	5	N.D.[e]	—	—
	15	3.36	4.94×10^{-8}	6.87×10^{-8}
	25	N.D.	—	—
	35	N.D.	—	—
10	5	N.D.	—	—
	15	0.54	—	—
	25	N.D.	—	—
	35	N.D.	—	—

[a] Samples were collected from microcosms and inoculated into reaction vials containing basal-salts solution of the same salinity as the microcosms.
[b] Mean of duplicate flasks per treatment.
[c] Obtained from mean culturable colony count.
[d] Obtained from acridine orange direct microscopic count.
[e] None detected as compared to killed controls.

pattern, with maximum populations at lower and higher NaCl concentrations (Fig. 6). When no NaCl was added, a large difference, of approximately 3 $\log_{10}$, between total and culturable cell counts was detected.

Uptake of ^{14}C-amino acids by *V. cholerae* in microcosms at different concentrations of NaCl or $MgCl_2$ showed that heterotrophic activity was affected (Table 3). Maximum uptake of amino acid mixture occurred in the presence of the intermediate, or control, $MgCl_2$ concentration, i.e., 7.74 g/1. When the $MgCl_2$ concentration was increased or decreased, uptake decreased. A similar uptake pattern was observed in microcosms adjusted to different NaCl concentrations (Table 3). With increasing or decreasing NaCl concentration, compared to the intermediate concentration, uptake decreased.

Uptake values per cell were largest in control microcosms, i.e., those with 17.09 g NaCl/1 (Table 3). With either increasing or decreasing NaCl concentration, the uptake per total cell and culturable cell decreased.

The ratio of the amount of incorporation of amino acid mixture to amount respired was found to be influenced by NaCl and $MgCl_2$ concentration (Table 3). In microcosms prepared with concentrations of NaCl and $MgCl_2$ of 17.09 and 7.47 g/1, respectively, lowest respiration to incorporation ratios were detected. Only in those flasks which received no NaCl was this ratio greater than 1.8, in-

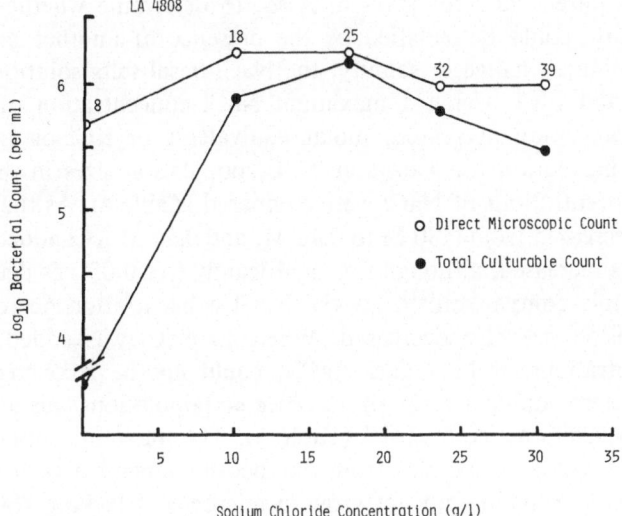

Fig. 6. Effect of sodium chloride concentration on the growth of *Vibrio cholerae* LA 4808 in microcosms. Numbers indicate corresponding salinity. (From Ref. 6.)

Table 3. Uptake of ^{14}C-amino acids by *Vibrio cholerae* in basal-salts amended with selected concentrations of sodium chloride and magnesium chloride

Salt Concentration (g/l)	Mean Uptake Rate ($\mu g l^{-1} hr^{-1} \times 10^{-2}$)	Uptake Per Cell ($\mu g l^{-1} hr^{-1} \times 10^{-6}$)	Uptake Per Culturable Cell ($\mu g l^{-1} hr^{-1} \times 10^{-6}$)	Resp./ Incorp.
NaCl				
0	7.30 ± 0.40^a	5.96	(1.46×10^{-2})	1:5.3
10.25	16.61 ± 3.21	3.69	8.29	1:1.7
17.09	12.74 ± 1.56	4.63	7.45	1:1.8
23.93	10.67 ± 0.49	3.56	6.53	1:1.5
30.76	5.33 ± 1.26	1.18	7.03	1:0.6
$MgCl_2{}^b$				
0	4.36 ± 0.39	2.91	4.95	1:1.1
4.641	10.65 ± 3.62	3.04	5.19	1:1.0
7.74	14.02 ± 2.41	5.97	9.39	1:3.3
10.83	11.11 ± 6.19	4.44	7.22	1:1.3
13.92	8.25 ± 1.65	1.74	5.53	1:1.1

^{a} Mean ± standard deviation
^{b} MgCl$_2$ added as MgCl$_2 \cdot$ 6H$_2$O

dicating the presence of physiologically stressed cells[17].

Since an effect on the *V. cholerae* populations was induced by varying NaCl concentration, an additional series of microcosms, employing a chemically-defined basal-salts mix, containing no added Na$^+$, was used to determine whether *V.*

cholerae required Na$^+$ for growth. Also, to determine whether a Na$^+$ requirement, if any, could be satisfied by the presence of another monovalent cation and to minimize change in salinity, the NaCl-basal-salts solutions were amended with KCl and LiCl. Using a maximum NaCl concentration of 0.30 M, as the NaCl concentration decreased, molar equivalents of KCl or LiCl were added.

After incubation for 4 days at 25°C, population sizes in the microcosms of varying concentrations of NaCl were compared (Table 4). As the NaCl concentration was decreased from 0.30 M to 0.10 M, and 0.20 M KCl added, the *V. cholerae* populations increased, although not significantly (p ≤ 0.05), as determined by Duncan's multiple comparison[21]. As the NaCl concentration decreased to 0.01 M, the population size also decreased. When no NaCl was added, *V. cholerae*, at the concentrations of LiCl and MgCl$_2$, could not be recovered by plating.

The heterotrophic activity of *V. cholerae* populations was also affected when NaCl concentrations were varied (Table 5). The maximum uptake of ^{14}C-amino acids was detected in samples from microcosms amended with 0.1 M NaCl and 0.2 M KCl. *V. cholerae* did not grow in microcosms lacking NaCl, but amended with LiCl, thus uptake rates could not be determined.

Since *V. cholerae* did not grow in microcosms amended with LiCl, to evaluate the influence of Na$^+$, K$^+$, and Li$^+$ on the activity of *V. cholerae*, a washed cell suspension was employed and uptake of ^{14}C-amino acids mixture determined (Table 6). Using freshly cultured *V. cholerae* cells, mean uptake was found to increase with decreasing NaCl concentration and increasing LiCl concentration, until a concentraion of 0.20 M NaCl and 0.10 M LiCl was reached. The lowest uptake rate was determined in systems without added NaCl. Similarly, the highest ratios of respiration to incorporation were detected in NaCl-deficient systems.

When NaCl and KCl were used to amend the basal-salts solution, relatively

Table 4. *Vibrio cholerae* population sizes in microcosms amended with selected concentrations of NaCl, KCl and LiCl

Microcosm Containing				
NaCl (Molar)	KCl (Molar)	LiCl (Molar)	Mean Log$_{10}$ Culturable count/ml	Mean Log$_{10}$ Total cell count/ml
0.30	0	0	5.550 ± 0.045[a]	5.821 ± 0.030
0.15	0.15	0	5.584 ± 0.028	5.947 ± 0.005
0.10	0.20	0	5.778 ± 0.035	6.000 ± 0.029
0.05	0.25	0	5.640 ± 0.041	5.808 ± 0.028
0.01	0.29	0	5.480 ± 0.056	5.687 ± 0.149
0	0.30	0	N.D.[b]	N.D.
0.15	0	0.15	N.D.	N.D.
0.10	0	0.20	N.D.	N.D.
0.05	0	0.75	N.D.	N.D.
0.01	0	0.29	N.D.	N.D.
0	0	0.30	N.D.	N.D.

[a] Mean ± standard error.

[b] None detected.

Table 5. Uptake of ^{14}C-amino acid mixture by *Vibrio cholerae* cultured in microcosms amended with selected concentrations of NaCl, KCl and LiCl[a]

NaCl (Molar)	KCl (Molar)	LiCl (Molar)	Mean Uptake Rate (μg/l/hr $\times 10^{-2}$)	Uptake Rate Per Culturable Cell (μg/l/hr)	Uptake Rate Per Total Cell Number (μg/l/hr)	Resp./ Incorp.
0.30	0	0	4.29	1.21×10^{-7}	6.48×10^{-8}	1:0.56
0.15	0.15	0	1.11	2.89×10^{-7}	1.25×10^{-8}	1:0.81
0.10	0.20	0	12.60	2.10×10^{-7}	1.25×10^{-7}	1:1.18
0.05	0.25	0	1.73	3.96×10^{-8}	2.69×10^{-8}	1:8.16
0.01	0.29	0	1.29	4.27×10^{-8}	2.65×10^{-8}	1:5.16
0	0.30	0	N.D.	—	—	—

[a] Samples for uptake studies were collected from the microcosms following the four-day incubation period and inoculated into reaction vials containing the basal-salts solution with salinity adjusted to that of the microcosm from which the inoculum was collected.

Table 6. Effect of sodium, lithium and potassium on uptake of ^{14}C-amino acids by *Vibrio cholerae*[a]

Molar NaCl	Quantity of Added LiCl	KCl	Mean Uptake Rate (μg/l/hr $\times 10^{-2}$)	Respiration: Incorporated
0.30	—	—	4.18	1:1.2
0.295	0.005	—	5.80	1:1.3
0.25	0.05	—	8.83	1:1.2
0.20	0.10	—	9.18	1:1.2
0.15	0.15	—	8.20	1:1.2
0.15	—	0.15	3.76	1:1.0
0.05	—	0.25	3.29	1:0.86
0.01	—	0.29	3.92	1:0.42
0.005	—	0.295	2.34	1:0.34
0.0005	—	0.2995	1.51	1:0.16
0	—	0.30	1.40	1:0.14

[a] Uptake was determined employing cells cultured in tryptic soy broth and washed five times in basal-salts solution containing no added Na^{+}.

large uptake rates were obtained (Table 6). In these systems, amino acid uptake decreased with decreasing NaCl concentraion, although the differences were not as great as in the NaCl-LiCl systems. Maximum uptake was obtained at 0.01 M NaCl and 0.29 M KCl. In the NaCl-KCl systems, respiration to incorporation ratio was 1:1, in the presence of 0.15 M NaCl and 0.15 M KCl. At all other concentrations, however, this ratio was greater than 1.0, indicative of stressed cells[17].

When *V. cholerae* was inoculated into culture tubes containing different substrates and different salt concentrations, it was evident that both the type of substrate and salt concentration influenced growth of *V. cholerae* (Table 7). Culture tubes containing a combination of 1% (w/v) glucose and 0.05% (w/v) yeast ex-

Table 7. Growth of *Vibrio cholerae* in basal-salts solution with 1% (w/v) glucose and 0.05% (w/v) yeast extract as the growth substrate and amended with selected concentrations of NaCl, KCl and LiCl

Added Salt(s) Concentration (Molar)		Incubation Time (Days) Before Growth					
		1	2	4	8	10	14
NaCl							
0.30		+[a]	+	+	+	+	+
0.20		+	+	+	+	+	+
0.10		+	+	+	+	+	+
0.075		+	+	+	+	+	+
0.05		+	+	+	+	+	+
0.025		+	+	+	+	+	+
0.01		−[b]	+	+	+	+	+
0		−	−	−	−	−	−
NaCl	*+ KCl*						
0.03	+ 0	+	+	+	+	+	+
0.20	+ 0.10	+	+	+	+	+	+
0.10	+ 0.20	+	+	+	+	+	+
0.075	+ 0.225	+	+	+	+	+	+
0.05	+ 0.25	+	+	+	+	+	+
0.025	+ 0.275	−	+	+	+	+	+
0.01	+ 0.29	−	−	−	−	−	−
0	+ 0.30	−	−	−	−	−	−
NaCl	*+ LiCl*						
0.30	+ 0	+	+	+	+	+	+
0.20	+ 0.10	+	+	+	+	+	+
0.10	+ 0.20	+	+	+	+	+	+
0.075	+ 0.225	+	+	+	+	+	+
0.05	+ 0.25	+	+	+	+	+	+
0.025	+ 0.274	+	+	+	+	+	+
0.01	+ 0.29	−	+	+	+	+	+
0	+ 0.30	−	−	−	−	−	−
NaCl	*+ Sucrose*[c]						
0.13	+ 0	+	+	+	+	+	+
0.10	+ 0.55	+	+	+	+	+	+
0.06	+ 0.125	+	+	+	+	+	+
0.04	+ 0.160	+	+	+	+	+	+
0	+ 0.190	−	−	−	−	−	−

[a] + = growth as indicated by turbidity.

[b] − = no growth.

[c] Sucrose was added to maintain osmotic pressure.

tract was used to demonstrate the influence of salt concentration of growth of *V. cholerae*.

In all tubes amended with only one salt, i.e., NaCl, growth occurred, although the lag time increased at the lower NaCl concentrations (Table 7). When 0.01 M NaCl was added, the lag period, before detectable growth of *V. cholerae* occurred, was between 24 and 48 hr. As the NaCl concentration was increased to 0.025 M, the lag period decreased, with growth detected after incubation for 24 hr at

25°C. Similarly, at all higher NaCl concentrations tested, growth occurred within 24 hr. However, in tubes containing no added NaCl, no growth of *V. cholerae* was evident during the 14-day test period.

Cutlures in which NaCl and KCl were present yielded results similar to those amended with NaCl alone (Table 7). At higher NaCl and lower KCl concentrations, growth of *V. cholerae* occurred within 24 hr. Only when the added NaCl and KCl concentrations were reduced to 0.025 M and 0.275 M, respectively, was the lag period extended. Culture containing 0.30 M KCl and no added NaCl failed to demonstrate growth of *V. cholerae*.

When cultures were amended with a combination of NaCl and LiCl, the growth pattern of *V. cholerae* was also similar to that obtained when only NaCl was added (Table 7). *V. cholerae* grew in all concentrations of LiCl tested, provided NaCl was also added. There was, however, an extended lag period when 0.01 M NaCl was added.

In all salt concentrations tested, if 1% (w/v) tryptone was employed as a substrate, detectable growth occurred within 24 hr. This was not true, however, with 1% (w/v) glucose or 0.05% (w/v) yeast extract added as sole substrate. No detectable growth occurred during the 14-day test period without addition of NaCl and both glucose and yeast extract. To determine if the growth patterns, obtained when varying concentrations of salts and different substrates were employed, arose from alteration of osmotic pressure, the test systems were amended with NaCl and sucrose to maintain an osmotic pressure equivalent to that of 0.13 M NaCl[17]. As observed above, if tryptone was employed as substrate, growth occurred if NaCl was added, regardless of concentration. No growth occurred with 1% (w/v) glucose as the substrate. However, with 1% (w/v) glucose and 0.05% (w/v) yeast extract as substrate, growth occurred within 24 hr, if also amended with NaCl. Without added NaCl, no detectable growth of *V. cholerae* occurred during incubation at 25°C for 14 days. A specific requirement for Na^+ is therefore suggested.

From the results of the studies of salinity effects, the hypothesis that *V. cholerae* is an autochthonous organism of estuarine and brackish water systems[10] is reinforced and emphasizes the need for an ecological approach in evaluating the role of *V. cholerae* in nature and in human disease. Under simulated environmental conditions, both Ol and non-Ol serovars behaved almost identically (Table 1). That is, *V. cholerae* LA 4808, a clinical isolate from a patient who became ill following ingestion of improperly prepared seafood; *V. cholerae* CA 401, a clinical isolate; and V-69, an Ol serovar from the environment but not associated with disease, all responded similarly.

A recent investigation into the ecological relationships of *V. cholerae* in aquatic systems in Kent, England, was carried out by West and Lee[22], using growth chambers *in situ*. They showed that the growth pattern for *V. cholerae* in chambers was similar to that obtained in the microcosms employed in our study and reported here. Therefore, based on the results of this study and previous work done in our laboratory[4, 5, 6, 9], it is concluded that, under a proper regime of nutrient, temperature, and salinity, *V. cholerae* is clearly capable of growth and survival in the natural aquatic environment.

In surveys carried out during the winter months, when the temperature is reduced, the occurrence of *V. cholerae* in aquatic environments of the temperate zone is apparently severely restricted[4, 10]. Hypotheses that have been put forward to explain the apparent disappearance of allochthonous bacteria, especially human pathogens, from an aquatic system usually involve a "die-off" induced by low temperature. However, as indicated by results obtained for microcosms incubated at 10°C (Fig. 2), *V. cholerae* can exist for extended periods of time, although often below detectable levels, as measured by plating or by direct microscopic observation[5]. It is possible that the few viable cells, i.e., "surviving" cells adsorb to surfaces of the container, in the laboratory, or to natural substrates, in the environment[23] and remain until favorable growth conditions return. It is also possible that viable organisms simply do not grow on any of the plating media used, without pre-treatment of the sample. Very recent work in our laboratory shows that viability of *V. cholerae* is maintained up to eight days, when suspended in filtered Chesapeake Bay water at 10°C, when monitored by direct counting procedures, without loss of O1 antigen (Fig. 7).

The influence of salinity on survival of *V. cholerae* in microcosms incubated at 10°C is unequivocal, based on its survival for up to 42 days at a salinity of 25 ‰ but not at 5 ‰[5]. Thus, in those aquatic systems in nature in which *V. cholerae* in known to be present, a seasonal distribution of this organism can be explained by "overwintering" in waters within an optimal salinity range for *V. cholerae*. In an estuary or brackish water area, these requirements can easily be met.

Results of experiments designed to detect a requirement for Na^+ by *V. cholerae* further support the hypothesis that the natural habitat of *V. cholerae* is estuarine or brackish[10]. The requirement for Na^+ cannot be met by addition of K^+ or Li^+, demonstrating a clear specificity of the requirement for Na^+ (Tables 4-7).

The requirement for Na^+ demonstrated by many marine bacteria has been well established, notably by the elegant research of MacLeod and his co-workers[17-20]. The obligate requirement for Na^+ is considered to be a differentiating characteristic useful in separating marine and estuarine bacteria from those of freshwater habitats[18]. In a recent report on the effect of Na^+ on growth patterns of a marine bacterium, Gow *et al.*[17] demonstrated that as the Na^+ concentration was decreased to near the minimum required to support growth, the major influence observed on growth was an extended lag period, prior to growth of the organism. Also, when no Na^+ was added and, therefore, the concentration was less than the minimum required, no growth occurred.

V. cholerae responds to various concentrations of NaCl similar to the marine bacterium, *Alteromonas haloplanktis* 216, studied by Gow *et al.*[17]. Using 1% (w/v) glucose and 0.05% (w/v) yeast extract as substrate, effect of specific ions on the growth of *V. cholerae* was tested and, at the lower NaCl concentrations, i.e., less than 0.01 M, the time required before growth occurred increased (Table 7). Also, in the absence of added NaCl, no growth of *V. cholerae* occurred. In systems receiving 1% (w/v) tryptone as substrate, growth occurred in the presence or absence of added NaCl, indicating that a sufficient quantity of Na^+ is available in tryptone to support growth of *V. cholerae*. A quantitative analysis of tryptone[24] demonstrates that, by weight, tryptone contains approximately 2.7% Na^+.

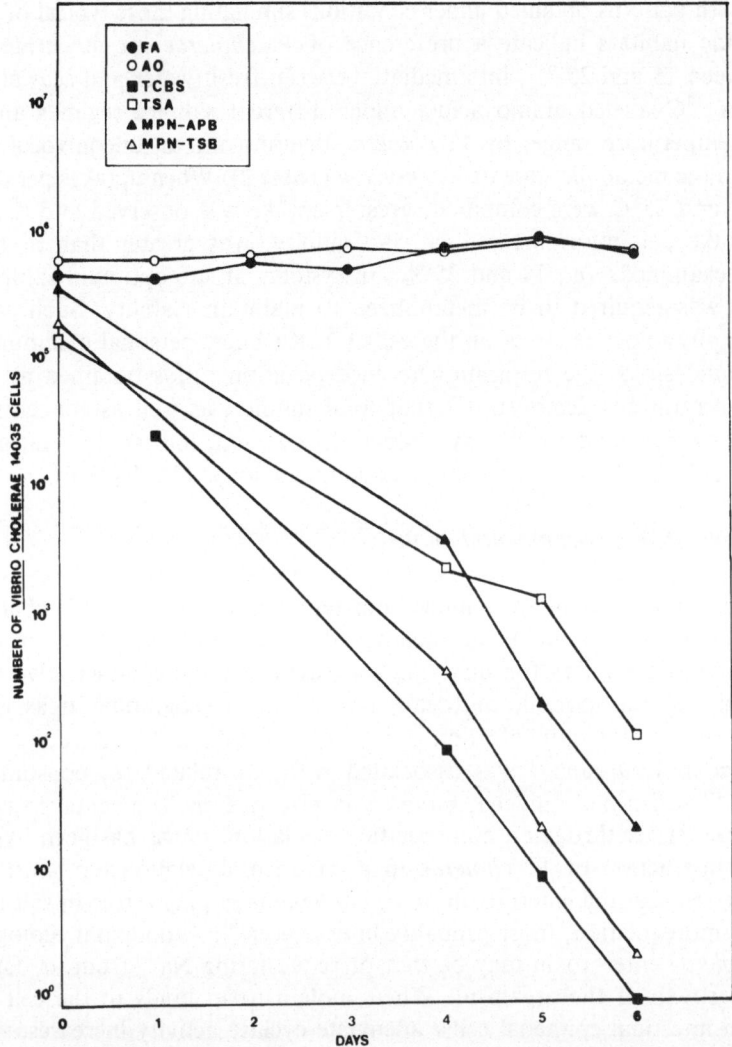

Fig. 7. Comparison of recovery and detection of *Vibrio cholerae* ATCC 14035 by immunofluorescent antibody and epifluorescent microscopy (FA), acridine orange direct count (AO), direct plating on Thiosulphate Citrate Bilesalt Sucrose (TCBS) agar and Trypicase Soy agar (TSA), and counting by a most probable number procedure in alkaline peptone water (APW) and Trypticase Soy broth (TSB) when suspended in filter-sterilized Chesapeake Bay water.

Thus, sufficient Na$^+$ is present in a medium prepared with 1% (w/v) tryptone (Difco), i.e., approximately 0.012 M Na$^+$, to support growth of *V. cholerae*. Since tryptone alone supported growth of *V. cholerae*, whereas glucose alone did not unless yeast extract was also present, it appears that *V. cholerae* may require one or more vitamins or other factors for growth, in addition to having a requirement for Na$^+$.

Growth patterns obtained under conditions simulating those typical of estuarine and marine habitats indicate a preference of *V. cholerae* for moderate salinity, i.e., between 15 and 25 ‰, intermediate between fresh water and seawater. Also, uptake of ^{14}C-labeled amino acids, under different salinity regimes and within a given temperature range, by *V. cholerae* demonstrate an unequivocal effect of salinity on the metabolic state of *V. cholerae* (Table 2). When uptakes per culturable cell at 20 and 25°C were compared, greater uptake was observed at 5 ‰ salinity, since uptake per culturable cell, at 5% salinity, was greater than at the other salinities examined, i.e., 15 and 25 ‰, in systems of sub-optimum salinity, more substrate was required to be metabolized to maintain viability. Such conditions suggest a physiological stress on the cells (D. Kushner, personal communication).

An analysis of the respiration to incorporation ratios obtained at different ionic concentrations demonstrates that total salinity, as well as concentration of specific ions, can render cells physiolocgically stressed, indicated by ratios greater than 1.0 (17; D. Kushner, personal communication). (Tables 3-6).

Interactions with environmental biota

Taking into account the salinity and temperature data for *V. cholerae* and considering it to be an indigenous member of the bacterial community of estuarine systems with a capability for surviving for extended periods under adverse conditions, many of the sporadic outbreaks of cholera in geographic areas without a known focus or source of infection can now be accounted for. A recent outbreak of cholera in Louisiana[1] was associated with, or related to, consumption of shellfish. Shellfish may, indeed, serve as an effective environmental reservoir for *V. cholerae*, either through a non-specific association, or, as has been hypothesized[9], by interaction of *V. cholerae* in a commensal relationship. Furthermore, it is suggested that the enterotoxin of *V. cholerae* may play a role in salt tolerance and/or osmoregulation, most probably in crustacea[9]. A potential ecological role of *V. cholerae* enterotoxin may be that of sequestering Na^+ from its commensal host for growth of the organism. When cholera toxin binds to the cell receptor of human intestinal epithelial cells, adenylate cyclase activity increases, which increases the level of cyclic 3', 5'-adenosine monophosphate (AMP). The increase in cyclic AMP activity results in an efflux of Na^+ and other electrolytes from epithelial cells, along with quantities of water, producing the symptoms associated with disease, i.e., cholera, in humans. Should cholera toxin affect epithelial cells of crustacea similarly, but less drastically, *V. cholerae*, in association with crustacea, would provide for itself a means for obtaining sufficient quantities of Na^+ from its host, should the salinity of the environment fall below that required for its survival and growth.

To illuminate the relationships between *V. cholerae* and estuarine biota, studies of the relationship of adult and immature copepods to *V. cholerae* has been examined[25]. Copepods collected by hand-trawl with a plankton net (No. 20, 77 μm mesh size) from waters of the Patuxent River, Sunderland, MD (salinity [S], 2 ‰); the Chesapeake Bay near Solomons Island, MD (S, 15 ‰); the Chesapeake Bay near Annapolis, MD (S, 22 ‰) and the Buriganga River, Dacca, Bangladesh

(S, 0.2 ‰) were exposed, under controlled conditions in the laboratory, to various strains of bacteria (Table 8).

The copepods were washed four times with water taken from the same collection site. Water used in the experiments was filter-sterilized by passage through an 0.22 μm pore-size filtration system (Millipore Co., Bedford, MA). Dead copepods were prepared by placing a glass flask containing 100 ml of water and copepods in a freezer at -60°C for 30 min. In the experiments, *ca.* 500 washed copepods were placed into each of several two-liter flasks containing 500 ml of filter steriliz-ed river or bay water. For experiments using *V. parahaemolyticus*, the salinity of the water was adjusted to 30 ‰ by addition of NaCl. Where indicated, flasks were inoculated with each bacterial strain to a final concentration of *ca.* 10^4 colony-forming units (CFU)/ml. Dead bacteria were obtained by heating a suspension of cells in phosphate-buffered saline for 15 minutes in a water bath set at 54°C. Death was indicated by the loss of cell motility in hanging-drop preparations observ-ed by light microscopy and lack of growth on gelatin agar. In selected flasks, a non-axenic algal culture, *Pseudoisocrysis* sp., was added to a final concentration of 10^3 cells/ml to serve as food supply for the live copepods. Addition of the algal culture did not result in an increase in the number of copepods in the flask.

The following flask combinations were prepared for each experiment: (a) live copepods, live algae, live bacteria; (b) live copepods, live bacteria; (c) live copepods, dead bacteria; (d) dead copepods, live bacteria; (e) live algae, live bacteria; (f) live bacteria; (g) live copepods, live algae.

After inoculation, flasks were incubated, under static conditions, at ambient temperature (23-26°C) for 336 hr. For sampling, five copepods were removed, along with 2 ml of water, and homogenized manually in a teflon-tipped tissue grinder (Wheaton Scientific, Millville, NJ) until all copepods were completely and

Table 8. Source of strains used in copepod experiments

Species	Strain No.	Source
V. cholerae 01 Classical Inaba	CA 401	Clinical isolate from Calcutta, India (1953)
V. cholerae 01 El Tor Ogawa	D-18050	Environmental isolate from river water, Dacca, Bangladesh (1980)
V. cholerae non-01	OSU 116	Environmental isolate from algae, Tillamook Bay, Oregon (1980)
V. parahaemolyticus	TK 18136	Environmental isolate from brackish water, Teknaf, Bangladesh (1980)
E. coli	E/C 744	Environmental isolate from river water, Dacca, Bangladesh (1980)
Pseudomonas sp.	PS 11361	Clinical isolate from ICDDR, B hospital, Dacca, Bangladesh (1981)

uniformly disintegrated. After appropriate decimal dilutions in phosphate-buffered saline had been prepared, 0.1 ml aliquots of each dilution were spread onto duplicate plates of selective medium. Thiosulphate Citrate Bile salts Sucrose (TCBS) agar (BBL Microbiology Systems) was used for *V. cholerae* and *V. parahaemolyticus*, MacConkey agar (Difco) for *E. coli* and Muller-Hinton agar (Oxoid, Columbia, MD) for *Pseudomonas* sp. Viable, culturable, heterotrophic bacteria were enumerated using plate count agar (Difco) amended to contain 1% NaCl (wt/vol). All plates were incubated at 35°C for 18 hr.

In addition, five copepods were removed from each flask, using wide-bore glass pipettes to avoid damage to the copepods as much as possible. Copepods were fixed in Bouin's solution (26) and prepared for electron microscopy.

Both non-Ol and Ol serovars of *V. cholerae* increased in number up to 100-fold in the presence of live copepods, compared with cells in the presence of cold-killed copepods. Figs. 8 and 9 illustrate the phenomenon observed when *V. cholerae* CA 401 was added to a Patuxent River water sample (S, 2 ‰). In the presence of cold-killed copepods, *V. cholerae* counts rose form 1.45×10^4 CFU/ml to 3.02×10^6 CFU/ml, within 36 hr, then fell to below detectable numbers by 144 hours. The viable, heterotrophic plate count remained around 10^6 CFU/ml for the first 36 hours, gradually rising to *ca*, 1 log increase before the sampling was terminated at 144 hr. The source of these bacteria was presumably in the gut of the cold-killed copepods.

In contrast, *V. cholerae* counts increased in the presence of live copepods, i.e., from 4.30×10^4 CFU/ml to 1.99×10^8 CFU/ml, within 36 hr and did not decrease to below detectable numbers until after incubation for 336 hr. The

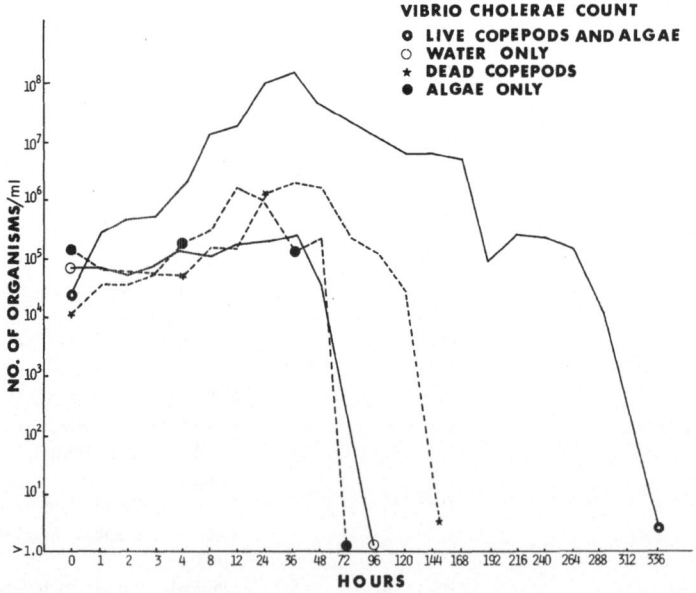

Fig. 8.   Growth of *Vibrio cholerae* CA 401 in flasks of Patuxent River water in the presence of live copepods and algae, dead copepods, and algae. (From Ref. 25.)

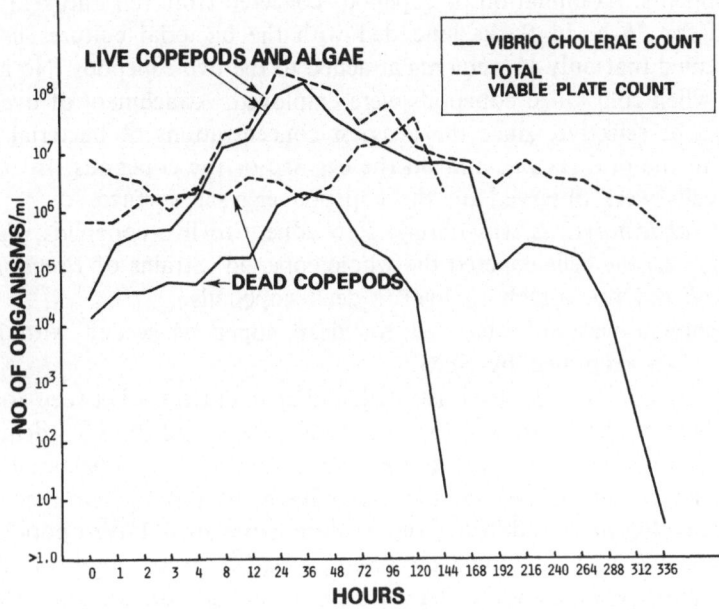

Fig. 9. Count of *Vibrio cholerae* CA 401 and total viable plate count in Patuxent River water in the presence of live copepods and algae, and dead copepods. (From Ref. 25.)

viable, heterotrophic plate count increased similarly as the *V. cholerae* count.

The contribution of a non-axenic algal culture and copepod gut flora to the plate count was not apparent until the numbers of *V. cholerae* decreased, near the end of the experiment. Appropriate controls showed that extended survival of *V. cholerae* CA 401 was associated with the presence of live copepods. Similar results were obtained with all other strains of *V. cholerae* and water samples when tested over a shorter incubation period of 36 hr. Thus, a striking trend towards increased cell number and survival of *V. cholerae* in the presence of live copepods was observed.

Studies were also made using water collected from the Buriganga River, Dacca, Bangladesh, employing an incubation period of 36 hr. In these experiments, *V. parahaemolyticus* demonstrated *ca.* a single log increase in numbers in the presence of live, but not when incubated in the presence of dead, copepods for 12 hr. Little change in count was detected when the experiments were repeated with incubation for 36 hr.

The strain of *Pseudomonas* sp. increased in population size in the presence of both dead and live copepods. Results obtained in control flasks indicated that these increases were not associated with copepods. Interestingly, the counts of *E. coli* were higher at 12 hr (1.91×10^5 CFU/ml) and 36 hr (4.91×10^5 CFU/ml) in the presence of dead copepods compared with 12 hr (8.40×10^4 CFU/ml) and 36 hr (7.30×10^4 CFU/ml) in the presence of the live copepods.

SEM revealed that the washing procedure for cleaning freshly-caught copepods effectively removed surface bacteria prior to contamination with test strains in

292

the experiments. Examination of copepods collected from the Patuxent River and incubated for 36 hr in flasks amended with the bacterial cultures used in this study revealed that only *V. cholerae* attached to the live copepods. No attachment was seen when cold-killed copepods were employed. Attachment of live copepods appears to be selective, since the heaviest concentrations of bacterial cells were observed in the oral region, and on the egg sac of the copepods. In some cases, dividing cells were observed on the copepod egg sac surface.

V. parahaemolyticus was observed to adhere to live copepods, but without selectivity, i.e., the cells covered the whole copepod. Strains of *Pseudomonas* sp. and *E. coli* did not attach to live or dead copepods.

Attachment was not observed for dead copepods seeded with heat-killed bacteria, when examined by SEM.

Previous studies have demonstrated similar interactions between zooplankton and members of the genus *Vibrio*. The study of Sochard *et al.*[27] demonstrated, by culture on marine agar 2216, that marine copepods carry a bacterial flora both on their surface and in the gut, the predominant bacterial group being members of the genus *Vibrio*. In addition, the predominance of a *Vibrio* population with zooplankton has been described by Simidu *et al.*[28], who found differences between the generic composition of bacteria from zooplankton and seawater samples.

Thus, it can be concluded that a significant association exists between *V. cholerae* and live copepods, with selective attachment taking place on the copepod surface. An interesting aspect of our observations is the lack of attachment of these strains to dead copepods. If chitin is the important factor in attachment by chitinolytic vibrios, as suggested by results of studies with *V. parahaemolyticus*[7], it might be expected that *V. cholerae* would adhere to dead copepods equally well as live copepods. This was not observed and the possibility that live copepods excrete growth-promoting or chemical attractant compounds specific for *V. cholerae* warrants investigation. In addition, the outermost surface of copepods is covered with an epicuticle of waxes[29]. The importance of this layer in primary attachment of chitinolytic vibrios to copepods is not known, although its net charge has been suggested as a limiting factor for attachment[7].

The attachment phenomenon observed to occur between *V. cholerae* and live copepods has ecological, as well as epidemiological, significance. Since *Vibrio* species produce an active chitinase, it is suggested, from the results of the present study and studies of the adsorption of *V. parahaemolyticus* to chitin particles and copepods[7] that a primary role of vibrios could be the colonization and initiation of degradation of chitinous material in aquatic ecosystems. Such a role has been postulated by Hood and Meyers[30], who demonstrated the role of *Vibrio* species in chitin turnover and metabolism in marine crustaceae.

Concluding remarks

Traditionally, cholera epidemiologists considered that the only reservoir of *V. cholerae* was the human intestine and that survival of the organism outside the human body was brief[31], a supposition that is no longer justified. A single case of cholera in Texas in 1973[32] was followed in 1978 by an outbreak involving

11 persons in Louisiana[1]. The phage types of the Texas and Louisiana isolates were identical, implying that the causative organism had been able to survive in the Gulf Coast environment between outbreaks[1]. More recently, studies have demonstrated the ability of non-toxigenic *V. cholerae* strains to survive and multiply in aquatic ecosystems in England[22]. Thus, data have accumulated supporting the original hypothesis of Colwell *et al.*[10] that *V. cholerae* is an autochthonous member of natural aquatic ecosystems.

In addition to growth of *V. cholerae* in association with planktonic copepods, the seasonality of cholera outbreaks in endemic areas, such as Bangladesh, may well be related to this association and to temperature and salinity responses demonstrated by *V. cholerae*. Almost every year in Bangladesh, an epidemic of cholera commences in September or October. According to Oppenheimer *et al.*[33], the zooplankton population decreases during the monsoon season (May-July) in response to a reduction in nutrient concentration in the water and a result of the heavy influx of rain water, which also alters the salinity. Subsequently, the zooplankton population increases during August and September, being preceded by a phytoplankton bloom. An increase in the copepod population is invariably paralleled, or shortly followed by, the appearance of cholera cases, initiating the annual epidemics which occur in Bangladesh. Colonization of copepods and other chitinous zooplankton may explain, in part, why *V. cholerae* is abundant in the water at the same time that the zooplankton are abundant.

A serious question currently under study in this laboratory is the infrequent isolation of *V. cholerae* serovar Ol from environmental samples during the inter-epidemic period in Bangladesh. A possible explanation lines in the demonstration of a "non-culturable state" for *V. cholerae* in which cells remain viable and substrate-responsive, but fail to grow on routine laboratory media (Xu, H.-S. N. Roberts, and R. R. Colwell, work in progress). This finding throws doubt on the efficacy of the alkaline-peptone water and TCBS agar isolation regime, originally developed for clinical specimens, but currently employed for environmental samples. It is possible that *V. cholerae* may be present ubiquitously and continuously in brackish and freshwater environments during the months of the monsoon, when nutritional conditions of the environment change. Under such conditions, *V, cholerae* cells may become unculturable, hence not detected by isolation techniques currently employed in clinical laboratories. In this state, it is hypothesized that *V. cholerae* may survive attached to copepods and subsequently multiply and outgrow in the water column and on the copepod surface, when conditions revert to optimum at the end of the monsoon period and the start of the cholera epidemic season.

Clearly, the implications of the association between *V. cholerae* and planktonic copepods and the physico-chemical parameters of the aquatic environment on the epidemiology of cholera will remain speculative until field studies, designed to detect and assess the significance of "non-culturable" *V. cholerae* cells, are completed. Work is in progress, as part of a collaborative University of Maryland-World Health Organization study, to elucidate the ecology of *V. cholerae* (Huq, A., P. A. West, and R. R. Colwell, work in progress).

If *V. cholerae* is, in fact, an indigenous member of the bacterial community of estuarine systems, possessing the ability to survive for extended periods under adverse conditions, many of the limited outbreaks of cholera in regions of no known, or apparent, human source of the causative agent can be explained.

Based on results reported herein, *V. cholerae* is concluded to be, as hypothesized by Colwell *et al.*[10], an indigenous member of the bacterial community of estuarine systems, evident not only from its requirement for Na^+ for growth, but also by its obvious preference for a salinity regime typical of brackish water areas and estuaries. It is important to note that the distribution of *V. cholerae* would not be limited to estuaries, since the requirement for Na^+ can be spared if a sufficiently high nutrient concentration is present[5, 6]. Results of this study demonstrate the usefulness of combined laboratory and field studies in gaining an understanding of the role(s) of *V. cholerae* in the natural environment.

This work was supported, in part, by grants from the National Science Foundation, DEB-77-14646; the National Institutes of Health, R22-AI-14242; the National Oceanic and Atmospheric Administration, NA81AA-D-00040 and NA79AA-D-00128; World Health Organization, C6/181/1.

We are indebted to Dr. P. A. West for careful reading of the manuscript.

REFERENCES

1. Blake, P. A., D. T. Allegra, J. D. Snyder, T. J. Barrett, L. MacFarland, C. T. Caraway, J. C. Feeley, J. P. Craig, J. V. Lee, N. D. Puhr, and R. A. Feldman. 1980. Cholera - a possible endemic focus in the United States. N. Engl. J. Med. **302**: 305–309.
2. Blake, P. A., M. L. Rosenberg, J. Bandeira Costa, P. Soares Ferreira, C, Levy Guimaraes, and E. J. Gangarosa. 1977. Cholera in Portugal, 1974. I. Modes of transmission. Am. J. Epidemiol. **105**: 337–343.
3. Dutt, A. K., S. Alwi, and T. Velauthan. 1971. A shellfish-borne cholera outbreak in Malaysia. Trans. R. Soc. Trop. Med. Hyg. **65**: 815–818.
4. Kaper, J. B., H. Lockman, R. R. Colwell and S. W. Joseph. 1979. Ecology, serology, and enterotoxin production of *Vibrio cholerae* in Chesapeake Bay, Appl. Environ. Microbiol. **37**: 91–103.
5. Singleton, F. L., R. Attwell, S. Jangi, and R. R. Colwell. 1982. Effects of temperature and salinity or *Vibrio cholerae* growth. Appl. Environ. Microbiol. **44**: 1047–1058.
6. Singleton, F. L., R. W. Attwell, M. S. Jangi, and R. R. Colwell. 1982. Influence of salinity and nutrient concentration on survival and growth of *Vibrio cholerae* in aquatic microcosms. Appl. Environ. Microbiol. **43**: 1080–1085.
7. Kaneko, T. and R. R. Colwell. 1975. Adsorption of *Vibrio parahaemolyticus* onto chitin and copepods. Appl. Environ. Microbiol. **29**: 269–274.
8. Kaneko, T., and R. R. Colwell. 1978. The annual cycle of *Vibrio parahaemolyticus* in Chesapeake Bay. Microb. Ecol. **4**: 135–155.
9. Colwell, R. R., R. J. Seidler, J. Kaper, S. W. Joseph, S. Garges, H. Lockman, D. Maneval, H. B. Bradford, N. Roberts, E. Remmers, I. Huq, and A. Huq. 1981. Occurrence of *Vibrio cholerae* serotype Ol in Maryland and Louisiana estuaries. Appl. Environ. Microbiol. **41**: 555–558.
10. Colwell, R. R., J. Kaper, and S. W. Joseph. 1977. *Vibrio cholerae*, *Vibrio parahaemolyticus*, and other virios: occurrence and distribution in Chesapeake Bay. Science **198**: 394–396.
11. Kosinski, R. J., F. L. Singleton, and B. G. Foster. 1979. Sampling culturable heterotrophs from microcosms: a statistical analysis. Appl. Environ. Microbiol. **38**: 906–910.
12. Singleton, F. L., R. W. Attwell, M. S. Jangi, and R. R. Colwell. 1981. Influence of salinity, nutrient concentration and temperature on growth and survival of *Vibrio cholerae*. *In* Proc. 17th Joint Conference on Cholera. The United States-Japan Cooperative medical Science Pro-

gram, National Institutes of Health, Baltimore, MD. October 25–28, 1981.

13. Daley, R. J. and J. E. Hobbie. 1975. Direct counts of aquatic bacteria by a modified epifluorescent technique. Limnol. Oceanogr. **20**: 875–882.

14. Francisco, D. E., R. A. Mah, and A. C. Rabin. 1973. Acridine orange epifluorescence technique for counting bacteria in natural waters. Trans. Amer. Microscop. Soc. **92**: 416–421.

15. Hobbie, J. E., R. J. Daley, and S. Jasper. 1977. Use of Nuclepore filters for counting bacteria by fluorescence microscopy. Appl. Environ. Microbiol. **33**: 1225–1228.

16. Hobbie, J. E. and C. C. Crawford. 1969. Corrections for bacterial uptake of dissolved organic compounds in natural water. Limnol. Oceanogr. **14**: 528–532.

17. Gow, J. A., R. A. MacLeod, M. Goodbody, D. Frank, and L. DeVoe. 1981. Growth characteristics at low Na^+ concentration and the stability of the Na^+ requirement of a marine bacterium. Can. J. Microbiol. **27**: 350–357.

18. MacLeod, R. A. 1965. The question of the existence of specific marine bacteria. Bacteriol. Rev. **29**: 9–23.

19. MacLeod, R. A. and E. Onofrey. 1957. Nutrition and metabolism of marine bacteria. III. The relation of Na^+ and K^+ to growth. J. Cell Comp. Physiol. **50**: 389–401.

20. MacLeod, R. A. and E. Onofrey. 1963. Studies on the stability of the Na^+ requirement of marine bacteria. pp. 481–489. *In*: Symposium on Marine Microbiology, C.H. Oppenheimer (ed.). Charles C. Thomas, Springfield, Illinois.

21. Ott, L. 1977. *An Introduction to Statistical Methods and Data Analysis*. Wadsworth Publishing Co., Inc., Belmont, Calif.

22. West, P. A. and J. V. Lee. 1982. Ecology of *Vibrio* species, including *Vibrio cholerae*, in natural waters of Kent, England. J. Appl. Bacteriol. **52**: 435–448.

23. ZoBell, C. E. 1943. The effect of solid surfaces on bacterial activity. J. Bacteriol. **46**: 38–59.

24. Anon. 1972. *Difco Manual of Dehydrated Culture Media and Reagents for Microbiological and Clinical Laboratory Procedures*, 9th (ed.), Difco Laboratories, Detroit, Michigan.

25. Huq, A., E. B. Small, P. A. West, M. I. Huq, R. Rahman, and R. R. Colwell. 1983. Ecological relationships of *Vibrio cholerae* with planktonic crustacean copepods. Appl. Environ. Microbiol. **45**: 275–283.

26. Baker, J., R. 1958. *Principles of Biological Microtechniques*. John Wiley and Sons, Inc., New York.

27. Sochard, M. R., D. F. Wilson, B. Austin, and R. R. Colwell. 1979. Bacteria associated with the surface and the gut of marine copepods. Appl. Environ. Microbiol. **37**: 750–759.

28. Simidu, U., K. Ashino, and E. Kaneko. 1971. Bacterial flora of phyto and zooplankton in the inshore water of Japan. Can. J. Microbiol. **17**: 1157–1160.

29. Hickman, C. P. 1967. Biology of the invertebrates. C. V. Mosley Co., St. Louis, Missouri.

30. Hood, M. A. and S. P. Meyers. 1977. Microbiological and chitinoclastic activities associated with *Penaeus setiferus*. J. Oceanograph. Soc. Japan. **33**: 235–241.

31. Felsenfeld, O. 1974. The survival of cholera vibrios, PP. 359–366. *In*: D. Barua and W. Burrows (ed.). *Cholera*. W. B. Saunders, London.

32. Weissman, J. B., W. E. DeWitt, J. Thompson, C. N. Muchnick, B. L. Portnoy, J. D. Feeley, and E. J. Gangarosa. 1974. A case of cholera in Texas, 1973. Amer. J. Epidemiol. **100**: 487–498.

33. Oppenheimer, J. R., M. G. Ahmad, A. Huq, K. A. Haque, A. K. M. A. Alam, K. M. S. Aziz, S. Ali, and A. S. M. Haque. 1978. Limnological studies of three ponds in Dacca, Bangladesh J. Fisheries **1**: 1–28.

Bacterial Diarrheal Diseases, eds., Y. Takeda, T. Miwatani, 297-308.
Copyright © 1985 by KTK Scientific Publishers, Tokyo.

PATHOGENESIS OF *VIBRIO PARAHAEMOLYTICUS*

Takeshi Honda, Yoshifumi Takeda and Toshio Miwatani

Department of Bactriology and Serology, Research Institute for Microbial Diseases, Osaka University, Yamada-oka, Suita, Osaka 565, Japan

Vibrio parahaemolyticus was first isolated by Fujino *et al.*[1] in 1950 as a causative bacterium of food poisoning. Since that time, this organism has been isolated very frequently from cases of food poisoning accounting for about 40 - 60% of all cases in Japan. Table 1 summarizes data on cases of food poisoning in Japan from 1968 to 1974 reported by the Ministry of Health and Welfare. *V. parahaemolyticus* was the bacterium most frequently isolated, followed in order by *Staphylococcus*, *Salmonella* and enteropathogenic *Escherichia coli*. A few fatal cases of *V. parahaemolyticus* infection have been reported every year and the mortality is about 0.04% (Table 1).

V. parahaemolyticus is also reported to be an important cause of traveller's diarrhea. Results of our study of causative bacteria of this diarrhea in patients who had just come back from abroad are shown in Table 2 Stools of patients were collected at Osaka Airport Quarantine Station and promptly examined. As shown in Table 2, enterotoxigenic *Escherichia coli* was the most frequently isolated, followed in decreasing order by Salmonella and *V. parahaemolyticus*. About 13% of the cases were due to *V. parahaemolyticus*.

Clinical features

The incubation periods in *V. parahaemolyticus* infection is 3 -24 hours, usually being about 10 -15 hours. The main symptoms are diarrhea and abdominal pain. Patients may also show fever, vomiting, nausea and general fatigue. The frequency of diarrhea is usually less than 10 times a day, but in some cases it is more than 20 times. The diarrhea is watery, mucus, bloody or mucus and bloody. A few cases show dehydration, collapse and cyanosis, and the case fatality is 0.04%. *V. parahaemolyticus* infection is usually a self-limiting disease and clinical symptoms last 1 - 2 weeks.

Cardiovascular symptoms have not been claimed in *V. parahaemolyticus* infection, but there are several reports indicating cardiovascular disturbances. Since the thermostable direct hemolysin produced by Kanagawa-phenomenon positive strains of *V. parahaemolyticus* is cardiotoxic, as described later, it is assumed that this hemolysin is responsible for the cardiovascular symptoms. Takikawa[2]

298

Table 1. Bacterial food poisoning in Japan (1968–1974).

Causative bacterium	Number of cases	% of total cases	Number of death	Mortality (%)
Vibrio parahaemolyticus	43,247	36.1	17	0.04
Staphylococcus	30,985	25.8	6	0.02
Salmonella	23,144	19.3	23	0.10
Enteropathogenic *Escherichia coli*	10,100	8.4	2	0.02
Clostridium botulinum	65	0.05	12	18.45
Other bacteria	12,367	10.3	1	0.01
Total	119,908	—	61	0.05

Table 2. Bacteriological examination of travellers' diarrhea at Osaka Airport Quarantine Station (1979–1981)

	1979	1980	1981	Total
Number of stools examined	819	1,186	977	2,982 (100.0%)
Number of positive cases	362	565	486	1,413 (47.4%)
Enterotoxigenic *E. coli*	120*	249	225	594 (19.9%)
Salmonella	128	199	138	465 (15.6%)
V. parahaemolyticus	118	155	120	127 (4.3%)
Shigella	29	43	55	82 (2.7%)
NAG *vibrio*	22	37	23	3 (0.1%)
V. cholerae	0	1	2	

*Data from May to December.

administered living cells of *V. parahaemolyticus* to a volunteer and observed a significant change in the blood pressure: the maximum blood presure decreased to 77 mmHg on the first day of infection and returned to 136 mmHg after 4 days. Significant decrease in blood pressure in severe cases of food poisoning due to *V. parahaemolyticus* was also reported by Saito[3].

We compared the electrocardiograms of patients during acute gastroenteritis due to *V. parahaemolyticus* and after recovery[4]. The T wave was significantly lower during the disease than after recovery. The P wave was also wider and higher during the disease and became normal on recovery. Typical changes in electrocardiograms from chest leads of one of the patients are shown in Fig. 1. Changes in the T wave were very clear: during the disease, the T wave not only became lower but also became biphasic in the V_2 and V_3 leads.

The titer of antihemolysin (antibody against the thermostable direct hemolysin) increased in about 37% of the patients[5]. The height of the T wave in electrocardiograms showed a positive correlation with the antihemolysin titer of convalescent sera of the patients (Fig. 2.).

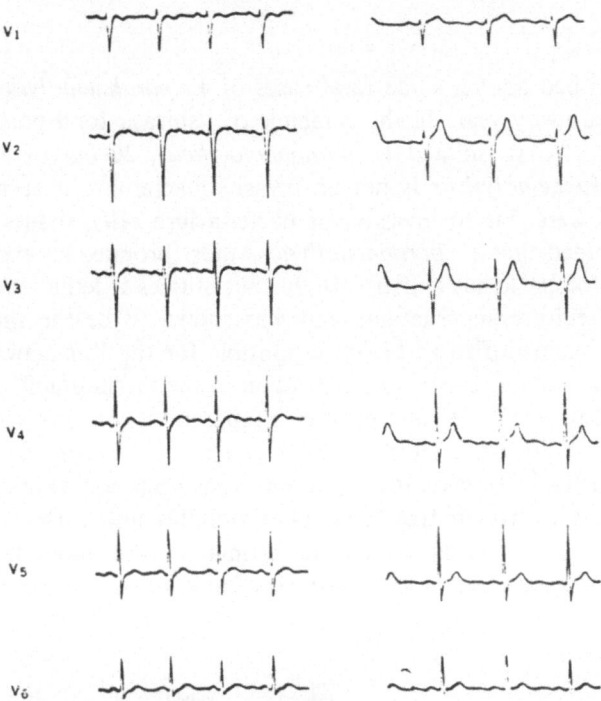

Fig. 1. Electrocardiograms (chest leads) of a patient suffering from severe diarrhea due to *V. parahaemolyticus* infection. Left and right columns show records during and after the disease, respectively. (From Ref. 4.)

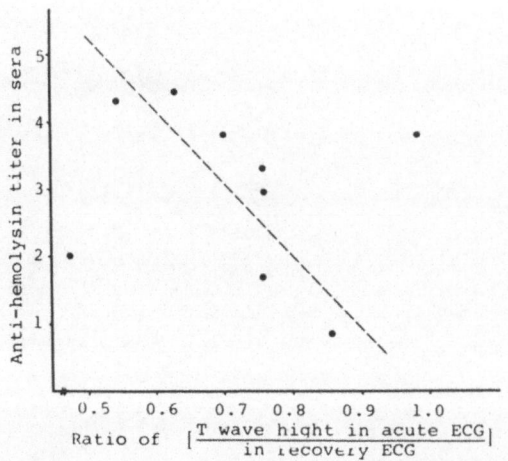

Fig. 2. Correlation of the height of the T wave in electrocardiograms and the antihemolysin titer in convalescent sera of patients.

Lethal activity of V. parahaemolyticus and cardiotoxicity of thermostable direct hemolysin

As described above, some fatal cases of *V. parahaemolyticus* infection have been reported every year. In the epidemic of "shirasu food poisoning", in which Fujino *et al.*[1] first isolated *V. parahaemolyticus*, 20 out of 272 patients died. Since *V. parahaemolyticus* is not an invasive bacterium, it seemed unlikely that these deaths were due to invasion of bacteria into cells, tissues or organs. Thus it was concluded that *V. parahaemolyticus* most produce an exotoxin(s) that was responsible for its lethal activity. In further studies a lethal toxin was found in the cell-free culture supernatants and was shown to be the thermostable direct hemolysin[6, 7], identified as being responsible for the Kanagawa phenomenon[8].

There are several reports of purification of the thermostable direct hemolysin[6, 9-12]. The homogeneity of our purified preparations was shown by conventional polyacrylamide disc gel electrophoresis (Fig. 3A), SDS-polyacrylamide disc gel electrophoresis (Fig. 3B) and analytical ultracentrifugation (Fig. 4). The purified hemolysin was a protein free from phospholipids and carbohydrates with a pI of about 4.2. The molecular weight was estimated to be about 42,000 by gel filtration. The biologically active himolysin was found to be composed of two identical

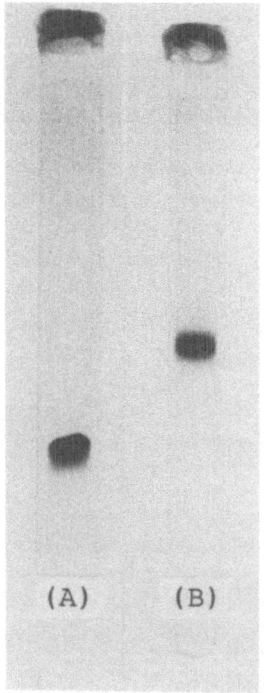

(A)   (B)

Fig. 3.   Conventional(A) and SDS-(B) polyacrylamide gel disc electrophoresis of the purified thermostable direct hemolysin.

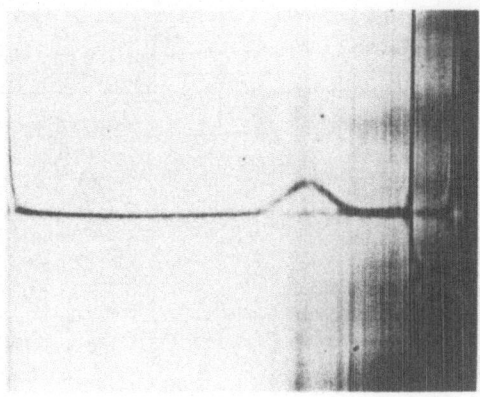

Fig. 4.   Pattern on analytical ultracentrifugation of the purified thermostable direct hemolysin. (From Ref. 6.)

subunits of approximately 21,000 daltons[13]. Analysis of its amino acid composition[6, 10, 12] showed that the hemolysin was an acidic protein, and the amino acid sequence of its N-terminal region was determined[12].

The purified hemolysin showed various biological activities, such as hemolytic activity, cytotoxicity to various culture cells, enteropathogenicity and lethal activity in small experimental animals[14]. Among these biological activities, we investigated the lethal activity in particular.

The purified thermostable direct hemolysin had strong lethal activity in mice and rats. As shown in Table 3[6] intravenous injection of 5 μg of the hemolysin killed mice in less than 1 minute, and even 1 μg of the hemolysin killed mice within 20 minutes. Intravenous injection of 10 μg of the hemolysin killed rats in about 2 minutes.

Since the rapid death of animals suggested that the hemolysin affected some vital organs of the animals, such as the central nervous system or cardio-vascular system, we examined the electroencephalograms and electrocardiograms of rats before and after injection of purified thermostable direct hemolysin[7]. Typical results of these experiments are shown in Fig. 5. In a rat (445 g) injected intravenously with 15 μg of the purified hemolysin the electrocardiogram exhibited a distinct increase in amplitude about 30 seconds after the hemolysin injection and beating of the heart stopped after about 30 seconds whereas the electroencephalogram remained normal until 80 seconds after the injection. An example of further analysis of electrocardiograms is shown in Fig. 6. In this experiment, a rat weighing 448 g was injected intravenously with 7.5 μg of the hemolysin at 0 time. About 15 seconds later, the P wave became wider and higher than normal, suggesting changes in conduction of intra-atrial impulses. At about this time the voltage of QRS increased and ST-T changed, suggesting changes in conduction of intra-ventricular impulses of electrical activation. About 17 to 18 seconds after the injection, the PQ interval became longer, suggesting inhibition of atrioventricular conduction. Then about 41 seconds after the injection, the pattern

Table 3. Lethal activity of the thermostable direct hemolysin on intravenous injection.

	Amount of toxin injected (μg/animal)	Survival time after injection
Mice	10.0	35.5 ± 4.8^a sec
	5.0	49.0 ± 8.4
	2.5	561.2 ± 368.8
	1.0	1121.5 ± 291.0
	0.5	no death
Rat	25.0	1.87 ± 0.22^b min
	10.0	2.15 ± 0.36
	7.5	7.00 ± 1.53
	5.0	180.00 ± 174.00
	2.5	no death

[a] Values are means $\pm$ S.D. for 10 mice.
[b] Values are means $\pm$ S.D. for 5 rats.

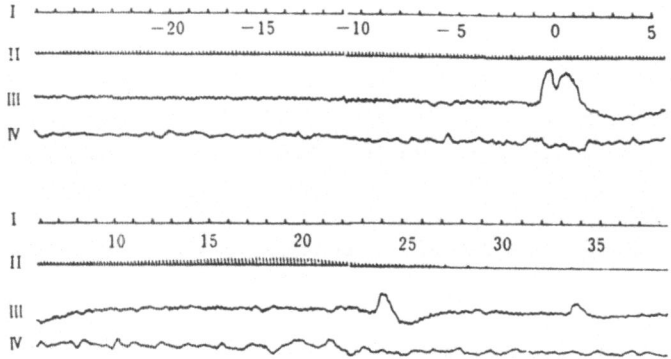

Fig. 5. Electrocardiogram and electroencephalogram of a rat injected with the purified thermostable direct hemolysin. The hemolysin was injected at 0 time. Line 1, time in seconds; line II, electrocardiogram with a unipolar chest lead around the apex of the heart; line III, electroencephalogram with a lead from the hippocampal area; line IV, electroencephalogram with a lead from the motor area. (From Ref. 7.)

showed change of the exciting foci in the ventricle and the heart rate decreased due to reduced excitation of the heart muscle. Ventricular flutter developed about 50 seconds after the injection and the heart stopped after 148 seconds.

Since these data suggested the cardiotoxicity of the thermostable direct hemolysin, we studied the effect of the hemolysin on cultured heart cells with which there was no possibility that the hemolysin could affect the heart through either the nervous or vascular system[7, 15]. When ventricular tissue from the heart of mouse fetuses of 14 - 16 days old was cultured in Eagle's minimum essential medium supplemented with 10% fetal bovine serum at 36°C under an atmosphere of 5% CO_2 in air, the cells beat spontaneously and regularly. When 1 - 1.5 $\times$ 10^6 cells were seeded into dishes, a large cell cluster of 2 - 4 mm diameter contain-

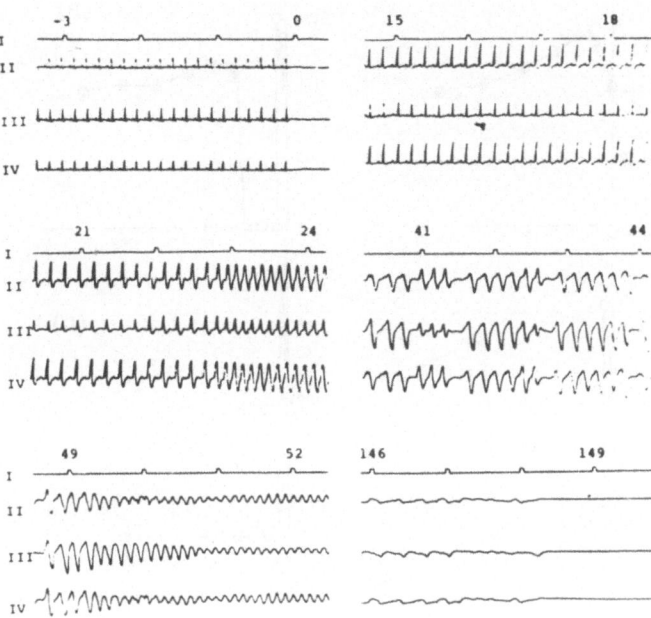

Fig. 6. Electrocardiograms of a rat injected with the purified thermostable direct hemolysin. The hemolyisn was injected at 0 time. Line I, time in seconds; line II, lead from a combination of electrodes in the right and left fore legs; line III, lead from a combination of electrodes in the right fore leg and left hind leg; line IV, lead from a combination of electrodes in the left fore leg and left hind leg.

ing more than 10^5 cells was obtained after cultivation for 1 day. All the heart cells in the cell cluster beat synchronously and regularly at 100 - 180 beats/min and this rate was maintained for at least 24 hours. The effect of the purified thermostable direct hemolysin on the beating of a cell cluster of cultured heart cells is shown in Fig. 7. On addition of 0.05 µg/ml of the hemolysin to medium the beating increased slightly, but it returned to normal within 10 minutes (Fig. 7A). On addition of 0.1 µg/ml of the hemolysin, the beating was first rapidly stimulated and then stopped suddenly within 1 minute. Then 6 minutes after the addition of the hemolysin, the beating suddenly started again at the normal rate and remained unchanged during further observation (Fig. 7B). Similarly, on addition of 0.2 µg/ml of the hemolysin, the beating first increased, then stopped and then started again (Fig. 7C), but the interval between the time of stopping and of starting again was longer than that on addition of 0.1 µg/ml of the hemolysin. On addition of 1 µg/ml or more of the hemolysin to the medium, the beating also increased and then stopped abruptly, and then almost all the cells rapidly disintegrated (Fig. 7D). Stimulation, stopping and recovery of the beating were observed repeatedly on repeated addition of the purified thermostable direct hemolysin to the medium.

An electrophysiological study on rabbit heart muscle in a perfusion system also showed the cardiotoxicity of the hemolysin[16]. Figure 8 shows the effect of

304

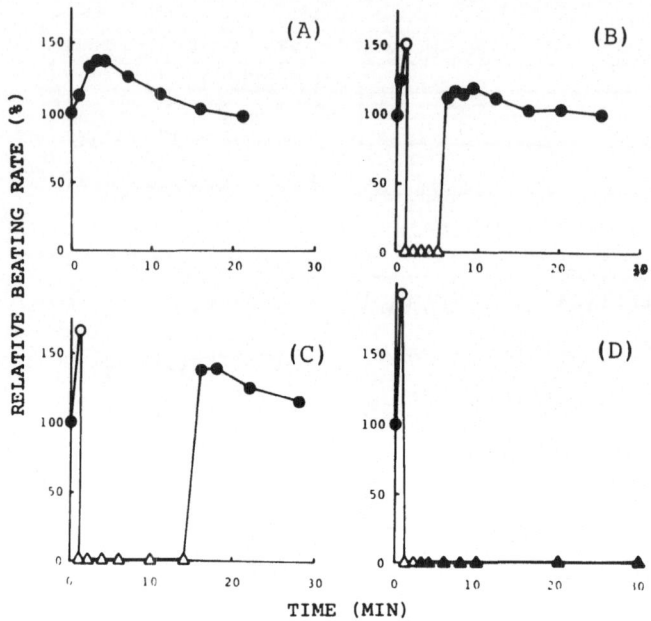

Fig. 7.   Effect of the purified thermostable direct hemolysin on the beating of myocardial cell clusters cultured in vitro. Mouse heart cells were cultured and the various amounts of the hemolysin indicated below were added to the medium at 0 time. The beating of cell clusters is expressed as percentage of that observed in the absence of the hemolysin. The concentrations of the hemolysin in the medium were : (A) 0.05 μg/ml; (B) 0.1 μg/ml, (C) 0.2 μg/ml and (D) 1 μg/ml. • Normal beating; ○, weaker beating; △, no beating but no cell disintegration; ▲, disintegration of the cells. (From Ref. 7.)

the hemolysin on the action potential of the sino-atrial node recorded with a microelectrode. At a dose of 2.5 μg/ml, the hemolysin caused reduction of the maximal diastolic potential, indicating membrane deporalization. The spontaneous action potential stopped about 10 minutes after hemolysin administration. After that time, although there was no spontaneous action potential, a single electrical stimulas could induce an action potential, as shown in the panel 4 of the upper row of Fig. 8. These data suggest that the hemolysin did not injure the mechanism generating the action potential, but damaged the autonomy of pace maker cells. From these and other reported data[17], we propose the mechanism for the lethal toxicity of the thermostable direct hemolysin shown in Fig. 9.

Activity of V. parahaemolyticus to cause diarrhea

Zen-yoji et al.[11] injected the thermostable direct hemolysin into ligated rabbit ileal loops and found that injection of 500 μg of the hemolysin caused accumulation of turbid, bloody fluid in the loops. Consistent with this, Obara et al.[18] reported that the hemolysin caused diarrhea in suckling mice. More recently, Miyamoto et al.[10] reported that as little as 125 μg of the hemolysin caused fluid accumulation in rabbit ileal loops. From these data, it has been suggested that the thermostable direct hemolysin is an important factor in causing

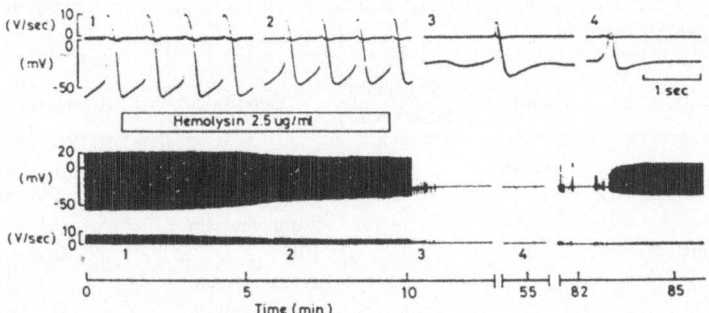

Fig. 8. Effect of the purified thermostable direct hemolysin on the action potential of the sino-atrial node. Fast speed original action potentials are shown in the upper row. The action potential shown in panel 4 of the upper row was elcited by a single electrical stimulus. Numbers in the upper row correspond to those in the lower row. A continuous tracting of the change of the action potential and the maximum rate of rise of the action potential in response to 2.5 μg/ml of hemolysin are shown in the lower row.

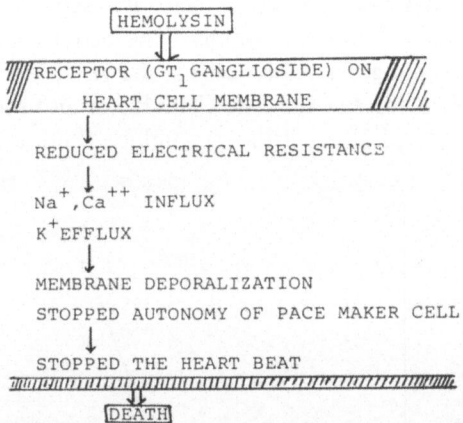

Fig. 9. Proposed mechanism of the lethal toxicity of the thermostable direct hemolysin.

gastroenteritis due to *V. parahaemolyticus* infection. However, the activity of the hemolysin in causing diarrhea with rather high doses may be explained by its cytotoxic activity observed with various cultured cells, such as FL cells, HeLa cells and human intestinal cells CCL-6[19].

The data shown in Table 4 indicate that antihemolysin (antibody against the purified thermostable direct hemolysin) did not prevent fluid accumulation in rabbit ileal loops caused by living cells of *V. parahaemolyticus*. These data suggest that a factor(s) other than the hemolysin is responsible for fluid accumulation induced by living cells of *V. parahaemolyticus*.

Previously, we reported the isolation and partial purification from the culture supernatants of *V. parahaemolyticus* of a factor, that caused morphological changes of Chinese hamster ovary (CHO) cells in a similar manner to that caused by cholera

Table 4.   Effect of antihemolysin on fluid accumulation in rabbit ileal loops induced by living cells of
V. parahaemolyticus.

Bacterium	Strain	Kanagawa phenomenon	Conditions[a]	FA ratio (ml/cm) ± SD[b]
V. parahaemolyticus	OP-286	+	PBS	0.59 ± 0.14
			Normal serum	0.53 ± 0.18
			Antihemolysin	0.59 ± 0.25
V. parahaemolyticus	9B-2R	−	PBS	0.60 ± 0.18
			Normal serum	0.51 ± 0.20
			Antihemolysin	0.50 ± 0.29

[a] Bacterial cells were suspended in heart infusion broth containing 0.5% NaCl and adjusted to a density
giving an absorbance of 100 (about 10^9 cells/ml) in a Klett-Summerson photometer (filter #66). Then
0.5 ml of the bacterial suspension was mixed with 0.5 ml of either phosphate buffered saline, pH 7.2 (PBS),
normal serum or antihemolysin (diluted 3-fold with PBS before use), and 1 ml of the mixture was injected
into a ligated ileal loop of a rabbit. Rabbits were kept at room temperature for 16 hours.
[b] Fluid accumulation was expressed as the FA ratio (ml of fluid/cm of loop length).

enterotoxin[20]. The partially purified CHO factor was separated from the hemolysin
by hydroxylapatite column chromatography. The activity of the CHO factor in
causing morphological changes of CHO cells is shown in Fig. 10. The CHO factor
is less potent than cholera enterotoxin. The CHO factor also showed skin permeability activity, but at a dose of 20 μg it did not induce fluid accumulation in ligated

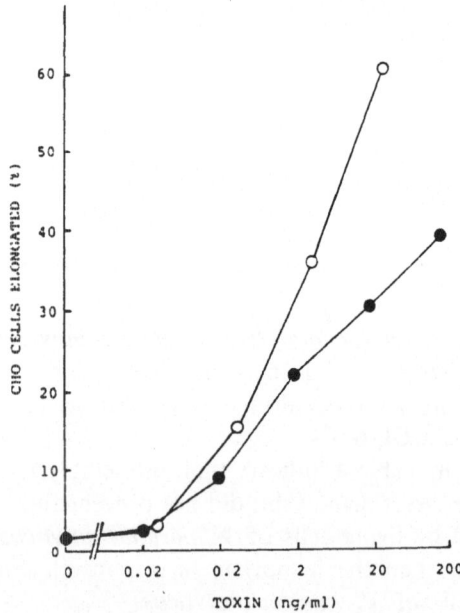

Fig. 10.   Effect of partially purified CHO factor on the morphology of CHO cells. The activity of
the partially purified CHO factor (•) and cholera enterotoxin (○) involved in changing CHO cells
from an oval to spindle shape was assayed.

rabbit ileal loops. Therefore, further studies are necessary to clarify the role of the CHO factor in the pathogenesis of *V. parahaemolyticus* infection.

REFERENCES

1. Fujino, T., Y. Okuno, D. Nakada, A. Aoyama, K. Fukai, T. Mukai, and T. Ueno. 1953. On the bacteriological examination of shirasu-food poisoning. Med. J. Osaka Univ. **4**: 299–304.
2. Takikawa, I. 1958. Studies on pathogenic halophilic bacteria. Yokohama Med. Bull. **7**: 313–322.
3. Saito, M. 1967. Clinical features of gastroenteritis due to *Vibrio parahaemolyticus* (in Japanese). pp. 295–310. *In*: *Vibrio parahaemolyticus* II. Fujino, T. and Fukumi H. (eds.). Naya Shoten, Tokyo.
4. Honda, T., Y. Takeda, T. Miwatani, K. Kato, and Y. Nimura. 1976. Clinical features of patients suffering from food poisoning due to *Vibrio parahaemolyticus* - especially on changes in electrocardiograms (in Japanese). J. Jap. Ass. Infect. Dis. **50**: 216–223.
5. Miwatani, T., J. Sakurai, Y. Takeda, S. Sugiyama, and T. Adachi. 1976. Antibody titers against the thermostable direct hemolysin in sera of patients suffering from gastroenteritis due to *Vibrio parahaemolyticus* (in Japanese). J. Jap. Ass. Infect. Dis. **50**: 46–51.
6. Honda, T., S. Taga, T. Takeda, M. A. Hashibuan, Y. Takeda, and T. Miwatani. 1976. Identification of lethal toxin with the thermostable direct hemolysin produced by *Vibrio parahaemolyticus*, and some physicochemical properties of the purified toxin. Infect. Immun. **13**: 133–139.
7. Honda, T., K. Goshima, Y. Takeda, Y. Sugino, and T. Miwatani. 1976. Demonstration of the cardiotoxicity of the thermostable direct hemolysin (lethal toxin) produced by *Vibrio parahaemolyticus*. Infect. Immum. **13**: 163–171.
8. Sakurai, J., A. Matsuzaki, Y. Takeda, and T. Miwatani. 1974. Existence of two distinct hemolysins in *Vibrio parahaemolyticus*. Infect. Immun. **9**: 777–780.
9. Sakurai, J., A. Matsuzaki, and T. Miwatani. 1973. Purification and characterization of thermostable direct hemolysin of *Vibrio parahaemolyticus*. Infect. Immun. **8**: 775–780.
10. Miyamoto, Y., Y. Obara, T. Nikkawa, S. Yamai, T. Kato, Y. Yamada, and M. Ohashi. 1980. Simplified purification and biophysiochemical characteristics of Kanagawa phenomenon-associated hemolysin of *Vibrio parahaemolyticus*. Infect. Immun. **28**: 567–576.
11. Zen-Yoji, H., Y. Kudoh, H. Igarashi, K. Ohta, and K. Fukai. 1974. Purificaiton and identification of enteropathogenic toxins "a" and "á" produced by *Vibrio parahaemolyticus* and their biological and pathological activities. pp. 237–243. *In*: International Symposium on *Vibrio parahaemolyticus*. Fujino, T., Sakaguchi, G., Sakazaki, R., and Takeda, Y. (eds.) Saikon Publishing Co., Tokyo, Japan.
12. Zen-Yoji, H., Y. Kudoh, H. Igarashi, K. Ohta, K. Fukai, and T. Hoshino. 1975. An enteropathogenic toxin of *Vibrio parahaemolyticus*. pp. 263–272. *In* Proc. lst Intersect. Conf. IAMS. Vol. 4. Hasegawa, T. (ed.), Science Council of Japan. Tokyo.
13. Takeda, Y., S. Taga, and T. Miwatani. 1978. Evidence that thermostable direct hemolysin of *Vibrio parahaemolyticus* is composed of two subunits. FEMS Microbiol. Letters **4**: 271–274.
14. Miwatani, T., and Y. Takeda. 1976. *Vibrio parahaemolyticus* - a causative bacterium of food poisoning. Saikon Publishing Co., Tokyo, Japan.
15. Goshima, K., T. Honda, M. Hirata, K. Kikuchi, Y. Takeda, and T. Miwatani. 1977. Stopping of the spontaneous beating of mouse and rat myocardial cells in vitro by a toxin from *Vibrio parahaemolyticus*. J. Mol. Cell. Cardiol. **9**: 191–213.
16. Seyama, I., H. Irisawa, T. Honda, Y. Takeda, and T. Miwatani. 1977. Effect of hemolysin produced by *Vibrio parahaemolyticus* on membrane conductance and mechanical tension of rabbit myocardium. Jap. J. Physiol. **27**: 43–56.
17. Takeda, Y., T. Takeda, T. Honda, and T. Miwatani. 1976. Inactivation of the biological activities of the thermostable direct hemolysin of *Vibrio parahaemolyticus* by ganglioside G_{Tl}. Infect. Immun. **14**: 1–5.
18. Obara, Y., S. Yamai, T. Nikkawa, Y. Miyamoto, M. Ohashi, and T. Shimada. 1974.

308

Histopathological changes in the small intestine of suckling mice challenged orally with purified hemolysin from *Vibrio parahaemolyticus*. pp. 253–257. *In*: International Symposium on *Vibrio parahaemolyticus*. Fujino, T., Sakaguchi, G., Sakazaki, R., and Takeda, Y. (eds.) Saikon Publishing Co., Tokyo, Japan.
19. Sakurai, J., T. Honda, Y. Jinguji, M. Arita, and T. Miwatani. 1975. Cytotoxic effect of the thermostable direct hemolysin produced by *Vibrio parahaemolyticus* on FL cells. Infect. Immun., **13**: 876–883.
20. Honda, T., M. Shimizu, Y. Takeda, and T. Miwatani. 1976. Isolation of a factor causing morphological changes of Chinese hamster ovary cells from culture filtrate of *Vibrio parahaemolyticus* Infect. Immum. **14**: 1028–1033.

Auther Index